Motherland Herbal

ALSO BY STEPHANIE ROSE BIRD

*The Healing Tree: Botanicals, Remedies, and Rituals from
African Folk Traditions*

African American Magick: A Modern Grimoire for the Natural Home

*The Healing Power of African-American Spirituality: A Celebration of
Ancestor Worship, Herbs and Hoodoo, Ritual and Conjure*

365 Days of Hoodoo: Daily Rootwork, Mojo & Conjuration

Earth Mama's Spiritual Guide to Weight Loss

The Big Book of Soul: The Ultimate Guide to the African-American Spirit

A Healing Grove: African Tree Remedies and Rituals for Body and Spirit

*Light, Bright, and Damned Near White: Biracial and
Triracial Culture in America*

Four Seasons of Mojo: An Herbal Guide to Natural Living

Sticks, Stones, Roots & Bones: Hoodoo, Mojo & Conjuring with Herbs

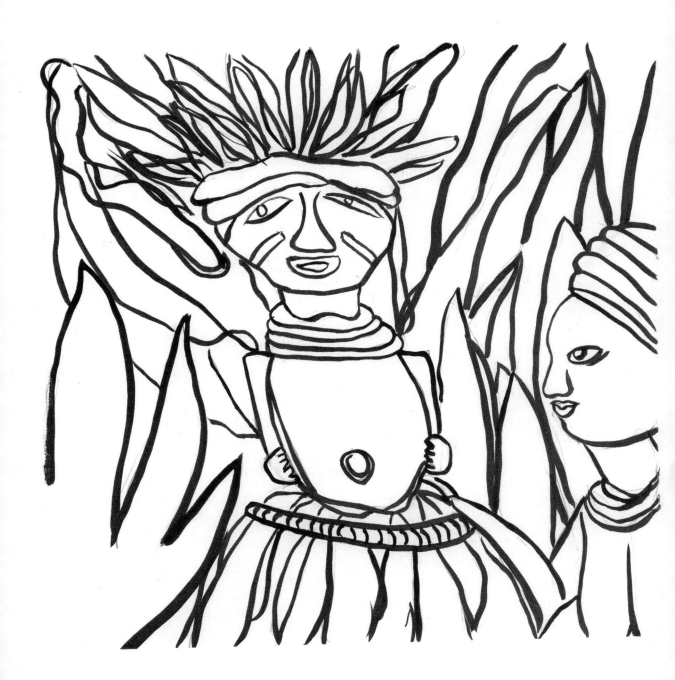

Motherland Herbal

The Story of African Holistic Health

STEPHANIE ROSE BIRD

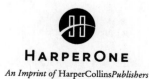

HarperOne
An Imprint of HarperCollinsPublishers

MOTHERLAND HERBAL. Copyright © 2024 by Stephanie Rose Bird. All rights reserved. Printed in the United States of America. No part of this book may be used or reproduced in any manner whatsoever without written permission except in the case of brief quotations embodied in critical articles and reviews. For information, address HarperCollins Publishers, 195 Broadway, New York, NY 10007.

HarperCollins books may be purchased for educational, business, or sales promotional use. For information, please email the Special Markets Department at SPsales@harpercollins.com.

FIRST EDITION

Designed by Bonni Leon-Berman
All illustrations created by the author.
Photograph on p. 107 © monique delatour/Shutterstock.
All other photographs courtesy of the author.

Library of Congress Cataloging-in-Publication Data has been applied for.

ISBN 978-0-06-330804-6

24 25 26 27 28 LBC 5 4 3 2 1

Akin to Aya (the fern), we have soared
when difficulties arose and searched out the Sun
when clouds made it hard to see the light of the Sky.

This book is dedicated, with love, to the Bird Flock.

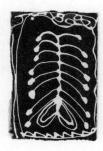

CONTENTS

Part I. Our Herbal Beginning   1

CHAPTER 1: Our Herbal Healing Ways: The Key Concepts   3

CHAPTER 2: Planting with Spirit / Harvesting Ashe: The Magical and Physical Seed   19

CHAPTER 3: Elbow Grease: Tools and Equipment for Working Roots   37

Part II. The Story of Herbs   47

CHAPTER 4: Osayin's Calabash: Spiritual Plants and Mystical Natural Products   49

CHAPTER 5: Getting to the Root: Roots, Bulbs, Tubers, and Health   75

CHAPTER 6: Harvesting the Grasslands: The Plains, Savanna, and Prairie   95

CHAPTER 7: Where There Is a Will, There Is a Way: Plant Life on Arid Land   119

CHAPTER 8: The Healer's Heart: Matters of Heart and Blood   139

CHAPTER 9: *Funfun* Health: Medicines of the Swamps, Mangroves, Lakes, and Seas   167

CHAPTER 10: The Sacred Wood   195

CHAPTER 11: Dudu Awo (Black Secrets)   233

Part III. Wisdom of the Directions: Navigating the Web of Herbal Life   265

CHAPTER 12: The Web of Life   267

CHAPTER 13: Spring into Ritual: Rain, Thunder, the Water Element, and Flowers   315

CHAPTER 14: Summer of Vibrant Health   371

CHAPTER 15: Harvesting Autumn   407

Acknowledgments   *437*

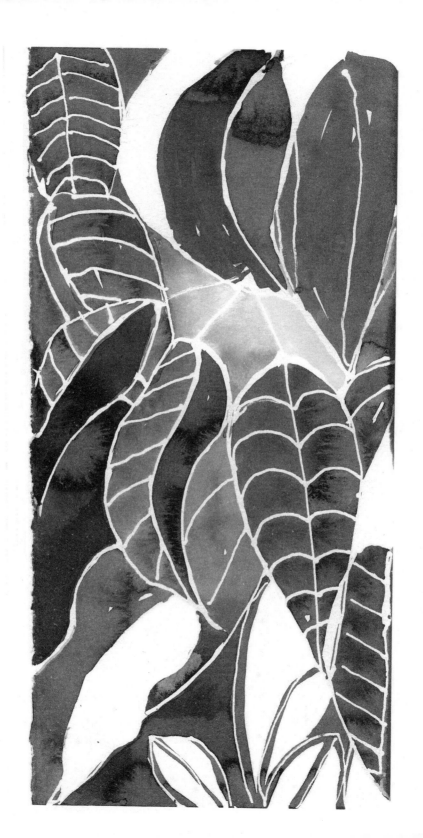

PART I

Our Herbal Beginning

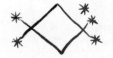

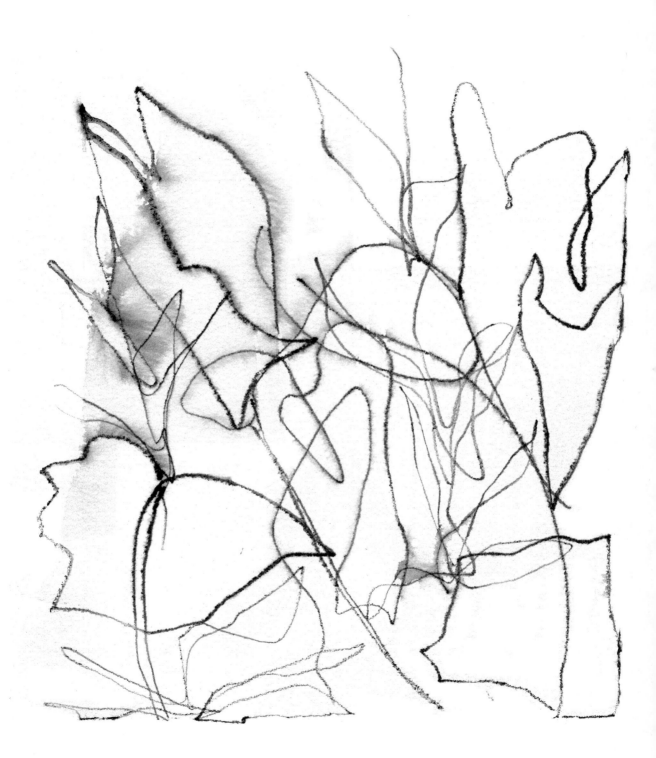

CHAPTER 1

Our Herbal Healing Ways

THE KEY CONCEPTS

FOLK MEDICINE HAS COME FULL CIRCLE. In ancient times it was *the* definitive word of the high priestess. Then in the modern era, wives' tales and even midwives' valuable work itself was replaced by biomedicine dispensed by mostly white, male doctors. All too often this type of medicine was out of our realm, spiritually, geographically, and financially. Even the *New England Journal of Medicine* has reported on the fact that often disease and ailments are misunderstood and thus go untreated in the African American population. Beyond studies or research, this is due to a healing language barrier. It comes as no surprise. Rather than sulk or complain, our response has been to use this as fuel for the persistence of tradition and the determination to heal ourselves.

Today, earth wisdom of the common folk—folk wisdom or mother wit, as it is commonly called in the African American community—is once again garnering the recognition it deserves. Indeed, it is through language, Grandma's story, tribal storytelling, the lore of the folk, that we begin to build a repertoire of readily available, inexpensive, natural health remedies. This understanding is compiled through an in-depth understanding of our immediate environment, which consists of plants, animals, minerals, the elements, particular weather conditions, and the spirit beings that create or destroy. Our healing landscape is not an apothecary stocked with dried herbs, capsules, and pills. Western medicines are just isolated parts of a much richer whole. The healing landscape is the earth as well as the ancestors, nature spirits, and spirit guides that bring it to life. By and large, this medicine is brewed at the hearth, in a womb-like cast-iron pot, created by mothering hands and a full heart aching to heal.

This collection of earth wisdom stemming from folklore goes further than simply treating illness. I have avoided the staggering statistics that prepare us for ultimate doom. The term *sickening* makes sense: it is a term aptly suited to the health predicament in which many find themselves. If you are wrapped up in sickness, perceiving yourself as ill, how can health prevail? Sick thinking does nothing for the spirit except to weaken it. In fact, while I will share ways various people approach illness and disease, my primary concern is with instilling wellness. It is the capacity to build a well society that will inevitably enable us to continue to survive—strong in mind, body, and spirit.

MOTHERLAND HERBAL: THE STORY OF AFRICAN HOLISTIC HEALTH shares earth wisdom from across Africa and the African diaspora. While many books have been written on the herbal wisdom of various groups of people, this is one of very few inspired by Africa. At times this story has seemed too huge to dare pen. The plants and the ways they are used medicinally in Africa and the diaspora could fill entire volumes. I have often asked myself, How dare I attempt to squeeze herbal wisdom from the Motherland into a single volume? The answer is that even though this is only the beginning of this story, it is a story that urgently needs to be written. As an African American herbalist who grew up surrounded by the forest in an active farming community, I knew I was uniquely qualified to attempt such an endeavor. Ultimately, this is only the beginning—the beginning of the telling of our herbal healing story, a story without a feasible ending.

As people continue to move across geographic, economic, and social boundaries, our ability to develop and share healing stories will grow and expand along with the journey. If there must be an end, let us hope it comes near the time that African healing wisdom is welcomed into the larger global circle of complementary and alternative medicines (CAM), integrative health, and alternative health practices. The African, Caribbean, and African American healing ways belong alongside the Native American Beauty Way, Australian Aboriginal Dreamtime medicine, Western herbalism, Chinese medicine, Ayurveda, and all the other systems recognized as contributing to the health of earth's people. Then and only then will the healing story be complete.

Meanwhile, I have compiled our unique approach to harvesting and dispensing healing medicines from the natural world. I do not believe in supplements as much as enriching the diet with whole foods, hand-processed herbs, and nutritious drinks. In this book, supplements are mainly provided by spiritual development, exercise, and creativity. This is not a medicine book in the Western concept of the word; it is holistic healing, thus it addresses each realm of health: mind, body, and spirit.

The holistic approach naturally lends itself to storytelling, which is why the griot (African storyteller) is held in high esteem. Through my own personal stories, the stories told by various individuals in their own words, regional folklore, and the story of how Black people interact with herbal medicines on both sides of the Atlantic, a picture develops of indigenous African healing ways. These stories come from the desert, forest, savanna, mountainous regions, islands, cities, and towns with heart. You will learn how the elements, spirits, and deity can contribute to healing. This calabash of ingredients is brimming. The stock made from the contents of the calabash will continue to be refined over the years, yielding a delectable stew. The promising cast-iron stockpot crammed with African healing ways is here, bubbling across boundaries, eager for the opportunity to nourish your soul.

African herbalism is a little-understood and seldom-discussed topic. Part of the difficulty arises with semantics and the scarce use of the term *herbalism* to describe African healing traditions. Most African healers are specialists engaged in various professions that combine herbalism with other forms of therapy. Priests/priestesses, Kumina practitioners, shamans, witch doctors, mother healers, bush doctors, hunters, medicine men, balm yard healers, midwives, sangomas, Obeahmen and Obeahwomen, Myal mediums, and diviners are all adept herbalists. Regular people, without specialized titles, have long understood the transformative powers and therapeutic abilities of djembes (talking drums), spirit dancing, singing, chanting, shouting, and making art. The marriage of art with healing isn't necessarily called music, dance, or art therapy; in Africa and the diaspora, it is considered community ritual and ceremony. Terminology aside, the arts like herbalism have been used therapeutically in Africa and elsewhere over the centuries.

The Healing Traditions of Africa in the Caribbean and Americas

Motherland Herbal explores the herbalism of Africa and within the African diaspora—not just herbal folklore, myths, and exotic ingredients from far away. African diasporic healing includes Vodou of Haiti, Candomblé of Brazil, Santería of Puerto Rico and Cuba, as well as the bush medicines of Jamaica and Trinidad. In the United States, the venerable history of herbalism and natural cures of Hoodoo and the Gullah people are discussed. Professor Sharla Fett of UCLA sheds light on this heritage in her book *Working Cures: Healing, Health, and Power on Southern Slave Plantations*.[1] Professor Fett reminds us of the Southern healing traditions practiced by enslaved Africans that include midwifery, herbalism, and the healing of the body, mind, and spirit. Fett puts these traditions into a sociocultural context, demonstrating how these institutions were tools of self-determination. It is midwifery that has been one of our more prominent holistic healing activities. According to midwife informants practicing in the early twentieth century, midwives not only delivered babies but also discussed nutrition with their clients, tried to make the home environment as clean and comfortable as possible for the mother and child, and some even provided homespun consul and acted as liaisons between welfare organizations and the community.[2]

When I was growing up in rural South Jersey, my family and I lived at the end of a dirt road in a segregated town. We were five miles from town, which was customary at that time in that area of New Jersey for Black folks and other people of color. We were also fifteen miles from the nearest hospital. My mother died from an embolism when she was in her early fifties. According to my family's account, she struggled for her life for almost half an hour as the family tried to help her in the best ways they knew, thinking it was simply an asthma attack—after which time the paramedics came and tried to revive her to no avail. We were stunned because my mother regularly saw her family physician. It was difficult to understand how a condition such as a blood clot went undetected.

---

1   Sharla Fett, *Working Cures: Healing, Health, and Power on Southern Slave Plantations* (Chapel Hill: Univ. of North Carolina Press, 2002).
2   These accounts of midwives' roles in the community as holistic health advisors as well as birth assistants come from numerous sources. Some of the more widely read include Loudell F. Snow, *Walkin' Over Medicine* (Boulder, CO: Westview Press, 1993); Debra A. Susie, *In the Way of Our Grandmothers: A Cultural View of Twentieth-Century Midwifery in Florida* (Athens: Univ. of Georgia Press, 1988); and Katherine Clark and Onnie Lee Logan, *Motherwit: An Alabama Midwife's Story* (New York: E.P. Dutton, 1988).

There was not just the fear of being unable to get treatment in time because of geography or uncaring doctors. There was, and to some extent remains, a suspicion of what the white doctors might do to harm the patient: theories of deadly medicines being given as experiments abound. This could appear to be a paranoid conspiracy theory were it not for well-documented cases of African American men with syphilis given no treatment.

Anthropology, human development, and pediatrics professor and author Loudell Snow describes these grim experiments:

"It is best to keep in mind the infamous Tuskegee Syphilis Study before deriding such belief.[3] The Public Health Service funded the study, which began in 1932 and continued until 1972. It included a large sample of poor African American men infected with syphilis; they were not educated about the true nature of their disease but were told that they had 'bad blood,'[4] the folk term covering a variety of problems. And they were left untreated so that researchers might have an opportunity to observe the natural course of the disease until 'end point,' that is, autopsy."[5] The large sampling of Black men numbered four hundred. As though deception were not bad enough for the men directly affected, some of their wives, mates, children, and grandchildren also contracted syphilis from the untreated men who sought treatment. Their number is estimated at fifty women and children (the seventeen children and two grandchildren had congenital syphilis).[6]

CANCER TOOK MANY MEMBERS OF my family, including my beloved father, grandmother (his mother), and her sister, my great-aunt. My father and grandmother were great believers in herbal/natural remedies and instilled these beliefs in me. My grandmother did not seek biomedical treatment or tests until she was at the end stages of her cancer. Likewise, my father refused follow-up biopsies until it was too late. I recall stories that indicate that there was a great deal of fear about cutting or surgeries at the hands of doctors because it was believed that the act of cutting and the removal of tissue itself would make an illness worse.

My father and grandmother lived at home with their cancer, drinking vegetable and

---

3   This is a reference to the fear of doctors and their biomedicines by African Americans.

4   James H. Jones, *Bad Blood: The Tuskegee Syphilis Experiment: A Tragedy of Race and Medicine* (New York: The Free Press, 1981).

5   Jones, *Bad Blood: The Tuskegee Syphilis Experiment.*

6   Janette Y. Taylor, "Talking Back: Research as an Act of Resistance and Healing for African American Women Survivors of Intimate Male Partner Violence," *Women & Therapy* 25, no. 34 (2002): 145–60; published simultaneously in the anthology *Violence in the Lives of Black Women: Battered, Black, and Blue,* ed. Carolyn M. West (Philadelphia: Haworth Press, 2002), 145–60.

fruit juices and taking tonics, minerals, and other natural supplements, many of which I developed for my father to augment his mainstream care. The two did their best to go about a "normal life" at home as much as possible and, eventually, combined biomedicine with natural medicines to alleviate their symptoms. Meanwhile, until the end of their lives on this earth, they sought out alternative treatments that could offer relief if not a cure.

My uncle, who I speak of frequently, was my father's brother. He did exactly as my father and his mother, though he had HIV, not cancer. He took whole foods as medicines, especially soul foods like collard greens, yams, beans and rice, and herbal and mineral supplements, and he sought out the assistance of fellow Babalawo (keepers of secrets, also called priests of Shango). He went deep into the spiritual dimension customary in various ATRs (African traditional religions, non-Abrahamic faiths of Africa's indigenous people), whereas my father delved deeper into Christianity. My uncle performed and participated in rituals and ceremonies. Moreover, he used djembes (African talking drums) therapeutically. I credit these alternative therapies with extending his life and enhancing his lifestyle during his illness. He lived with HIV for fourteen years before it developed into AIDS. He was very reluctant to take biomedicines, fearing that the HIV and AIDS were the creation of scientists who wanted to wipe out the Black race. He could not trust Western medicine with that belief firmly rooted.

Today, my aunt on the same side of the family struggles with mental and physical illness. I have observed her utilizing dance that merges liturgical and spiritual dance therapeutically. She is heavily dependent on spirituality, manifested in Holy Scripture, for her mental and physical well-being. Whereas there are some rather simple, well-known pharmaceuticals that would probably alleviate her symptoms, she clings instead to her own unique combination of movement, spirituality, and home remedies to provide relief. One of her ailments is a severe joint problem that affects her hips. While it once seemed as though a drug like CELEBREX would be the ultimate treatment to alleviate her symptoms, new findings are coming to light that suggest this drug has serious side effects that were not previously revealed to users of the pharmaceutical.

My uncle and father carried their beliefs into the twenty-first century. The fact that Black community members were forced to live so far from town and it took such a long time for paramedics to come to help my mother did not help the already well-placed suspicions of mainstream medical establishment. My father, I am sad to say, died in 2004 of lung cancer, and his brother died a few years before him of AIDS.

It is notable that my uncle fit the profile of many African Americans who become involved with wellness, holistic health, and natural remedies, especially men. My uncle was a Black Power civil rights activist during the 1960s and 1970s. For my uncle and many African Americans who choose natural remedies and complementary therapies over biomedicines and mainstream doctors, the choice reflects a quest for self-determination and empowerment. Engaging in CAM is frequently connected to activism in the Black community.

AS A PEOPLE, WE HAVE traditionally communicated and lived with other groups of people and continue to look at neighboring cultures for inspiration and wellness information. Dr. Faith Mitchell's book *Hoodoo Medicine*[7] highlights the cooperation between African, Native American, and European cultures in the development of African American healing systems. Mitchell discusses the open-mindedness displayed by our people during challenging times and our willingness to respect and incorporate the traditions of others into our own corpus of healing knowledge. The blending of medical and spiritual dimensions in herbalism has been and continues to be an important hallmark of our culture.

Nowhere in the diaspora is the amalgamation clearer than in Jamaica. Many Jamaicans attribute their African heritage to the Twi people of the Akan group, whose beliefs are discussed at length in part III. Some Jamaican words are closely aligned with Twi language, including *duppy*, which in Twi is *adope*, meaning "spirit." There is also indigenous culture incorporated into Jamaica courtesy of the Taino people. Apart from Twi, there is a recognized Kikongo contingent also from West Africa. There is a large helping of European blood, from the British particularly, though some also from the Portuguese and other cultures. There is a South Asian, Hindu influence as well as Jamaicans who trace some of their heritage to China. According to Arvilla Payne-Jackson and Mervyn C. Alleyne, in their dense study of Jamaican healing traditions, *Jamaican Folk Medicine: A Source of Healing*,[8] Jamaican healers—whether they are considered Obeahmen or Obeahwomen, Myal mediums, Revivers, Kumina practitioners, balm yard healers, or mother healers—consider the

---

7   Faith Mitchell, *Hoodoo Medicine* (Columbia, SC: Summerhouse Press, 1999).
8   Arvilla Payne-Jackson and Mervyn C. Alleyne, *Jamaican Folk Medicine: A Source of Healing* (Jamaica: Univ. of the West Indies Press, 2004).

wisdom of ATRs, European herbalism, India's Ayurveda, and Chinese medicine in their unique fusion of multicultural folk medicine.[9]

Elsewhere in the Americas the stew is equally rich. According to Margarite Fernández Olmos and Lizabeth Paravisini-Gebert in *Creole Religions of the Caribbean: An Introduction from Vodou and Santería to Obeah and Espiritismo*, "Santería or Regla de Ocha, Regla de Palo, and the Abakuá Secret Society follow the traditional African approach of dynamic and flexible cultural borrowing and merging, a resourceful and creative strategy common in African, where religious ideas travel frequently across ethnic and political boundaries."[10]

My own work, *Sticks, Stones, Roots & Bones: Hoodoo, Mojo & Conjuring with Herbs,*[11] revolves around Hoodoo, as it is the magical herbal tradition in the United States that embodies the essence of African healing wisdom that I am most familiar with. I will use the terminology of Hoodoo—for example, *rootwork*—as a synonym for herbalism because that is the way the practice has been described in the United States by African Americans historically.

Though initially it may elicit a flinch, objective use of the term *witch doctor*, stripped of religiosity and negative stereotypes, aptly fits African herbalism as well, since it suggests a spiritual and physical connection. A green witch knows her herbs and uses them to heal body, mind, and spirit in the same way a doctor utilizes biomedicines to treat illness and disease. The African American rootworker does not simply heal a sore throat; she examines environmental issues, spiritual matters, overall health, and the psychological state of her client.

In *The Healing Wisdom of Africa*, Malidoma Patrice Somé, a Dagara from Burkina Faso, states:

> *According to indigenous African philosophy, you cannot just give an aspirin or cook up an herbal recipe for healing. There are two things at work. One is the knowledge of the spiritual nature of the plants and the second and more important is the knowledge of the energetic configuration and the identity and purpose of the person being treated.*[12]

---

9   Payne-Jackson and Alleyne, *Jamaican Folk Medicine*.
10   M. Fernández Olmos and L. Paravisini-Gebert, *Creole Religions of the Caribbean: An Introduction from Vodou and Santería to Obeah and Espiritismo* (New York: New York Univ. Press, 2003), 24.
11   Stephanie Rose Bird, *Sticks, Stones, Roots & Bones: Hoodoo, Mojo & Conjuring with Herbs* (Saint Paul, MN: Llewellyn Worldwide, 2004).
12   Malidoma Patrice Somé, *The Healing Wisdom of Africa: Finding Life Purpose Through Nature, Ritual, and Community* (New York: Jeremy P. Tarcher / Putnam, 1999).

This book celebrates the ways people of African descent conceive of healing with herbs. Even though Africa and the African diaspora are huge places, conceptually, African herbal healing has a very specific language that brings these places closer together until it almost acts as a singular practice. While there are numerous groups of people with distinct languages, cultural practices, and worldviews in Africa and the diaspora, this book examines the qualities that unify our vision of health and healing. I call these fundamental qualities the key concepts of African herbal healing ways: (1) animism, (2) spirit, (3) ashe, (4) holism, and (5) the role of the seasons on health.

Animism

Animism is the foundation on which most earth-based spirituality and "natural" healing traditions are built. An animistic vision of the world is one where nature is viewed as a vibrant living force. Our creator, ancestors, spirits, sustenance, and hope for the future are alive in nature.

Animism is not abstract. If you comb through personal memories, you are bound to find a moment when animism has colored your vision or shaped experiences. I can still vividly remember such a day that occurred fifteen years ago. It was eerie. We were in front of what seemed to be an endless procession of cars at my mother's funeral. Dad looked up to the sky on that crisp autumn day; an ironic grin crossed his full lips, and then suddenly tears rolled down his ruddy cheeks. "It's such a beautiful day," he said quietly and then more loudly, "such a beautiful day." Tears also filled my eyes. I looked to the stark, cloudless sky and, strangely enough, I had to agree with Dad: what a beautiful day it was.

Perhaps the reason Dad and I could see the mixed blessing through our mutual pool of tears was that we not only grasped animism conceptually but we were certain that Ma's spirit had returned to earth and was now completely free to exist among the clouds, trees, and lakes. She had become a part of the beauty of that day. This is something I internalized and also expressed as a visual artist—painting landscape as though it were animated with spirit. Animism encourages us to take care of the land because it is a way of taking care of our people simultaneously.

Animism, the idea that nature is alive with spirit, is a unifying belief within both my Native American and West African heritage. Engagement with animism was an everyday occurrence living on that slim track of the Pine Barrens of southern New Jersey called Alloway, because the spirit of the Nanticoke Lenni-Lenape people enriched our lives with beauty and grace. During each season we couldn't help but recognize the presence of their spirit living in nature. Rumbling and roaring as they passed under our ice skates below the frozen lake. Within the breezes that swung the sweet-smelling laurel blossoms back and forth, releasing their delicate scent into the spring air. Through the call and answer of the bullfrogs from their tree stumps during the dog days of summer, and most of all, we recognized their lights flickering through the brightly hued forests of fall as they traveled on the backs of fireflies.

In an animistic view of the world, there is an important purpose for us once we journey into the realm of the spirit. We continue to be honored by our family and ancestors. Even in death, we continue to have a vital role in our communities. We live free of the constraints that society, or even a corporeal body, previously had. Animism allows us to meld with the seasons, becoming as one with our environment. In traditional West Africa, the concept of animism is central, particularly among the Yoruba. Many African Americans are descendants of the Yoruba, thus their cosmology colors our thoughts.

Spirit of Egun, Ghede, and Others

Traditions aside, it remains challenging living in a society fixated on clearly delineated boundaries. Crossing boundaries is a normal part of my life, as it is for many multicultural people. We speak various tongues, whether it is an officially recognized language or a tribal, Creole, patois, or perhaps colloquial language of our homes and neighborhoods that differs from what is taught in schools. As we travel through life communicating with various people in ways that seem most appropriate, tightly fixed spaces become alien.

When my people were enslaved and brought to the United States, they quickly learned that speaking of spirit was a "no-no." Eventually, African traditional religions were made illegal in the United States and parts of the Caribbean; colonialist incursions have been made in various parts of Africa as well.

Still, there remained a cultural standpoint that healing from plants was sacred and that, because of this, plants themselves were imbued with spirit. Quimbois, Obeah, Shango, Vodou, Myal, Hoodoo, Lucumí, and Regla de Ocha (the religion of the orishas, hard-to-define beings who live in the past, present, and future) continue because they fill a vital function in Black society: the ability to address the spiritual realm, the environment, and the physical in a manner that reflects traditional African healing ways.

Rather than communicate this belief with one another or with other cultures, enslaved Africans adapted their language to the Christian or Islamic faith of the dominant cultures. Prayers were incorporated into healing work that maintained various elements of African traditional spirituality (ATRs); in the Americas and Caribbean especially, scripture from the Holy Bible masked the ATRs in the Christian cloak of either the Protestants or Catholics, whose religions were more acceptable. Rather than describing herbs as being imbued with spirit or a healer as being connected to the spirit of nature, the connections were described as coming from God. In this way healing remained sacred work but it was communicated in acceptable language. Sharla Fett condenses this type of translation of plants and healers as doing spiritual work in her book *Working Cures:*

> *A spiritual orientation toward the local landscape defined the herbal practice of enslaved communities. The herbalism of Southern Black people, it can be argued, expressed a sacred worldview as clearly as singing, praying, or dancing. As they gathered, administered, and taught about botanical medicines, enslaved African Americans enacted a relationship with the land that was both practical and spiritual.*[13]

When you think of spirit, I am sure healing, prayer, invocation, and the church quite naturally come to mind. Like most Africans and African-descended people, my family has close ties to organized religions, and in fact, my maternal grandmother was a spiritualist minister of a Holiness church. My second father, however, was a Babalawo of Shango. My uncle, who became my spiritual padrino of sorts, was a drummer and a well-respected priest who did healing energy work.

He became one of the most influential figures in my spiritual life. After observing me from childhood, he was convinced that I was a child of Oshun, orisha of love and sensuality. When I grew up, it became clear to him that, rather than being born of Oshun, I was instead daughter of Yemaya-Olokun, orishas of the upper and lower sea. I feel this relationship to mothering, nurturing, and water keenly and share that infinity in this book.

Mostly my clan is Methodist, Baptist, Pentecostal, and Muslim, thus I grew up with organized religion of diverse types as a spiritual foundation. ATRs, like that of the Yoruba

---

13 Fett, *Working Cures*, 76.

people, were the original path of African people before conversion to Christianity or Islam. Therefore animism and the sacred vision of plants are highlighted in *Motherland Herbal*.

Spirit is also the ghede in Haiti and Vodou and egun in parts of West Africa and in the path of Ifá. Both of these words for spirits refer to the spirit of the ancestors—those who have passed on. We realize that these spirits are a guiding force in our healing practices. We listen to them in our dreams and invite their energy to bless herbal blends so that they are imbued with their spirit. This is a very important facet of African-inspired healing work and holistic health. It is important to preserve and disseminate these older ways of thinking as they form the crux of a distinctive approach. African herbalism helps us maintain a spiritual connection with our planet as well as contact with the ancestors and the community.

Ashe

Ashe is a very important West African concept, vital to the understanding and practice of African nature-based healing. Ashe is harvested from the coming together of diverse natural materials—water, stones, flowers, berries, rocks, fire, tree bark, and their attendant folklore. To heal people, their environment, ancestors, or attendant spirits, African people have traditionally combined the use of herbs, floral waters, incense, candles, and spiritual washes beautifully with prayer and invocation. It is easy to contemplate the meaning and power of ashe when we look inside a mojo bag or at an African figurative sculpture, or contemplate the stories of Osayin, Oya, Oshun, or Yemaya-Olokun, as we will do later on. Within each is a confluence of power and a distinctive approach to collecting, maintaining, and dispersing that energy. African people have a lengthy history of showing that, to be whole and healthy, we need to work closely with nature's gifts.

> **I believe in God, only I spell it N-A-T-U-R-E.**
> —*Frank Lloyd Wright, American architect*

Organic is a word we hear tossed about with increasing frequency. My relationship to the divine, earth, and the ancestors is organic and fluid. It is also a gift since I am not bogged down by strict dogma or a singular vision. I embrace the plurality of the divine as it manifests in the feminine. For me, divine is . . . well, simply divine.

Quite often throughout this book, I will mention the gods and goddesses, for they grace

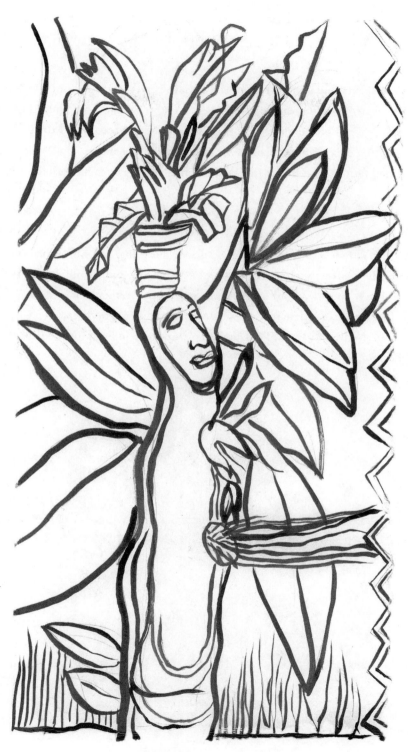

Democratic Republic of the Congo power figure

my life with health and spiritual well-being. I have been moved in tender ways by the Great Goddess, heard her whisper, roar, moan, laugh, and cackle. I recognize her smile in the sun-dappled leaves of the forest. I float, held only by her breath as I drift in the ocean. I feel her shifting energy in correlation with the stages of the moon. I will guide you through recipes, meditations, and rituals that facilitate magical engagement with the divine through herbs.

Holism

Holism does not view illness as being localized, but rather examines the other facets that may upset the system, such as events that occur in the community, home, workplace, or social circles. It considers multiple systems in the body rather than a localized complaint. Holistic healers are the shamans, priestesses, midwives, and herbalists whose work focuses on the mind, body, and spirit. Holistic herbalism exists in both the medical and the spiritual dimension.

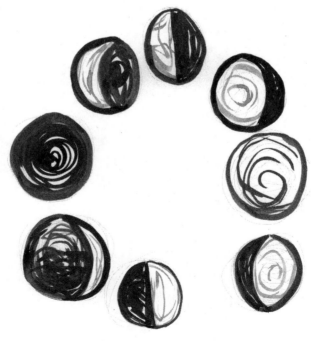

Moon phases

Much is made of the fact that shamans, conjurers, rootworkers, and so-called witch doctors treat problems of the spirit. The spirit is not nebulous; instead, it is contained within the body and affects the mind. It is easy to consider the healing ways of Africans and other indigenous people as the origin of holistic healing. Medicine people have always treated the mind, body, and spirit, which is the essence of holism, yet heretofore African practitioners and their descendants have been largely excluded from the holistic health conversation. No more.

As an African American holistic guide, *Motherland Herbal* is focused on health, maintenance, wellness, the environment, and prevention rather than illness. This guide seeks to unify various cultural traditions and African heritage with contemporary healing wisdom from around the world. Appreciation for nature, the environment, community, ancestors, the home, and yourself are considered throughout this book.

Seasonal Healing

Finally, you will notice that the practical segment of this book focuses on the seasons. *Motherland Herbal* works with seasonal observances, the herbs and foods of each harvest, as well as seasonal magical traditions in the way of the indigenous people who inspired it. The seasons affect our lives, and in order to address our health holistically, we need to work in accord with them. *Motherland Herbal* also considers the seasons in relation to the stages of life, beyond simply being times of year. This brings the story full circle.

- Winter is dedicated to the elders, ancestors, dreaming, and remembrance.
- Spring focuses on birth, children, renewal, detoxification, and cleansing.
- Summer is devoted to youth, love, pregnancy, and growth.
- Fall revolves around changes, beauty, middle age, and prevention.

Living close to the earth, paying attention to the changing of the seasons, seasonal observances, and community harvest is central to becoming involved in herbalism in a practical way. Relax and enjoy the journey toward good health!

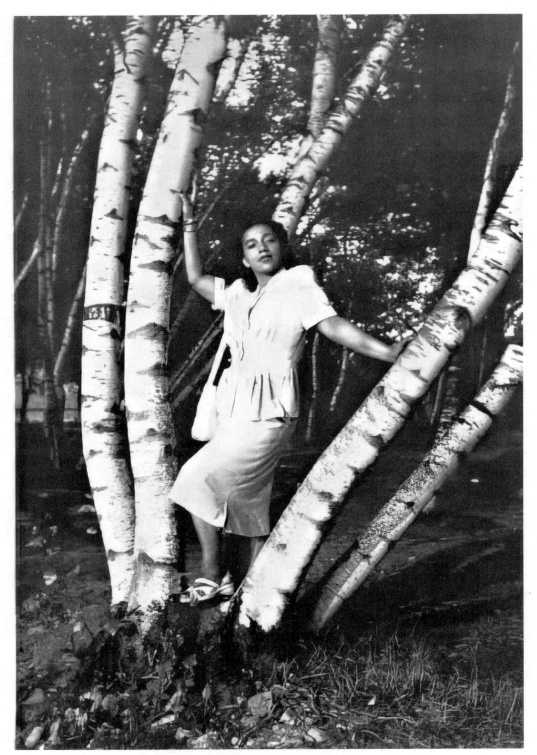

Daddy's mother, Grandma Lucille, as a young woman

CHAPTER 2

Planting with Spirit / Harvesting Ashe

THE MAGICAL AND PHYSICAL SEED

MY PARENTS HAVE PASSED ON, but they are alive in my spirit. Though their parents were from the South, both of them were raised in North Jersey. For reasons unbeknownst to me, they decided as a young couple not to repeat the experience of their upbringing with their own children. They moved us to the country, and although we hated it at first, I realize it has made me who I am. My childhood experiences have inspired my painting, poetry, and writing. In large part, it is those experiences in my youth that are the impetus for this herbal guide.

My mother and father seemed to adapt to country living almost too easily. We quickly went from renting a small cottage by the lake to living off the land for nearly two years as my father built our home from the ground up. Before I knew it, Dad was hunting deer, fishing, and gardening, not just for fun but also as the mainstay of our sustenance. We supplemented this with buying milk, eggs, and a half side of beef and similar foods from local farmers who were also my parents' friends. The gardening is something my father did until shortly before his death. The same holds true for my mother. My mother had an incredible green thumb and could take tomato plants from seed to flower to fruit indoors—off-season, mind you—without the assistance of grow lights.

When you are a teenager, the most important thing seems to be fitting in and being cool. I found my parents' homespun ways more than a little embarrassing. During the period when our house was being built, we lived in a log cabin with a fireplace and kerosene stove as the only sources of heat. We had no running water for nearly two years. This meant that we had to do a lot of physical work to accomplish ordinary tasks that most people take for granted. Like it or not, we had a window into the daily lives of those who had lived well before us as we walked in their shoes in some respects. I credit this with cultivating creativity and helping me understand how to live in accord with nature.

Between my parents and our grandfather, who was born on a slave plantation in 1890, I learned how to make organic fertilizer from ordinary kitchen refuse and from castoffs from fresh lake fish, as well as the right times for planting, how to harvest various fruits and vegetables, and how to preserve the harvest by freezing and canning. I even learned how to make fruit wine and moonshine, should push come to shove.

Since in many ways this book is a tribute to the ancestors and to those who have lived close to the land, part of its lesson is to encourage you to learn from your parents, even though it may seem "uncool." Learn from their parents if they are still around, and from the elders in your community. Appreciate cultural heritage, but also bring your own energy into traditions to help keep them alive and up-to-date.

Growing one's food from seed to flower to fruit is one of life's more satisfying activities. The move I spoke of occurred when I was about seven. We moved from a stone's throw away from Manhattan two hundred miles away, to a place in rural New Jersey that is called the Delaware Valley. I grew up in Jersey-tomato-, blueberry-, and eggplant-growing country. Our school bus ride took us past numerous fields of various types of grain, sheep, horses, and cows. In fact, the county over from ours, Cumberland County, is one of the country's largest producers of eggplant. This was not idyllic in the least; there were practical and social difficulties. As African Americans, we were in an extreme minority. In the long run, this allowed me to have more time to commune with nature, observe my surroundings, and connect with my people, when the opportunity presented itself.

Whatever you planted seemed to bear fruit in southern New Jersey; no wonder it is called the Garden State. I have many memories of planting and growing and of the harvesting season.

Around 6:30 a.m. the foggy mist skips daintily over the silky green lake as we head over the dirt hill to Aunt Edith's place. Aunt Edith's house is freshly painted; the cinder blocks are now turquoise. Her yard dwarves the bungalow tucked beneath sweeping mimosa trees with their fringed pink and white delicately scented blooms. We plant things on her land; she has areas of land without trees—a rarity in our wet and wooded neighborhood.

Aunt Edith's favorite plants were pole limas.

Now, the bean in my hand mimics the yin/yang symbol, but in a dull, dry skin and creamy grayish-tan color. I remember how we'd start tillin' and weedin' before it got too hot, and when it did, the old folk drank beer and gave me a swig too, which went nicely with our salted Jersey tomatoes.

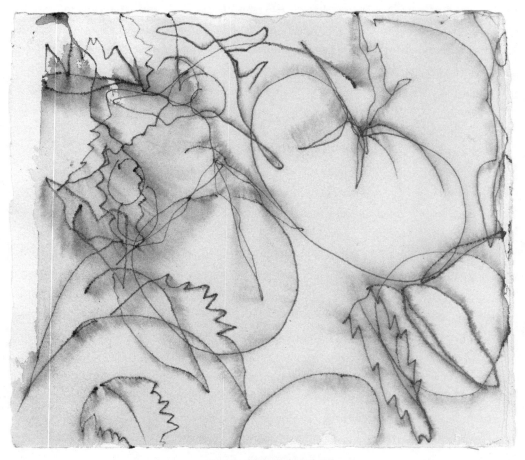

Mama's Jersey tomatoes

On weekends we'd wake even earlier to go to the larger fields used by various companies. We lived near the lands farmed by Green Giant, Hunt's, and other commercial produce companies. After the workings of their huge machines, so much was left behind to harvest. We'd go in and pick and pick and pick some more, till I thought or hoped I had cramps in my hands—bushels and bushels of beans. We were careful in case anyone official might see, but fortunately, they never did.

When we arrived at home, Ma had picnic tables set out in the front yard to make our work easier. It was time to put up (preserve) the harvest to see us through fall, winter, and into the spring. *Thwack!* The bushels of beans would hit the table hard. We'd begin our sorting and snapping of the string beans. This consumed the better half of the day. Then the next day, we'd put the beans "up," or preserve them, for winter.

Back in the present moment in suburbia, I hold my bean, remembering as I stroke it. It is a perfect teleport into my youth. Beginning to the left, and ending not quite right—the pod where egg and seed meet. Snap one, snap two, three, and four.

"Mommy, were you listening to me at all?" my daughter asks impatiently. Spread the soil and plant your seeds, girl . . . I dream on.

The water boils, and I let the snapped beans tumble free from their cobalt-blue Tupperware colander. Minced onions and garlic sizzle in the seasoned cast-iron skillet as I sprinkle on some dried cayenne, pepper, and coarse sea salt. A splash of apple vinegar followed by the cubed potatoes—*plop, splash*—on top of the green beans.

TODAY, EVEN THOUGH I LIVE in an urban suburb in Illinois, I am lucky to live on land with black, humus-rich soil, which we have enhanced with our own kitchen compost. The rich soil enables me to remain in touch with the Earth Mother through gardening; though my patch of earth is now small, it is still my own. On my land I continue to plant magical and literal seeds, hopes and dreams for the future as well as tributes to my people.

Living far away from the home of my family, paying these tributes is something that came to me intuitively. I recalled how many families had cemetery plots on their land. Being hundreds of miles away, it made sense to try to pay some sort of visual homage to my departed loved ones on my land. Richard Westmacott wrote one of the most in-depth books on the African American ways of gardening and maintaining yards. In *African-American Gardens and Yards in the Rural South,*[1] he highlights ways of gardening, tending land, and maintaining a yard that are distinctively African American. These include having transplanted plants from nearby forests such as dogwood trees, which is something my family did. My parents also transplanted mountain laurel, which grew profusely in the area. Planting memorial plants to pay tribute to someone you love who has departed this earth is another specific aspect of Black Southern gardens. The inclusion of symbolic magical talismans like seashells, coins, or other special objects as part of the garden decor is another feature, as is the utilization of rocks, particularly river rocks, alongside the pathway and bottles hung in trees as protective amulets. Robert Farris Thompson discusses the bottle tree phenomenon

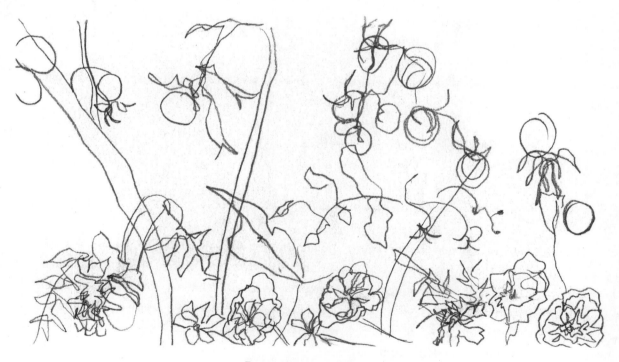

Tomatoes and marigolds

---

1   Richard Westmacott, *African-American Gardens and Yards in the Rural South* (Knoxville: Univ. of Tennessee Press, 1992).

in *Flash of the Spirit*,[2] along with the other ways people in the African diaspora go about imbuing their garden with spirit.

Westmacott also notes that in the Southern tradition, landowners often buried their deceased family members on the property, as I had also observed. This changes the character of the yard, making it part cemetery and part garden—bringing life and death together. Perhaps this story about my own garden will bring forth ideas for making your own spirit garden as a protective amulet to your home and tribute to your ancestors:

The Pathway Home

Ambling down the path, boxes and bags held snug, when the vision of a new home in the distance offsets my balance.

I pause.

A cursory glance over the barren gray dirt that someone thought was a yard, and a plan hatches:

- A couple of forsythia bushes over there.
- A smatter of deep purple Dutch iris here.
- Maybe some double-blooming raspberry-scented peonies right there.
- A cluster of sweetly fragrant lilies closest to the front door.

Ah, that would be a nice touch. At long last—a creative plan to fill the void.

We waddle back and forth—arms brimming with precious possessions. Just before dusk, with boxes, bags, paintings, sculptures, and tatty furniture tucked safely indoors, it is time to venture back outside. After living in the inner city with barely a tree over five years old, having a yard, however barren and small, is emancipation.

What would Mama think?

There is none of the bucolic splendor here that I grew up with. This tight and tidy brick two-flat is only a stone's throw away from the El tracks.

Once, the view from my bedroom window was of a verdant lake rimmed with sweeping

2   Robert Farris Thompson, *Flash of the Spirit* (New York: Vintage Books, 1984).

pines and sleepy willows. Now, I look out over the canyon created by the expressway and a river of ever-flowing, noisy vehicles.

As an artist, I realize the world is as beautiful as imagination permits.

I plow the soil diligently with my hand tools, flipping her over and over again with my pitchfork. Soon enough, it becomes evident that, like me, she is still very fertile. As I dig down deep, I find the soil to be as rich and black as a Yoruba queen. Within these dark depths, I plant an array of seeds and bulbs:

- Lullabies at night for the little one
- Sunny daffodils by day to light the way for the boys
- Purple pansies, Mama's color and flower in her memory
- Hope, for the healthy birth of the little girl growing within my still-flat belly
- Sunflowers, narcissus, and a variety of botanical tulips for my grandmothers
- Negro spirituals, as a tribute to Grandpop
- Shiny pennies are tossed for luck
- Yarrow for my ultra-strong great-grandma Louise
- Sensual Bourbonnais roses for my dear Aunt Rose
- Daily water and fire rituals for clarity, strength, and protection
- Aquilegia (Spring Song Columbine) for my second mum, Iris, who radiates gentility, power, and grace
- Rites of fertility, recipes for continued health, creativity, and the infinite capacity to love

All anchored by a round cairn of stone symbolic of my soulmate. All set behind a whitewashed picket fence that seemed to begin aging as soon as it was erected (sprinkled with gopher's dust to bar evil spirits from entry . . .), and so it went for over a decade.

The little one and I head up the path. Projects, chores, responsibilities, appointments, obligations, that heady scent of lilac, Bourbonnais roses, and the remaining narcissus muddle my thoughts. The path from home is not the straight walk it once was.

Today my path is strewn with leaves, stems, flowers, and looming shadows.

Veronica Speedwell leans over each side of the walkway gossiping with the little chrysanthemums. The peonies now need their own zip code, but at least the lilies keep to themselves. The black-eyed Susans are spreading everywhere, but the crone wort (*Artemisia vulgaris;* Where the hell did she come from?) thankfully is just as thick as she is tall. I hear her cackle coming and going, though sometimes it is just barely audible. She and her feathery leaves looking like helping hands and all. Tough sage green on top, tender, soft, and silver beneath, tassels above all, lending sultry airs all around.

Mysteriously, crone wort has taken up residence outside our front door. Where once there was order, plans, and direction to my garden, there is now a lush green space, whose semblance of order lies beneath, at the base of the garden, within the roots.

Buried remnants of well-laid plans intermingle with seashells and pennies from days of old. My garden is now a sanctuary. Birds, bees, children, and weary commuters find soul food and solace as they make their way through the world.

This place people used to call a yard is now more of a healer's thatch.

Approaching a wildflower prairie, this space is sheltered by a teeming forest of sunflowers with the crone wort and her stylish tresses acting as gatekeeper.

I could go on and on about my tangled mass of stems, overgrown perennials, strangling weeds, and stinging thistles. Most often, though, I just want to get home and latch that decrepit gate behind me.

No matter that, as of this spring, the elder boy towers over me and I feel the rustling of Oya's skirts as he passes in pursuit of hopes and dreams beyond my reach. Though they are gangly and a bit unruly, still, I know that as each child grows, the sunflowers will present their aspirations to the sun.

Our toddler and the newly transplanted French lavender, rose-scented geranium, geranium chamomile, and hyssop vie for the warming rays of the sun and merciful light along with a precious bit of space to call their own.

Stooping over to lessen the load, the reflection in the puddle reveals a wide-hipped, thick-legged Black woman, flicks of gray intermingled in her reddish-brown Afro.

She looks back at me with the fixed gaze of one who sees.

Time to stop overlooking the ancient wisdom that has taken root at my doorstep. Tonight I will cut some crone wort down for the first time. I'll rub her between my palms, inhale her camphor-like aroma deeply, and then place a bit of her green blood on my third eye to enhance my foresight. Next, I'll stuff the stems and leaves in a jar and drench them in safflower oil.

While I'm waiting for the crone to release her powers into the oil, I'll do another cutting.

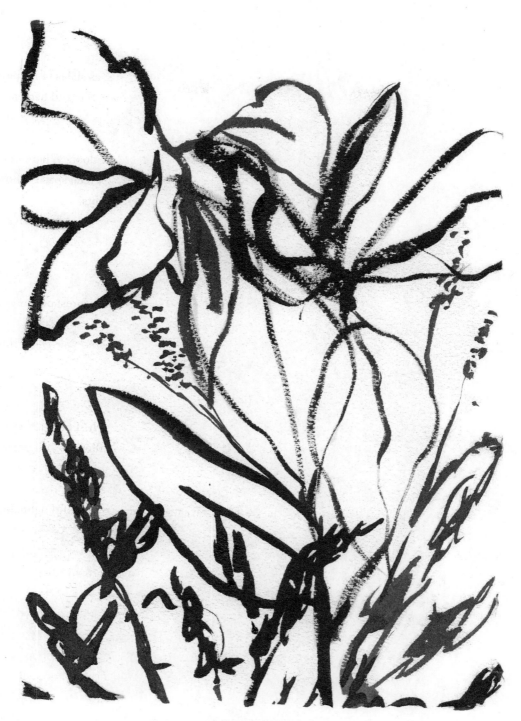

Lavendar and iris

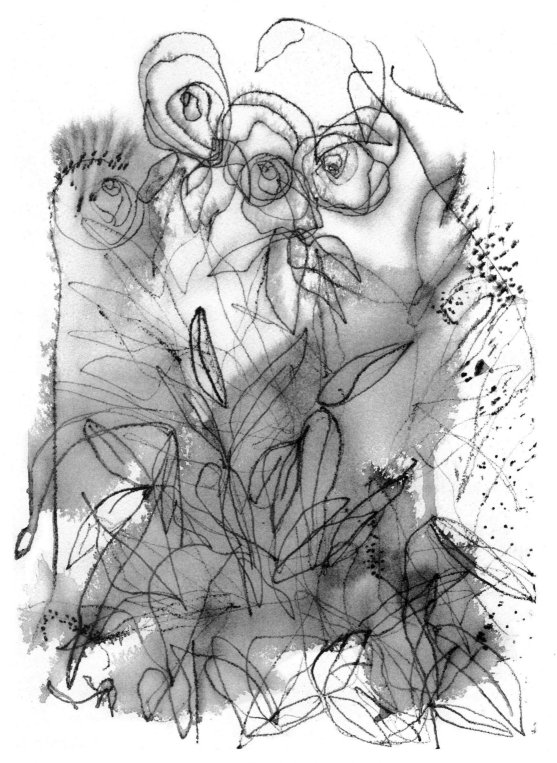

Healer's thatch

This bunch of the feathered hag will be braided, tied with hemp string, and once dried, she will be lit. The flames will be snuffed, so only her husky voice remains, to be waved over the doorstep that she faces and protects.

"Crone wort, bless this path, stoop, and entry and all those who cross this way," I implore in hushed tones by the light of the full moon. Once the moon completes her full cycle, I'll strain a bit of that precious green oil and pour it on my naked body, letting it penetrate my tired soul, aching joints and Earth-shaped belly. When I am healed, I'll work on my soulmate, my children, and perhaps others in need of her life juice.

Time to use what has been given and to realize that I am no longer a slender girl eagerly searching for homes on distant shores:

> Woman of the house
> Planter of seeds
> Tiller of dreams
> Too old to call maiden and too young to call crone

Creating a Spirit Garden

No one can tell you how to make your own spirit garden because all of the seeds for it are planted within your soul. I can make a few suggestions for your consideration as you plan such a garden.

- First and foremost, you need to allow yourself plenty of rest, *still time,*[3] and meditation so that you can tap into your intuition—your spirit within.
- Have a blank book in whatever pattern or style will inspire you to record recollections, dreams, and thoughts about your garden. Keep this and a pen handy, tucked away in a place that is easily accessible so that you can use it as the thoughts arise.
- If this is to pay tribute or remind you of someone you love who has passed on, try to think about the things, colors, sounds, textures, flowers, vegetables, fruits, and herbs

---

3   *Still time* is the time you set aside where you are not concerned about work, sustenance, your love life, family, or anything. It is simply time to be quiet and exist, observing what thoughts occur once your slate of thoughts has been wiped clean.

that person or animal enjoyed. Write these down in your spirit garden journal. Make plans to purchase seeds or harvest cuttings from a neighbor during planting season.

- Consider the zodiac—this was a huge pastime with our ancestors in the United States. Do you want to make certain beds in the pattern of your, another person's, or an animal's astrological sign? Consider the strengths and weaknesses of each sign.
- You could also work with a powerful African amulet like the ankh, symbol of everlasting life.
- Rather than plant in a pattern, you could simply mark out the pattern of the astrological sign, hex sign, or African amulet using stones.
- Collect textured materials to put in the garden, for example smooth sea glass,[4] patterned marbles, pieces of flat rounded glass,[5] charged quartz crystals, river rocks, or driftwood.

Points to Remember

- Quartz crystal makes your garden area conducive to vision quest, divination, and healing energy.
- River rocks invoke the spirit of Oshun, orisha of sensuality, beauty, and sexuality.
- Driftwood invokes the spirit of Yemaya-Olokun, mother orisha who nurtures and protects her children.
- Consider statuary. Some people like to put saints, the Virgin Mary, or the Virgin of Guadalupe in their gardens. Others prefer Earth goddesses from ancient Egypt like the Triple Goddess Symbol, Goddess of the Nile, or even a bust of Nefertiti. Still others have patrons whose energy they like to keep nearby. These include many different types of Buddhas, Saint Francis, Santa Barbara, Black Madonnas, Kwan Yin (Goddess of Compassion), and Lakshmi (Goddess of Prosperity, Sensuality, and Abundance).
- Borrowing from the Cayman Islanders and Southern African Americans, you could also try keeping a swept yard. This bears some resemblance in spirit to Japanese sand gardens. Cayman Islanders are known for drawing out wave patterns that can be seen

---

4   This is glass that has been smoothed by the ocean so that it has no rough edges.
5   These are sold at garden centers and craft stores for indoor gardening and candle environments.

in the moonlight. African American people sweep these types of gardens smooth with a brushwood broom. You could use your magical besom, which is the name witches use for brooms. The garden must be kept free of foot tracks and weeds; it is a labor of love. These types of gardens are still seen in parts of West Africa.[6] An area devoted to the swept yard will be especially appealing to those who enjoy a place of quiet contemplation but who may lack the green thumb for growing plants. A swept yard is covered in soil or you can bring in white sand and each week you sweep the yard (or even a small area of the yard) into subtle patterns to instill a feeling of inner peace.

- Finally, a great deal can be said by the selection of the plants themselves. Herbs are featured in the following chapters that enslaved Africans brought to the Americas and Caribbean. These include watermelon, okra, black-eyed peas, sesame, eggplant, yams, peanut, cantaloupe, and West Indian gherkin.[7] You can also use plants to symbolically suggest a person as I have done in the spirit garden shared on pages 24–29.
- There are infinite ways to create an African spirit garden. The main limitations are set by your imagination, so stay in touch with your intuition, angels, or muses; listen intently; and start with small, manageable increments that are easy to complete.

Creative Harvesting

Now, some people will become really intimidated by the idea of gardening, figuring they don't have enough land or any land of their own to plant in and till. For folks living in cities, apartments, and other tight spaces where land comes at a premium price, the primary source for gathering of herbs may well be specialty catalogs, health food stores, and online. Even within this commercial arena, the way you go about gathering is critical, and the relationships developed can be meaningful, educational, and fun. Things to look for:

- Are the herbs ethically harvested? (Be careful about barks and roots; some like echinacea are overharvested and face extinction.)
- Are the herbs organically grown? This is the safest method for personal care products and consumables.

---

6   Westmacott, *African-American Gardens and Yards.*
7   William E. Grimé, *Ethno-botany of the Black Americans* (Algonac, MI: Reference Publications, 1979), 19–63.

- Are the prices fair, without excessive markups? Do some research and price comparisons.
- Are the herbs usually in stock, available without delays?
- Is the source convenient and practical for you?
- Is a knowledgeable person available to answer your questions?
- Start out with a local shop if possible, but as you become comfortable with creating your own brews, branch out into wholesale. Buying herbs in bulk saves big bucks!

Other Suggestions for City Dwellers

- Look for freshness (bright color, no mold or mildew, strong scent) and expiration dates on herbs.
- Grow your favorite herbs in pots on the windowsill, terrace, or inside using grow lights.
- Visit your local farmers market, investigate organic whole-food co-ops, or drive outside the city to support roadside farm stands.

Your Herbs Will Find You

When you are starting as a gardener, you wonder, What should I plant? What will grow? With which herbs do I want to work? Herbs will show up for you, in your life, when you need them, how you need them. The herbs that have shown up for me at different times in my life are:

- Achillea, better known as yarrow, is one of my foundational plants, and as such, it is my stalwart friend and has not left me yet.
- Mugwort, from which I made many a smudge stick, was prominent when I needed it but has since faded back.
- Lamb's-quarter, a gentle reminder that weeds are good and useful.
- Poke, an African American healer's plant, has popped up out of nowhere in my backyard. Its presence is massive and comforting.
- Plantain is so plentiful here in the Midwest and so very practical.
- Soapwort, also called Bouncing Bet as in Betsy or Betty, is outside my writer's desk window. Each year its showing of flowers gets increasingly more massive. Bouncing

Bet reminds me to be authentic in my writing and daily life. It is the soapmaker's plant; *wort* means "herb."

A Note About Foraging

If you are fortunate enough to go foraging (gathering fresh herbs from the forest, fields, or other locales), make sure you have permission and are not harvesting on restricted land or harvesting a fragile or "at-risk" plant. Here is a working list of such plants archived by the United Plant Savers.[8] You will want to use these with a great deal of discernment if you are dealing with wholesalers or buying in quantity.

AT-RISK PLANTS

- American ginseng (*Panax quinquefolius*)
- Black cohosh (*Actaea [Cimicifuga] racemosa*)
- Bloodroot (*Sanguinaria canadensis*)
- Blue cohosh (*Caulophyllum thalictroides*)
- Echinacea (*Echinacea* sp.)
- Eyebright (*Euphrasia* sp.)
- Goldenseal (*Hydrastis canadensis*)
- Helonias root (*Chamaelirium luteum*)
- Lady's slipper orchid (*Cypripedium* spp.)
- Lomatium (*Lomatium dissectum*)
- Osha (*Ligusticum porteri, L.* spp.)
- Peyote (*Lophophora williamsii*)
- Slippery elm (*Ulmus rubra*)
- Sundew (*Drosera* sp.)
- Trillium, Beth root (*Trillium* sp.)
- True unicorn (*Aletris farinosa*)
- Venus flytrap (*Dionaea muscipula*)
- Virginia snakeroot (*Aristolochia serpentaria*)
- Wild yam (*Dioscorea villosa, D.* sp.)

8   https://unitedplantsavers.org.

TO-WATCH PLANTS

- Arnica (*Arnica* sp.)
- Butterfly weed (*Asclepias tuberosa*)
- Cascara sagrada (*Rhamnus purshiana*)
- Chaparro (*Castela emoryi*)
- Elephant tree (*Bursera microphylla*)
- Gentian (*Gentiana* sp.)
- Goldthread (*Coptis* sp.)
- Kava kava (*Piper methysticum*; Hawaii only)
- Lobelia (*Lobelia* sp.)
- Maidenhair fern (*Adiantum pedatum*)
- Mayapple (*Podophyllum peltatum*)
- Oregon grape (*Mahonia* sp.)
- Partridgeberry (*Mitchella repens*)
- Pinkroot (*Spigelia marilandica*)
- Pipsissewa (*Chimaphila umbellata*)
- Spikenard (*Aralia racemosa, A. californica*)
- Stoneroot (*Collinsonia canadensis*)
- Stream orchid (*Epipactis gigantea*)
- Turkey corn (*Dicentra canadensis*)
- White sage (*Salvia apiana*)
- Wild indigo (*Baptisia tinctoria*)
- Yerba mansa (*Anemopsis californica*)

Ancestor Harvest Offering

Before harvesting from your own garden or foraging in the wild, it is important to use rituals to ensure a good harvest and make offerings to the earth, thanking her for her fertility. Here is an offering to try:

Bring fresh fruit and vegetables of the season, a white pillar candle, and matches to a fresh water source (pond, river, stream, lake) close to you. Those without a body of water can still pay tribute using a portable fountain. Set out fruit special to your family or heritage. Clear a space down to the dirt for the candle. Light it. Begin your prayer of thanks. *I know that you were here in my beginning and that you will be here in the end. Blessed be. Thank you for always being with me, for influencing, shaping, and making me whole. Blessed be. I lay these fruits out for you to partake in the presence of our elixirs of life. Blessed be. I am yours; you are mine, in body, mind, and spirit. Blessed be.* Bow your head. Listen to the ancestors' response. When you are ready, extinguish the candle and take it with you, but leave the fruit out as food to the ancestors at the site.

Harvesting Leaves

Look for leaves of a consistent green color without brown or yellow spots. Harvest mid-morning, after the dew has evaporated. Gather leaves before the plant begins to flower. For plants such as basil or oregano with long growing seasons, pinch back tops to prevent flowering. (Flowering takes energy away from the main body of the plant.) Keep herbs separated by type; tie the stems loosely with twine or hemp string, together in a bundle. Until you are very familiar with all the herbs, it is best to label the bundles and date them as well. Hang them up to dry immediately after harvesting to prevent mildew or deterioration.

Hang herb bundles, stem up, in an area with good circulation away from direct sunlight. The ideal temperature for the first 24 hours is 90 degrees, followed by 75 to 80 degrees the rest of the time. Most herbal bundles will dry in 2 to 3 weeks. Petals and leaves should feel light, crisp, and paperlike. If there are small buds or tiny leaves, which may fall off during the drying time, create a roomy muslin bag to encase flowers and leaves; tie loosely with twine or hemp string at the stems. This is particularly important with seed-dropping plants such as fennel or sunflowers. When herbs are completely dry, store the whole leaf and stem away from direct sunlight in dark glass or stainless-steel airtight containers.

Harvesting Flowers

Select healthy flowers in the early afternoon during dry weather conditions. Flowers are extremely delicate. Take extra care not to bruise the petals; refrain from touching them. Cut them from the stem and allow the flowers to drop into a basket. Dry smaller, more delicate flowers such as lavender and chamomile whole; hang them upside down, tied with twine over a muslin cloth or large bowl, or wrap them loosely with muslin to retain the dried buds.

Use fresh flowers whenever possible. You may also freeze them in an ice-cube tray filled with spring water.

Harvesting Seeds

Collect seeds on a warm, dry day. Seeds need to dry in a warm, airy environment. Make provisions to catch the quickly drying seeds by placing a bowl or box underneath hanging plants.

Harvesting Bark

Bark peels easiest on damp days. Choose a young tree or bush, if possible one that has already been pruned, cut, or taken down naturally by wind or stormy conditions; this will prevent damage or even death to the plant. Stripping too much bark from a tree will kill it. A thoughtful approach to Mother Nature's gifts is essential. Bark may harbor insects or moss, so wash it first and allow it to dry flat on waxed paper in a location that is well-ventilated and away from direct sunlight.

Harvesting Roots

Roots are ready for collecting after autumn harvest. Dig up roots after their plant has begun to wither and die. Extract the whole root while trying not to bruise it. Like bark, roots need to be cleaned before they are dried; they also require ethical harvesting to yield ashe. Cut roots into small sections and dry them in an oven set between 120 and 140°F. Turn and check the roots regularly. They should feel light and airy like sawdust when fully dried. For marshmallow root, peel away the top layer of skin before drying in this manner.

Harvesting Berries

Use the same procedure as for bark, but remember berries and fruits take a long time to dry, about twice as long as leaves. You will know when they are fully dry because they will become very light and wrinkled, and will have reduced in size by nearly half. Turn them frequently and check for leaking juices. Replace the paper below them often to prevent the growth of bacteria or mold.

CHAPTER 3

Elbow Grease

TOOLS AND EQUIPMENT FOR WORKING ROOTS

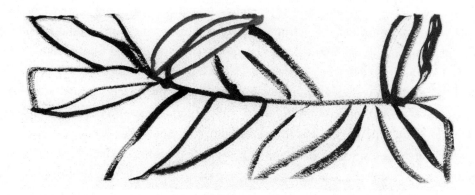

The Means of Working Roots

History and the cross-cultural use of herbs and aromatherapy are intriguing, yet in order to actually work with herbs (rootwork), practical hands-on information is required. The beauty of African aromatherapy and our herbalism is that they incorporate the best of both worlds—East and West come together, melding medicine with magical intent capable of touching the spirit realm.

In the next few pages you will find some of the most useful tools to help you in the journey toward practicing rootwork. Some of these ways and means will seem very African, whereas others will seem more Western. However you slice it, these tools will enable you to do rootwork.

Tools

Baskets—preferably sweetgrass[1] or other handwoven natural material for holding freshly harvested fruits, vegetables, and herbs.

Blender—glass or stainless-steel pitchers are preferred over plastic, as they can be thoroughly cleansed, whereas some residual matter may be retained in plastic, contaminating future blends. Blenders are used for thoroughly mixing and liquefying a variety of natural ingredients including vegetables, fruits, and grains.

Bottles and jars—very important pieces of equipment. I like using recycled bottles as much as possible for shampoo and conditioners. Mouthwash bottles, liquid dish detergent, shampoo and conditioner bottles, as well as lotion, yogurt, and baby food containers are all useful. At times you will want to make special blends as gifts or for your stores. There are plenty of specialty container suppliers who carry powder dispensers, spray-topped bottles, cologne bottles, flip-top bodywash bottles, and decorative jars with screw tops for this purpose. It's nice now and again to use decorative containers for yourself, especially the powder dispensers, since powders are important to African herbalism. Remember: when using recycled materials, it is very important to sterilize them first by boiling plastic containers and cleansing glass bottles with very hot soapy water; rinse and allow to dry before beginning. They can also be sterilized in a dishwasher if you have one.

Cauldron—this doesn't have to be fancy or bought from a specialty shop; a plain cast-iron Dutch oven will do. However, if you want to brew your potions in a proper cauldron, there are plenty of suppliers who carry them.

Charcoal blocks—buy these in quantity, as they are the most efficient way of burning lose herbal incense. Avoid those that contain saltpeter—it is toxic when burned. Pure bamboo charcoals from Japan are available and make a wholesome alternative.

Coffee bean grinder—an electric-powered tool with swiveling blades, the coffee bean

---

1   Sweetgrass baskets are made primarily by the Gullah people and sold at markets in Charleston, South Carolina, and other Low Country, Sea Coast Island locations. Some sweetgrass basket co-ops now also make these available online at virtual stores.

grinder is a convenient way to grind tough spices and roots compared to its ancestor the mortar and pestle, which requires hand-grinding and lots of elbow grease. (Watch out, though: really tough spices and roots do need to be ground by hand or they'll break your coffee grinder. Trust me, I've been through quite a few.) These are available at coffee shops, home improvement centers, department stores, and discount shops.

Double boiler—an indirect way of heating that prevents waxy mixtures like ointments and candle wax from cooking too quickly. A double boiler can be improvised by floating a stainless-steel bowl in water in a pot slightly larger than the stainless-steel bowl.

Droppers—essential for dispensing droplets of essential oils, fragrance oils, body fluids, or other precious liquids that you don't want to waste. Throughout the book, I ask that you drop in essential oils; this is the approach used by good perfumers, because it helps ensure that the oils don't clump up and instead disperse evenly.

Drying rack—an implement on which fresh herbs are hung by their stems and left to dry. It's also an attractive way to display and store dried herbs indefinitely.

Firepit—a miniature fireplace that is portable and generally kept on the patio. This is great for burning incense and fire rituals if you don't have a fireplace. These are growing in popularity, thus they are more widely available and are sometimes simply referred to as *patio fireplaces*. Look for these at your garden center, home renovation shops, sporting goods stores, and specialty shops.

Food processor—even a mini model without all the fancy attachments will do to blend and liquefy ingredients for personal care recipes.

Freestanding mixer—a convenient but not essential tool. Used for whisking and thoroughly blending ingredients while saving your personal energy.

Funnel set—used to prevent spills and to ease the transfer of liquids, oils, and powders from the bowl or pan to a small-necked bottle, referred to here as bottling.

Glass storage jars—used mainly for oil infusions and tinctures. Tinted-glass spring or cork tops work well. Don't forget to sterilize first.

Gloves—thick cloth gloves to protect the hands when harvesting berries, rose hips, roses, or other thorny branches; plastic gloves to keep your hands from contaminating herbal infusions, brews, decoctions, balms, salts, or other handmade herbal blends.

Grater, Teflon or stainless steel—these are recommended because they last longer and resist sticking and rusting. Mainly used for shredding beeswax and refining roots.

Juicer—creates fruit and vegetable juices.

Kerchief—these are made of simple cloth, plain or patterned, and they come in handy for keeping your locs, braids, or any type of hairstyle away from your brews and blends. Some ingredients you work with are damaging to the hair and irritating to the scalp, so it is good to protect your hair while working with herbs. It is also important to maintain the highest standard of cleanliness possible so that your herbal blends, brews, or potions are less likely to become contaminated by bacteria, dirt, or oils.

Kettle—to boil water used for infusing herbs.

Measuring spoons—preferably made of stainless steel with clearly marked measurements etched into the surface.

Mixing bowls—glass, ceramic, or stainless steel is recommended because they will not become stained from colorants, nor will they harbor bits of leftover ingredients once cleaned properly. Cleanliness is very important because dirty bowls or other equipment will introduce bacteria to your recipes, lessening their longevity and efficacy.

Mortar and pestle—this is a hand-grinding tool set, consisting of a bowl and a stick-like grinding tool that can be made of wood, marble, soapstone, or various other materials. In many ways a mortar and pestle is symbolic of the African community, and it is an essential tool of both cook and healer. Quite frequently when the African village is depicted in African stelae or other forms of art, the mortar and pestle is figured prominently because the set is considered an indispensable tool for sustenance. Mortar and pestles are used for food preparation, grinding flour from various grains to make bread, and most important to our discussion here, the mortar and pestle is used to hand-grind resins, tough spices, barks, roots, berries, grasses, leaves, and flowers. I recommend hand-grinding with a mortar and pestle over using a food processor or coffee bean grinder because the process allows the healer to become influenced by the healing spirit energy of the plant. The energy of the plant is released along with the aromatic oils of the plant that is being ground, diffusing this energy into the air and imbuing the environment and your soul with force and power.

Nonreactive measuring cups—both dry and liquid types. Pyrex, tempered glass, and stainless steel work best. Glass and stainless-steel measuring cups are easy to clean thoroughly, which prevents cross-contamination of ingredients from remnants of herbs and other debris.

Plastic bags—to temporarily contain spices or other dried materials that require an airtight storage.

Plastic caps—used for placing over the head and hair to trap body heat and encourage the penetration of conditioners and colorants, while keeping messy treatments off the neck and clothing.

Pot holders—quite a bit of herbal work involves heat; pot holders protect your hands from burning and are essential when working with infusions, decoctions, and other brews dependent on heat.

Pruning shears—it is good to have a sharp pair of heavy-duty shears for harvesting woody herbs, plants like roses that have thorns, evergreen branches, and other tough materials.

Scissors—you will need to have scissors on hand for cutting twine, string, cheesecloth, and leaves.

Splash-proof apron—highly recommended protection against the caustic sodium hydroxide used during cold-processed soapmaking. Also consider putting old clothes to use as smocks or work clothes.

Stainless-steel pans—those with heavy bottoms work best because they distribute heat evenly and resist burning and overheating. Most important, stainless steel stays inert, which prevents the contamination and depletion that are likely to occur while using cast iron, aluminum, or copper. Make sure you have tight-fitting lids handy as well; they help retain the medicinal qualities of the volatile oils. Otherwise, these precious substances evaporate. Stainless-steel **whisks** and **stirring spoons** are recommended for the same reasons.

Stirring wand—usually made of nonreactive glass or ceramic and used similarly to a cocktail stirrer to blend perfumes while discouraging cross-contamination.

Storage bins—used to hold dried herbs. Dark glass containers with spring tops or stainless steel are ideal. Keeping light away from the herbs helps them retain their medicinal qualities longer. Some folks store them in brown paper bags, particularly when they are being dried. This works well only if you don't have moths or other pests that might try to eat the herbs.

Stove or hot plate—for heating, drying, and simmering decoctions, potions, and brews.

Straining devices—cheesecloth (muslin) stretched over a preserve or other wide-necked jar and secured with a rubber band or twine, or what I prefer to use, a stainless-steel **sieve**.

Sun tea jars—glass or plastic jars used to brew herbs in sun or moonlight.

Thermometers—candy thermometers will work, and a meat probe will work as well, but these days soapmakers find clinical-grade infrared noncontact thermometers are the most useful.

Twine—good for tying herbs together at the stems before hanging to dry and for fixing muslin to jars for straining. Hemp string is an excellent alternative for strength and durability.

Ways of Rootworking

Freeing Up the Ashe

Once you have a good collection of tools, your means for rootworking, the fun is just about to begin. Ashe, the liquid essence of a tree, plant, root, flower, bud, berry, or leaf that contains healing energy, can be collected in various ways. To capture this precious energy, try some of the following traditional herbalism methods:

Agbo—African infusion method, by which a vegetable or fruit (called *aseje,* meaning "medicinal food") or herb is infused in water and then squeezed by hand to release the ashe.

Agunmu (pounded medicine)—this is an herbal substance including resins that are powdered on a grinding stone.

Decoction—made by extracting ashes from the tougher parts of the plant including the roots, bark, or berries, decoction is accomplished by simmering the tough parts of the plant in a covered pan of water over medium-low heat for 30 minutes to 5 hours depending on the toughness of the herb. Once this process is complete, the ashe is readily available for healing work in the brew, which is formally called a decoction.

Etu (burnt medicine)—slowly charring ingredients in a cast-iron or other heavy pot. The etu is then consumed as is or used in a body rub.

Infusion—can be either water-based or oil-based. Water-based infusions are teas containing ashe, also called *tisanes* or *brews*. Infusions are made by extracting the volatile oils of a plant in the following manner: pour boiling distilled water over the herb and keep it covered for 30 minutes to 1 hour. Heating in water for a longer time on a very low temperature on the stovetop infuses tougher herbs; the pot should be tightly covered to retain the healing medicine rather than allowing it to escape into the air.

Maceration—helps release the volatile oils and delicate scents of buds and flowers. To macerate buds, mash them up in a mortar with a pestle or pulse for 30 seconds in a mini food processor.

Oil-based infusion—extract the volatile oils from herbs by putting herbal materials into a sterilized (dry) container. Fill the jar to the top with loosely packed dried herbs and pour on your preferred oil such as olive, sunflower, sweet almond, or safflower oil, covering the plants completely and filling the jar to the top. Cover tightly, keep away from direct sunlight, and give the jar a whirl every day for 4 to 6 weeks (depending on desired strength).

Tincture—the extraction of healing medicines from herbs created by using 100-proof alcohols such as vodka, grain alcohol, rum, or ethanol. The concentrations of volatile oils are greater in tinctures than through infusion or decoction. The procedure is to fill a sterilized jar to the top with loosely packed herbal material. Be sure to use alcohol like vodka (do not use rubbing alcohol; it is too harsh and smells so strong that it will overpower any scents). Place on a sunny windowsill and swirl gently every day for 4 to 6 weeks. Strain off herbal material and pour into a sterilized tinted bottle. Cover with a cork or other tightly fitted top.

Specialties

Maceration—kin to tinctures, macerations can be created by following the above procedure but replacing the alcohol with different liquids. For example, vinegar makes an acidic extract. Macerated buds or flower petals added to vegetable glycerin make an emollient, scented extract; and honey poured over macerated buds or petals produces an edible emollient tincture that is delicately scented and terrific in love potions or in edible body rubs.

Maceration helps release the volatile oils and delicate scents of buds and flowers. To macerate buds, mash them up in a mortar with a pestle or pulse for 30 seconds in a mini food processor.

Magical Spirit Hand—Often a special hand that is different from the normal hand is used in the preparation and consumption of magical or spiritual medicines. This hand is typically the left hand, considered the magical hand, as many people are right-handed. As a lefty, I might add a note to others like me that you would want to switch to your right hand if utilizing this technique because that would be the special hand for you that is not used in mundane activity.

Toddies—Since the ancient African civilizations at Axum, Kush, Nubia, Khemet, and Egypt, African healers have combined herbal infusions with wine or other alcoholic beverages.

Spirit Works Within the Roots

Knowing the proper harvesting, drying, handling, and extracting techniques is essential to African herbalism but it is by no means the last word. The term *workin' roots* means that you should try to incorporate affirmations, incantations, and prayers if you wish or meditate as you work with herbs in order to access their spirit energy. Parts II and III of this book feature recipes combined with various types of magical work that will help you call up the ancestors or spiritual helpers to assist with healing work.

Speaking directly to the pot, fire, candle, and herb is also essential. Remember: rootwork has an animistic foundation. Animistic philosophy addresses each element or aspect of nature as being alive. Objects from nature are imbued with animism and ashe, so they have a universal energy force within them that connects us all like an umbilical cord. To simply *use* herbs, flowers, stones, bones, fire, or water without paying homage to their life force insults spirit. In Haiti, for example, spirits are believed to mount the human, helping them to carry out healing work. Healers under the influence of various lwas (spirits of the past, present, and future associated with Haitian Vodou) will fall into a trancelike state; some dance during healings while others sing or chant. In the United States many healers in the African American community commence their work with prayers, psalms, or song. Bringing together spirit with healing work is an exciting experience and it is also a distinctive aspect of ATR-inspired herbalism. To summarize, yes, there are tools, equipment, and methods, but there is also spirit, the spirit of nature, the ancestor spirits, and the spirit within your *self*. Be sure to remain attentive to your intuition as you work roots because often it is the way spirit communicates and assists with healing work.

PART II

The Story
of Herbs

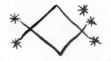

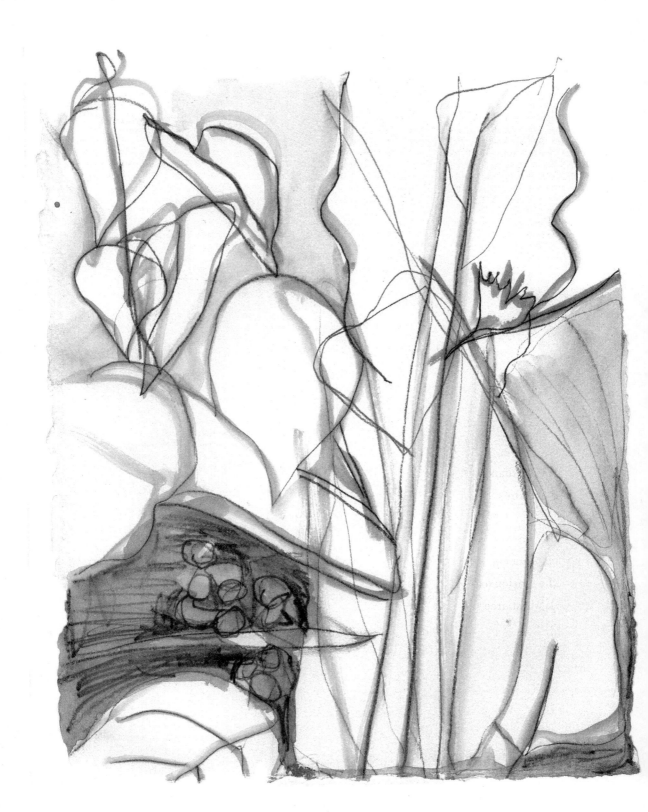

CHAPTER 4

Osayin's Calabash

SPIRITUAL PLANTS
AND MYSTICAL
NATURAL PRODUCTS

PLANTS AND NATURAL PRODUCTS IN FOCUS

- Calabash
- Cucumber
- West Indian gherkin
- Pumpkin
- Luffa
- Gourd
- Watermelon
- Muskmelon (cantaloupe)
- Calabash tree
- Okra
- Greens (mustard, collard, turnip)
- Callaloo
- Black-eyed peas
- Tobacco
- Honey
- Beeswax
- Propolis
- Royal jelly

ONE OF THE LARGEST AND more-studied ATRs is the earth-based faith of the Yoruba people called Ifá. Ifá's knowledge of traditional medicine is what enables people to become healers. Within Ifá is the knowledge of the foundation of all disease, the energy of the disease, and how to access natural, curative, protective, or preventive ashe from wherever it may exist to bring about wellness.[1] The knowledge of Ifá allows healers to understand the nature of plants and animals. Incantations or ashe words are a powerful component because words are understood to yield a great deal of power. Incantations and the ability to use divination to bring all this plant knowledge together create potent medicine that is distinctively West African. The body of Yoruba myths of creation is called Odù. The Odù includes the identification, uses, meanings, and secret words of the plants.

This practice manifests in many forms in the Black Atlantic as well. One tradition has been recorded in coastal plains of North Carolina, wherein ailments like burns are talked right out of the body. The practice called *talking fire out of burns* utilizes incantations that address deities similar to orishas, since orishas are actually angelic spirits. The incantations almost always invoke angels. Here is one:

> There came two angels from the north
> One brought fire; and one brought frost
> Go out fire and come in frost.[2]

The practice of talking fire out of burns stems from the same type of direct communication and understanding of the root of the ailment that is utilized in West Africa by those who know Ifá and in the United States by rootworkers.

---

1   M. A. Makinde, *African Philosophy, Culture, and Traditional Medicine* (Athens: Ohio Univ. Center for International Studies, 1988), 88.
2   Thomas Stroup, "A Charm from North Carolina and *The Merchant of Venice,* II, vii, 75," *Journal of American Folklore* 49 (1936), 266.

Meet Osayin

Ewe O, Ewe O
My plants; my plants!
—from the Odù of Ifá, the word of Osayin as told by
the griot

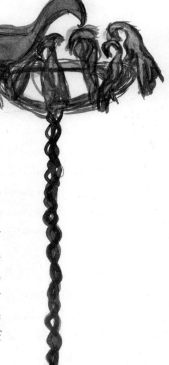

Osayin's staff

Practitioners of Ifá believe numerous orishas populate the world today. There is discussion and appreciation of about twelve orishas, but there are actually about six hundred. Intimate contact with orishas can bring about dramatic changes difficult for science to explain; you would do well to investigate them. A curious orisha happens to also be the patron of the herbal arts; his name is Osayin. Unlike most of the other orishas, whose birth is of orisha parents, Osayin sprang forth from the womb of Mother Earth herself like a seedling. He stayed hidden within the forests, and that way Osayin learned all there is to know about plants. Still, Osayin was the servant of Ifá and, as such, he taught herbalism to Ifá practitioners and to those knowledgeable of that particular path.

In these days we would call this orisha physically challenged. He is called lame, with one arm, a very large ear that does not hear at all, and a tiny ear that hears extraordinarily well. This orisha has a high-pitched voice that is difficult to listen to. Osayin is one-eyed and misshapen according to griots who teach us through oral tradition.[3] This complex orisha shows us what can become of greed and admonishes against hoarding our gifts. In modern language, his story is a cautionary tale to herbalists who become intoxicated with power, retaining it rather than sharing.

We know Osayin as the African Green Man, Yoruba orisha of herbal medicines of the

---

3   Olmos and Paravisini-Gebert, *Creole Religions of the Caribbean,* 50.

forest and bush, and patron of herbalists called *curanderos* by the African Brazilian people. Green is the color of health and healing in nature. Thanks to the chlorophyll that makes plants green, they are able to utilize the sun's energy to generate food in the process called photosynthesis. Photosynthesis converts carbon dioxide and water into carbohydrates, and oxygen is released in the process. Osayin, our Green Man, is orisha of wild-crafted herbs, berries, flowers, barks, and wood. His presence has always captivated my imagination because he is one of the chief orishas at the center of my world.

According to the griots, Osayin collected all the medicinal herbs of the forest as well as the knowledge of how to use them. As a spiritual herbalist, he tucked all of his botanicals and knowledge in a *güiro,* or calabash. There were numerous other orishas with characteristics helpful to the business of the world, but Osayin wanted to keep the knowledge of herbs out of their reach—high up in a tree, hidden in a calabash.

Oya, orisha of weather and changes, generated a huge wind, followed by a storm that knocked the calabash of herbal knowledge down to earth. She did this with the blessing of numerous orishas who desired herbal wisdom. In the Americas and Caribbean, in a path influenced by Ifá called Regla de Ocha, or Rule of the Orisha, Osayin is represented by the *güiro* (gourd) that hangs in the Santería ile or house-temple. Tribute must be paid to Osayin before his herbal medicine can be used in ceremonies, spells, and cures. Osayin's symbols include the gourd where his spirit resides and a twisted tree branch, as well as his color—green. In Catholicism, Saint Benito, Saint Jerome, and Saint Joseph represent his spirit.[4]

As herbalists, we celebrate the magic held within the calabash, but we also realize that this earth wisdom should be available to all—this is the lesson of Osayin and the calabash. With no choice left, Osayin's calabash of herbal information, recipes, rituals, and ceremonies for health and spiritual well-being is now open to all. If you dare to look deep within the calabash, who knows what might be waiting inside?

---

4   Olmos and Paravisini-Gebert, *Creole Religions of the Caribbean.*

Calabash Child

We begin our focus on individual herbs within the calabash because it has so many wonderful uses in African holistic health including the arts (especially music), divination, lifestyle enhancement as a tool, and health, as well as the stories that inform them. One West
African folk story shows us that there are truly surprising things held within the calabash
plant:

A royal couple is unable to have children. They have a sincere desire for a child; their
heart goes out to this wish each day. Meanwhile, their farms are doing exceedingly well
and are about ready for the harvest. The king's wife goes out to the fields to marvel at the
huge leaves and flowers of her plants. She notices something moving beneath a particularly
promising calabash plant. Lo and behold, it is a child, a beautiful little girl. This girl does
not have a human mother or father. She is born from within a calabash. When the king's
wife calls her Calabash Child, she rolls into a ball and becomes a calabash once more. Ex-
cited by the possibility of having a child of her own, Calabash Child or not, the king's wife
gives her a name to represent her extraordinary origins, Ifeyinwa ("nothing like a child"),
and brings her home. The king gives the girl a pet name of his own, Onunaeliaku ("born
to consume wealth"). He and his wife lavish the girl with love, attention, and gifts. Soon
enough, she becomes spoiled and is not nice to anyone. Naturally, everyone wants to call
her Calabash Child, but she is proud and haughty, especially after being adopted by royalty. She forbids anyone to call her Calabash Child. One day, when the king and his wife
are away on a trip, the servants dare to call the girl Calabash Child. They know she does
not like it, but her poor behavior toward the workers makes them eager for revenge. They
irritate her to no end by reminding her that she comes from within the calabash plant. The
girl tells her parents, and this causes the harshest punishment of all to be dispensed on
all participants in the taunting—death. With the offering of human blood spilled on her
behalf, Calabash Child becomes a girl made of flesh and blood.[5]

---

5   Told by Stephanie Bird, inspired by the telling by Buchi Offodile in *The Orphan Girl and Other Stories: West
African Folk Tales* (Brooklyn, NY: Interlink Books, 2001), 157–61.

Family Cucurbitaceae

It is easy to see the wonder and fear with which Osayin is viewed. Many of the life-sustaining herbs of Africa and the Black Atlantic are in Osayin's family—Cucurbitaceae. This family of plants includes:

- *Cucumis* (cucumber and melon)
- *Momordica charantia* (African cucumber)
- *Cucurbita* (pumpkin and marrows)
- *Citrullus vulgaris* (watermelon)
- *Luffa cylindrica* (vegetable sponge)
- *Lagenaria* (gourd)

The Four Great Cold Seeds of old *materia medica* (meaning the collected healing wisdom of the ages, derived from the Greek physician Pedanius Dioscorides, first century CE) were the:

1. seeds of pumpkin
2. seeds of gourd
3. seeds of melon
4. seeds of cucumber

These four great seeds were bruised and rubbed in water. An emulsion was formed. This healing formula was used to treat catarrhal infections, bowel disorders, and urinary infections. Next time you are cleaning a member of the great seed family, perhaps you should think twice before throwing away such a precious cache of healing medicines.

In terms of names, *pumpkin* is derived from the older name *pompion*. English melons were once called *millions*, hence the current name *melon*. Squash (*C. melopepo, C. ovifera, C. pepo*) are called *marrows* in England. Melons are very diverse. The largest, *Cucurbita maxima,* is a gourd; the smallest is the size of an olive. The shape can be globular, egg-shaped, spindle-shaped, or serpentine. The skin is netted, ribbed, furrowed, or smooth.

The flesh ranges from white to green to yellow to orange. The melon fruit is eaten or juiced. The root is used as a purgative. The active bitter principle in melon root makes an emetic.

Calabash (*Lagenaria siceraria*)

The calabash bottle gourd is not just a container for the orisha Osayin; it is also a useful tool. Bottle gourd has great symbolic importance to the Yoruba. *Lagenaria siceraria* are used as a float when fishing, and this may explain how the gourd was able to establish itself across the Atlantic Ocean. The Jamaican enslaved people were given an extremely small allotment of personal goods during the early 1700s; one of these items was the calabash, which they used as a cup, bowl, spoon, and musical instrument resembling a lute. The other two items were a mat to lie on and an earthen pot for cooking.[6] Numerous groups of transplanted African people used the small gourds as water cups and bottles and the large gourds as storage jars.[7] Pumpkins and squash were popularly used in the same manner as well.[8]

CREATING A GOURD BOTTLE OR VESSEL THE OLD-FASHIONED WAY

- Make a hole at whichever end you wish to use as the top of the vessel.
- Pour boiling water inside to dissolve the pulp.
- Extract the pulp.
- Rinse with sand.
- Rinse again with water.
- Repeat until clean.
- Dry and then use.

---

6   Grimé, *Ethno-botany of the Black Americans*, 12–13.
7   Grimé, *Ethno-botany of the Black Americans*, 137–38.
8   Grimé, *Ethno-botany of the Black Americans*.

THOMAS JEFFERSON REPORTS IN HIS *Notes on the State of Virginia* (1785) that enslaved people made banjos from large gourds with long straight necks on the plantations. The long-necked top was covered with rattlesnake skin, which would bring in some of the magical-spiritual ashe of the powerful snake. This type of instrument was probably used in ritual and ceremony. Mixed-raced people referred to as Creoles, as well as Blacks, were reported to use the gourds as vases, goblets, and soup tureens. In Ghana and other parts of West Africa, the gourd is used to make spoons, ladles, sieves, drinking utensils, and a *danka*, which is a vessel for holding water, palm wine, and other fluids useful to the community. The calabash is also used in ceremony, ritual, and ancestor veneration in some of the hunter-gatherer societies in East Africa. The calabash was used medicinally in Jamaica in a way similar to a Chinese medicine method called cupping. The calabash was sliced in half, pressed hard on the painful spot (cupping), and removed briefly before the cupping process was repeated.[9]

In *The Healing Drum: African Wisdom Teachings*, authors Yaya Diallo and Mitchell Hall share the soulful ways calabash are important to ceremony, ritual, and other community activities in the village of Fienso in the Republic of Mali. Diallo, who grew up there, reports that his people, the Minianka, would not till, sow, weed, or harvest the fields without music. Music accompanies and enhances the harmonious teamwork of the farmer.[10]

A couple of key instruments are created from the calabash gourd. The balafon is an instrument of the spirit realm, designed to communicate with the invisible world of the inner dimensions of our universe. Some call it an African xylophone. It has carved wooden keys mounted on a rectangular frame constructed of wood. Strung underneath the frames are a series of gourds with holes cut into their tops. The gourds act as resonators. Musicians hit the keys with two sticks with rubber wrapped on the ends. The balafon is a wind instrument and is also percussive. The tones have a quality that resonates with the water element in the human body, in the way rain and the sound of storms can bother, excite, and soothe our souls.

---

9 Grimé, *Ethno-botany of the Black Americans,* 12–13.
10 Yaya Diallo and Mitchell Hall, *The Healing Drum: African Wisdom Teachings* (Rochester, VT: Destiny Books, 1989), 80.

This instrument had divine inspiration. Kanté saw the balafon, which did not exist in our world, in his dream. He heard the sweet music and awakened to create what he saw. Kantè lived in the tenth century in the present-day Republic of Guinea. Today the balafon is played during ceremonies—both religious and funerary—and is used to call to snakes and reptiles. Because of its ability to draw snakes, balafon players wear protective amulets while playing.

A bafoko is a large calabash covered tightly with goatskin. In the middle of the calabash there is a circle of resin about four inches in diameter. Where the resin is located, there is a different tone than the uncovered calabash. The bafoko is played in ceremonies along with the balofon.

A string instrument called the bolon is based on the bafoko. A stalk of millet is inserted into the skin of the bafoko and is then attached inside the calabash. Two strings attach to the end of each millet stalk, rising above the skin and extending to the outside of the calabash. This instrument has a bass sound when plucked. It is played at funerals and various ceremonies.

Calabash are a truly remarkable container—pregnant with the possibility of numerous healing and household uses, while also making delightful music for the soul of humans, animals, and spirits.

Luffa cylindrica (Vegetable Sponge) aka Loofah

Luffa has to be harvested and eaten while it is very young to be palatable. A use for the mature luffa, and the one you may be most familiar with, is using it as an exfoliating scrub for the face or body. This is wonderful for scrubbing the heels, elbows, knees, and anywhere you have dry skin. On the face, use it gently to exfoliate, remove black and white heads, and add a healthy glow to the face. Some types of luffa are used for scrubbing pots and pans or as a dishcloth.

MAKING A LUFFA SPONGE

- Soak seeds overnight before planting to speed germination. Those who live in colder temperate zones should begin planting indoors in peat pots (luffa needs a long growing season).

- Plant outdoors in full sun, according to seed packet directions, as soon as there is no danger of frost, where your luffa has plenty of room to grow. You can use a trellis for small gardens. When female plants flower, fruit will soon follow.

- Allow to grow for several months; the outer part of luffa will become dry and the color will range from yellow to black when ready to pick.

- Cut fruit off with your penknife or gardening shears. Shake out the seeds and reserve them in a paper bag for next planting season.

- Peel the dried skin like you would peel onion skin. You can soak the luffa in water to make peeling easier.

- To clean, soak overnight in a solution of water with just a small amount of castile soap and bleach in a basin, sink, or bathtub.

- In the morning hang them in the sun to dry and bleach further.

- When dry, either use them whole or slice them down. (See soap recipe for sliced luffa on page 352.)

A Sponge Cucumber *Luffa operculata* Helps with Seasonal Allergies

Intrigued to find a member of the luffa family in my allergy medicine, I wanted to find out why. Recent evidence-based studies[11] suggest *Luffa operculata* reduces itching and runny noses as well as watering eyes experienced by sufferers of hay fever and similar upper respiratory disorders. It is efficient, well tolerated, and improves quality of life, with no reported side effects. It is combined with other natural ingredients and sold as a homeopathic treatment under the name Zicam.

---

11 R. L. Zhou and J. C. Zhang, "An Analysis of Combined Desensitizing Acupoints Therapy in 419 Cases of Allergic Rhinitis Accompanying Asthma," *Chung Kuo Chung Hsi I Chieh Ho Tsa Chih* 17, no. 10 (October 1997): 587–89; and M. Weiser, L. H. Gegenheimer, and P. Klein, "A Randomized Equivalence Trial Comparing the Efficacy and Safety of Luffa comp.-Heel Nasal Spray with Cromolyn Sodium Spray in the Treatment of Seasonal Allergic Rhinitis," *Forschende Komplementärmedizin* 6, no. 3 (1999): 142–48.

Pumpkin

The pumpkin is an herbaceous plant. *Cucurbita pepo*, called *apakyi* in Ghana, is also utilized as a container for storing clothing and selling *aboloo* (steamed cassava dough), and as a float for fishing. The pumpkin is revered in Africa since it can hold up to four gallons of water. Some of the pumpkin stem is used to make buttons.[12] Baby pumpkin is eaten, as well as the leafy shoots, which are called *krobonko*, and are served as a vegetable. The leaves of the pumpkin are making waves on both sides of the Atlantic in a dish called *egusi*. The outside is used while the inside is discarded.[13] Fluted pumpkin (*Telfairia occidentalis*) is foraged in Ghana where it grows in the forests. The seeds are roasted and eaten.[14] Pumpkin

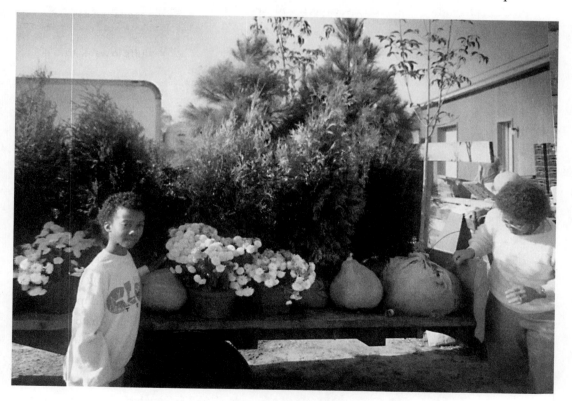

My sister Rene Louise and my ma, Margaret Marie, circa 1985

12 Daniel K. Abbiw, *Useful Plants of Ghana: West African Uses of Wild and Cultivated Plants* (London: Intermediate Technology Publications, 1995), 110.
13 Abbiw, *Useful Plants of Ghana*.
14 Grimé, *Ethno-botany of the Black Americans*, 53.

seeds contain 30 percent reddish fixed oil, traces of a volatile oil, protein, sugar, starches, and fiber. The seeds can be enjoyed roasted when ripe and must not be used if more than a month old. Pumpkin seed has been used medicinally and is a part of the official German Pharmacopoeia, 10th edition. The Commission E report of the American Botanical Council has approved the seeds for the treatment of irritable bladder. The seeds contain amino acids and cucurbitin. Consumption of pumpkin seeds may help reduce bladder stones in children.[15] The flesh of pumpkins and their relative squash are boiled, mashed, fried, and used in sauces or served with rice.

Pumpkin is very high in beta-carotene antioxidants believed to fight off numerous health problems including heart attacks, cancer, and cataracts.[16] Pumpkin seeds are an inexpensive, nutritious snack, a good source of protein, and a great way to enjoy multiple parts of the vegetable. Herbalists recommend pumpkin seed oil applied topically to the face or taken by the level teaspoon twice a day as a treatment for acne.

Watermelon

Though our juicy red watermelon, so beloved on Juneteenth and at our summer BBQs, was thought to be related to a South African citron melon, researchers from Washington University in Saint Louis, Missouri, now believe a Sudanese Kordofan melon (*C. lanatus*) may be the actual relative to what we enjoy. There has also been genetic research to support an interpretation of an Egyptian tomb painting that shows watermelon to have been enjoyed, just as we do, after meals in the Nile Valley as many as four thousand years ago. The latest research by Susanne S. Renner, honorary professor of biology at Washington University, suggests the related undomesticated cultivars of watermelon are from both West and Northeast Africa.[17]

Watermelons are almost always available in urban markets in season. There is an incredible variety in melons in terms of shape and size; some varieties are grown just for the seeds. Refreshing to both humans and animals, melons are a staple food in North Africa and parts of the Middle East. Burullus Delta Lake, east of the Rosetta channel of the Nile, is particularly noted for their watermelon, which is yellow inside. There are numerous crops in the northern hemisphere from May until November. The food value of watermelon, in

15 American Botanical Council, *The Complete German Commission E Monographs: Therapeutic Guide to Herbal Medicines, Expanded Commission E report* (Austin, TX: Boston Integrative Medicine Communications, 1999).
16 Jean Carper, *Food—Your Miracle Medicine: How Food Can Prevent and Cure Over 100 Symptoms and Problems* (New York: HarperCollins Publishers, 1993).
17 Talia Ogliore, "Seedy, Not Sweet," *The Source,* Washington Univ. in St. Louis, August 2022.

regard to the recommended daily value percentage for a 2,000-calorie-per-day diet, is 92 percent water, 45 percent fat, and 54 percent protein. The seeds contain citrulline, which is a performance-enhancing amino acid, as well as vitamin C, carotenoids, lycopene, and cucurbitacin.[18] The seeds are also used as a passable coffee substitute and to make beauty products, especially for the face.

Watermelon has high amounts of lycopene, glutathione, antioxidants, and anticancer compounds. The gorgeous pink fruit is mildly antibacterial, antiviral, and shows promise as an anticoagulant.[19] In Africa, ground melon seeds are used to make paste and to thicken stews. Watermelon is the most consumed melon in the United States. Forty-four states produce more than fifty varieties of this thirst-quenching treat.

Honeydew and Cantaloupe

True cantaloupe (*Cucumis melo* var. *cantalupensis*) only grows in a small part of Italy. What we refer to as cantaloupe is actually a muskmelon, an annual trailing herb with large palmately lobed leaves, tendrils, and a deep, bell-shaped corolla on the flowers. Muskmelon has blood-thinning capacity. Melon root is used as a purgative in some traditional medicine as well as an emetic. Orange-fleshed melons contain ample antioxidants.[20] Green honeydew is a useful way of replenishing moisture in the body and it quenches thirst during the heat of summer. One new area that is being investigated is the idea of melon as an antiplatelet aggregation and anticoagulant food (deterring blood clots).

Melon: Juicy Fruit from the Motherland for the Soul

Not long ago, middle-class Black people, as well as those aspiring to be so, shunned melon. This was in large part due to the days of the minstrel show, when products, advertisers, and actors denigrated African culture using the foods we brought with us to the New World like melons. African Americans depicted as low-class, "country" people, also called pickaninnies, were shown eating watermelon and spitting the seeds from gaps between their teeth.

Today, it is important to realize that eating melons in their myriad forms offers a way to stay connected with the unique aspect of our culture while also gaining enormous health benefits.

---

18 Fatima Hallal and Kerri-Ann Jennings, "The Top 9 Health Benefits of Watermelon," Healthline, February 23, 2023.
19 Carper, *Food—Your Miracle Medicine*, 487.
20 Carper, *Food—Your Miracle Medicine*, 482.

Melons, the juicy fruit, are healing in a holistic way, as they bring culture and nutrition together. No wonder they remain a central feature in our summer gatherings and celebrations.

Cucumber

Cucumbers are wonderful raw in salad, juiced alone or with other vegetables, or in cold soup. They seem to have a cooling effect and are recommended for summer and as an accompaniment to hot foods such as curries in a dish called raita that also contains yogurt.

Cucumber is used cosmetically in face masks, particularly to help revive tired eyes. Often two cooled cucumber slices are placed over the eyes to encourage rest and replenishment at home or day spas. They purportedly reduce dark circles around the eyes and help with puffiness. If the cucumber were well chilled, the cold temperature alone would help reduce puffiness in the way ice does, yet the smooth texture is more comfortable. Many people enjoy the thinner-skinned, seedless, hydroponically grown cucumber, also called the English cucumber, though it is now grown in many locations. The seeds do have benefits. Cucumbers contain antioxidants especially good at fighting skin cancer.[21]

West Indian Gherkin

Enslaved Africans brought this little cousin to the cucumber to the New World. Gherkin is believed to be a cultivated and altered form of the African species of *C. prophetarum* or *C. figarei,* even though they are both perennial and the Caribbean species is annual. It is a much-sought-after food, eaten raw, cooked, or pickled. Gherkins accompany meals, are a snack food, and are frequently pickled. The "juice," which is primarily vinegar, is used in the preparation of cold salads and consumed as a healthy drink.

Calabash Tree (*Crescentia cujete*)

The calabash tree is not in the *Cucurbitaceae* family, yet the shell of its fruit bears strong resemblance to the gourd. Calabash tree is a small tropical tree that grows up to twenty-five feet tall. It has rough bark and simple leaves. The shell of the fruit resembles that of a gourd and has the capacity to hold from one ounce to one gallon of liquid depending on the size of the fruit. They are used to hold water, rum, or broth. They are sometimes used as a pot for outdoor cooking. In Barbados, household implements like spoons, bowls, and utensils are

---

21 Carper, *Food—Your Miracle Medicine.*

made from the fruit.[22] The pulp has medicinal applications. In Suriname the fruit pulp is used to treat respiratory problems in traditional medicine and the shell holds powder and serves as a flask, washbasin, dish, or decoration when it is carved. The tree grows well in Jamaica. It is used there as a container and a pot. The flesh is used as a medicinal poultice. In Barbados, spoons, bowls, and utensils are made from the fruit. In the West Indies, buttons are made, as are cups, saucers, punch ladles, and spoons.

Osayin's Green Bounty

While the family *Cucurbitaceae* and the calabash tree fruit bring Osayin's calabash immediately to mind, there are a few other precious gifts that are of him as well. These soul foods include greens. Green is Osayin's color, and it also represents the verdant essence of Mother Earth. Osayin's array of greens represents fertility, vitality, and health. Greens also instill these traits in us, building our resistance to illness and strengthening our entire body system. In West Africa the preferred green is called bitter leaf, which is washed to remove its bitter taste. Cassava leaves are enjoyed, as are ewedu, red sorrel, yakuwa, and pumpkin leaves. Jamaica has made callaloo[23] a much-loved vegetable-and-seafood stew featuring their unique greens called variously dasheen, Chinese spinach, taro tops, or callaloo bush. In Africa and the diaspora, beet tops, kale, and spinach are some of the greens enjoyed.

While people once thought greens, such as collard, mustard, and turnip (tops), were a lowly food, now people all round the world celebrate the nutrient-rich gift of Osayin's greens. Greens are especially high in lutein, chlorophyll, and antioxidants. Lutein is the main antioxidant that helps the eyes. Greens are showing promise as a deterrent for macular degeneration. This ailment consists of a deterioration of the sensitive central region of the retina, which weakens the field of vision. Of all the green vegetables, kale is number one, collard greens are number two, and spinach is number three in terms of their concentration of lutein.[24]

---

22 A. C. Smith, "Angiosperm Evolution and the Relationship of the Floras of Africa and America," in *Tropical Forest Ecosystems in Africa and South America: A Comparative Review,* ed. B. J. Megers, E. S. Ayensu, and W. D. Duckworth (Washington, DC: Smithsonian Institution, 1973), 33, 49–61.
23 These have to be cooked in a special way because of their high calcium oxalate content.
24 James A. Joseph, Daniel Nadeau, and Anne Underwood, *The Color Code: A Revolutionary Eating Plan for Optimum Health* (New York: The Philip Lief Group, 1992), 112.

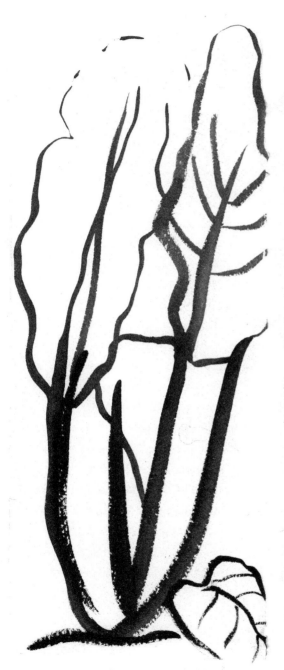

Chard from my garden

As you shall see later, collard, mustard, and turnip greens need not be overcooked or superfatted to be tasty. The soul food we enjoy is packed with antioxidant vitamins and minerals—especially wholesome when not overwhelmed by animal fat. In Asian cuisine, such as Thai food, collards and other greens are stir-fried, and they are delicious, showing there is no real need to cook the greens until they are dull and lifeless. Try your leafy vegetables such as collard, mustard, and turnip greens seasoned with apple cider vinegar and sautéed in olive or palm oil with onion and cayenne. If you want to cook them more in accord with tradition, which amounts to stewed greens, by all means drink the broth (*pot liquor*) for additional optimal health benefits. They can also be braised using a splash of avocado oil, a dash of sea salt, and apple cider vinegar; seasoned with freshly cracked pepper, cayenne flakes, and freshly crushed garlic; and simmered in a smidgen of vegetable broth or stock for 10-15 minutes. This retains their green color and freshness. Traditionally, our people have enjoyed cooking these vegetables in a cast-iron skillet. Cooking greens in cast iron and adding a dash of vinegar or splash of lemon makes them even richer in iron than they normally are. Some folks cook them with tomato, and the acidity interacts with the cast iron in the same way as vinegar or lemon, again enhancing their iron-rich quality. Greens are an excellent food for young people who are having growth spurts, as well as pregnant women and the elderly, because they are high in calcium.

Clean and Green

One of the reasons people often save greens—that is, collard, mustard, turnip, or even spinach and kale—for special occasions is the challenge of cleaning them. I remember my grandmother and mom soaking them overnight in the bathtub. Following in their footsteps, I have done this myself. Soaking your greens in the sink and adding vinegar to the water accelerates the cleaning process—no more overnight soaking. For those craving convenience, more and more shops are carrying pre-cleaned and chopped greens and spinach.

Another of Osayin's green wonders is okra.

Okra (*Abelmoschus esculentus L. Moench*), Also Called *Quiabo*, *Guimgombo*, *Ochroes*, *Gumbo*, and *Ocro*

I love the definition of a pod, as it relates to the amazing soul food okra. Synonymous with a cocoon, capsule, husk, or sheath, an okra pod encases many elements of African diasporic culture. Biologically, according to Merriam Webster, a pod is "an elongated dry fruit that develops from one or more carpels of a flower, splits open along a seam, and contains seeds that may be attached to the wall of the pod."

As interesting as it is poignant, it is believed that okra seeds, like rice, black-eyed peas, and watermelon seeds, were braided into enslaved Africans' hair. This allowed okra to serve as the pod or vessel, carrying this precious, soul-nourishing food source to make it with us to Brazil, the Caribbean, and the Americas.

Okra has pointed ridged green pods with a stem at one end. There are ample white seeds inside. The more they are chopped, the more thickening agent is released. Okra is best picked young, when they are less fibrous and more tender. The pod is eaten boiled or used as a stew thickener;[25] the leaves are used cosmetically for their softening ability, medicinally, and as a nourishing whole food. Okra is very high in the antioxidant alpha-lipoic acid.[26] A synonym for *okra* on both sides of the Atlantic is *gumbo*; even though it is spelled differently in West Africa than it is in the diaspora, the meaning is still the same. In *Africanisms in the Gullah Dialect*,[27] Lorenzo Turner identifies words from various African languages. In Gullah patois, for example, *gombo* is the word for *okra*. A complex, vitamin-rich vegetable that changes the quality of our beloved stew that also bears its name—gumbo!

25 Grimé, *Ethno-botany of the Black Americans,* 19.
26 Joseph, Nadeau, and Underwood, *Color Code,*117.
27 Lorenzo Dow Turner, *Africanisms in the Gullah Dialect* (New York: Arno Press, 1969).

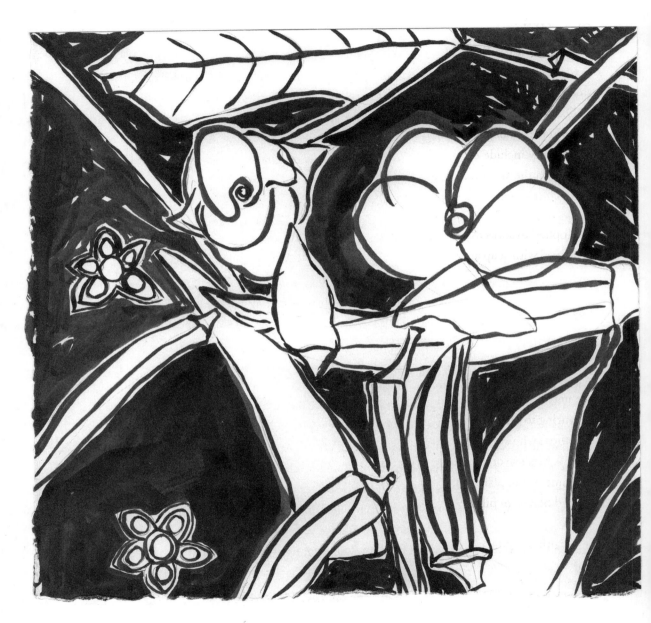

Okra

Okra (*Hibiscus esculentus*)

Cultivated in the Sudan, Guinea, and savanna-woodland countries of West Africa and used as a backyard crop, okra of this genus is eaten in soup or stews, sliced, dried, and stored. It is high in calcium and relieves constipation.[28]

Okra of either species, like the Cucurbitaceae family's squash, is rich in the antioxidant glutathione, among other healthy constituents. Some early uses recorded within the Gullah community include eating the blossoms and pods as well as the seeds. The blossoms are sautéed in the same way as squash blossoms. The roasted seeds make a coffee substitute. Okra blossoms are used in two types of poultices:

- Applied to sores that don't heal
- Mixed with soap and sugar and applied to wounds to speed healing[29]

Black-Eyed Peas

Black-eyed peas are actually legumes. They are also called cowpeas. In West Africa snacks called kosai and moyin-moyin are made of black-eyed peas. Black-eyed peas were so beloved by enslaved Africans that they brought them with them to the New World. The peas are nutritious, inexpensive, easy to grow, and easy to cook; they are sustainable and are nurturing to our soul (which is why they are called soul food). A large-scale study showed that those who eat beans every week were 40 percent less likely to die of pancreatic cancer.[30] This is because of the protease inhibitors in legumes.

Some of the places black-eyed peas are very popular include the Low Country in the United States, in pilau cooked by East Africans, and in India, Zanzibar, and Mauritius.

Health benefits per ½ cup:

- Protein: 7 grams
- Fat: 0 grams
- Carbs: 18 grams
- Fiber: 6 grams
- Sugars: 3 grams

---

28 Abbiw, *Useful Plants of Ghana*, 38.
29 Mitchell, *Hoodoo Medicine*, 84.
30 Carper, *Food—Your Miracle Medicine*, 258.

Black-eyed peas are a good source of complex carbohydrates, calcium, iron, vitamin A, magnesium, zinc, copper, manganese, and vitamin K. They contain antioxidants and flavonoids and are helpful for pregnancy health, weight management, increasing energy, reducing risk of diabetes, aiding digestion, and bone health.

Just as other legumes, they are considered around the world to be lucky charms. Black-eyed peas are a featured food for our New Year's meal. Black-eyed peas are thought to usher in silver money and are served with white rice, which symbolizes fertility and longevity, as well as stewed tomato, which is symbolic of love and sensuality. Corn bread accompanies the meal. As soul food, it was traditionally cooked with pork, though this is changing for health reasons. Today, many people enjoy this as a plant-based vegan meal for health reasons, chief among them is that vegan cooking reduces vein-clogging saturated fats. This meal, called Hoppin' John, is featured in part III.

Tobacco (*Nicotiana tabacum* L.)

Yes, this is a health book, so do not be fooled by seeing tobacco included. This entry is not intended to encourage smoking. This is to show the close connection between spirituality, ritual, ceremony, devotion, and healing with tobacco.

Tobacco in Traditional and Folk Medicine

Let us start with the aspect that is hardest to swallow—healing. Here are some medicinal applications from traditional medicine and folklore:

- Tobacco mixed with annatto is used to kill vermin and chiggers in ulcers.[31]
- As a treatment for colic, half a gill of rye whiskey and a pipe of tobacco was placed in a whiskey bottle. Tobacco was smoked from a pipe and the smoke was blown back into the whiskey bottle. The tobacco-infused whiskey was then shaken and drunk.[32]
- A white clay pipe aged and turned black with smoke was broken and pulverized to a fine powder. This powder was given for colic.[33]

31 M.-É. Descourtilz, *Flore pittoresque et médicale des Antilles* (Paris, 1821–1829 and 1833).
32 J. G. Hoffman, *Pow-Wows, Or, Long Lost Friend: A Collection of Mysterious and Invaluable Arts and Remedies for Man as Well as Animals* (Pomeroy, WA: Health Research Publishers, 1820), 16.
33 Hoffman, *Pow-Wows.*

- Pure tobacco smoke is used as an expectorant for the symptoms of colds.[34]
- The anodyne quality lends tobacco to treating headache, and it is used in that manner in Trinidad.[35]
- The eugenol constituent makes tobacco a useful febrifuge.[36]
- In terms of skin disease, tobacco contains propionic acid, a fungicide; isoeugenol serves as a fungistat; and the guaiacol it contains deters eczema.[37]

Brown Spirit Medicine

Tobacco is considered an offering to the ancestors in Native American culture. It has a lengthy history as a component of the shaman and sorcerer's medicine bag in the ancient empire of Songhay. Tobacco is carried in hunters' shirts along with their other natural amulets.

Tobacco is smoked in the form of a cigar in Haiti, Cuba, Puerto Rico, and elsewhere in the Black Atlantic during healing work, rituals, and ceremonies of various paths. As it is used elsewhere by indigenous people, tobacco is used by African people as an offering to deities and to the egun. The Yoruba take a tobacco-leaf-infused bath to invoke or honor the warrior orisha Ogun. Obatala is honored with a wild tobacco bath. Offerings to the orishas Elegba and Oya also include tobacco.

I frequently begin rituals, ceremonies, cleansing, and healing work with an offering to the egun of tobacco. I burn this as I would any loose incense on a hot charcoal. I also mix tobacco in various incense blends including kinnikinnick, which is a specialty thought to be of the Algonquin people. I recommend that you do the same and that you also place loose incense on the altar for the egun.

34 Payne-Jackson and Alleyne, *Jamaican Folk Medicine*, 156.
35 Payne-Jackson and Alleyne, *Jamaican Folk Medicine*, 163.
36 Payne-Jackson and Alleyne, *Jamaican Folk Medicine*, 164.
37 Payne-Jackson and Alleyne, *Jamaican Folk Medicine*, 166.

Honey: Sweet Spirit

Anthropologist Colin Turnbull describes intriguing accounts of Black folks interacting magically with honey. He shares observations of the honey dance and honey ritual of the Forest People, a group of small-stature people who reside in the Ituri Forest of the Congo. Turnbull reports that there were very special games during honey harvest season. Men would pretend to be honey gatherers, dancing in a long, sensual, curvilinear line. They would look up exaggeratedly as if searching for bees. The women were the honeybees. They would appear, singing in a soft, rhythmic buzz, buzz, buzz chant. The women would tap the men on the head and sparks would literally fly (this was a love and harvest ritual). There was a fire of special woods at the hearth for the occasions and indigenous leaves moistened so they would smoke rather than flame. The combination of flame and smoke billowed upward. Men would blow their honey whistles, while women clapped their hands and sang, hoping the calls would travel with the smoke, calling the bees to make more honey.[38]

The use of honey weaves a consistent thread through ancient Egyptian apothecaries, recipes, and rituals. Honey is an important ingredient in kyphi, unique Egyptian incense used to pay homage to the god Ra and goddess Isis that also contains dried fruit, red wine, and resins. Honey was used to mix a kohl solution to paint the eyes, used cosmetically in hair and facial care, and was a part of ancient Egyptian devotion.

In Mali, *soume* is an alcoholic drink derived from honey that is consumed from a calabash. Around the calabash and under the influence of *soume*, young people learn the secrets of their community. The elders gather around the *soume*-filled calabash to brag, remember, and gossip.[39]

The Samburu people of East Africa mix milk from their cattle with honey and pour it as a libation for spiritual blessing of the land. They pour blood from the cattle as well as honey as a libation in a land-cleansing rite. They have done this publicly in recent times as a gesture of peace with neighbors with which there have been land disputes.

The Bemba people of Zambia, in southern Africa, enjoy all the healing foods already mentioned, along with honey and grains, as an important part of their sustenance.

---

38 Colin Turnbull, *The Forest People: A Study of the Pygmies of the Congo* (New York: Touchstone / Simon & Schuster, 1962), 276–77.
39 Diallo and Hall, *Healing Drum*.

In the Black Atlantic, the honey orisha is Oshun, called Oxun in Brazil and Ochun in Cuba. Oshun is invoked to bring healthy children, easy childbirth, love, sensuality, beauty, refinement, and sweetness.

The people of Trinidad and Tobago use the honey of Oshun in blessings, rituals, and ceremonies. An offering is prepared along with water, brandy, olive oil, and sugar and is placed out in a calabash as an offering to Oshun during some Trinidad and Tobago thanksgiving rites:

- Devotees consume an offering that includes duck, honey, olive oil, sugar, and brandy.
- A libation of honey, lavender, brandy, and olive oil is poured in honor of Oshun, also called Goddess of Water Powers and sometimes referred to as Saint Philomene.
- A honey dressing is rubbed on a bamboo pole to invoke the spirit of Oshun.
- A table is laid with honey, a calabash, candles, grains, and flowers to honor Oshun.

Jewels of the Golden Hive
Our friends the bees produce many items of great use to the herbalist:

Beeswax—used to thicken creams, salves, balms, pomades, and soaps. Beeswax is also used on magical seals and practical seals to firmly close corked bottles of elixirs, potions, and brews.

Propolis—used by bees to seal the hive; bee medicine that protects them from bacteria, viruses, and fungi is used by people for the same reason.

Honey[40]—derived from various flowers and herbs; medicinal content various with the flower that is its source.

Raw honey—is straight from the beehive; though it may be strained, no heating is involved.

---

40 It is important to take note that honey is a serious allergen for some individuals; honey is contraindicated for nursing mothers and babies who are not yet immune to some of the bacteria it contains.

Royal jelly—as its name suggests, royal jelly is fed to the young larvae that eventually grow up to become queen bee. Royal jelly contains an antibacterial protein that Japanese researchers have named royalisin. Royalisin is rich in amino acids and is an effective deterrent for staph and strep species of bacteria.[41] Royal jelly shows potential as an antitumor substance. In Japanese research, royal jelly had a significant effect on treating sarcoma cells but no effect on leukemia cells in a lab test.[42]

Whipped honey—the naturally occurring glucose spontaneously crystallizes and the crystallization is controlled, yielding a creamy honey. This is a dense, rich honey product that can be spread on toast like peanut butter.

Commercial raw honey—has a minimum amount of processing. Honey is a part of story, song, dance, ritual, and economic opportunity for Africans and people of African descent. It is also a tasty way to sweeten teas and baked goods, allowing us to cut down on sugar consumption. Honey is sensual and is useful in lovemaking rites as an edible body balm. It is also an excellent cosmetic, making an easy facial that controls oily skin, a soothing instant lip balm, and a softening hair conditioner—go easy and rinse well, though! Here are some of the applications for honey:

- Apply topically.
- Apply to cracked lips as a healing balm.
- Apply to cuts as an antimicrobial and antiseptic.
- Add to tea or drinks by the level teaspoon for an energy boost.
- Take orally by the teaspoon with lemon to soothe a sore throat, cold, or cough.
- Take when you have a hangover; honey helps the liver with oxidation.
- Heart benefits are suggested from some tests that indicate increased antioxidants in blood, softened arteries, and lower cholesterol after the consumption of honey.

---

41 S. Fujiwara et al., "A Potent Antibacterial Protein in Royal Jelly: Purification and Determination of the Primary Structure of Royalisin," *Journal of Biological Chemistry* 265, no. 19 (July 5, 1990): 11333–37.
42 *Nippon Yakurigaku Zasshji*, *Folia Pharmacologica Japonica* 89 (February 1987): 73–80.

- Apply directly to the eyelids to treat inflammation and conjunctivitis.
- Apply directly to foot ulcers (diabetic); add a dressing and post-secondary dressings to keep honey from seeping.
- Apply topically directly to burns.
- Apply to wounds to speed healing and as a slight antiseptic.
- Use diluted with distilled water as a douche to treat vaginal yeast infections.
- Apply to meat to soften the texture while cooking (marinate) and to fight foodborne pathogens; it is thought that honey traps free radicals within meat as it cooks.

We close this chapter and Osayin's calabash for now, sealed with honey, the natural product that is a supreme mind, body, and spirit healer.

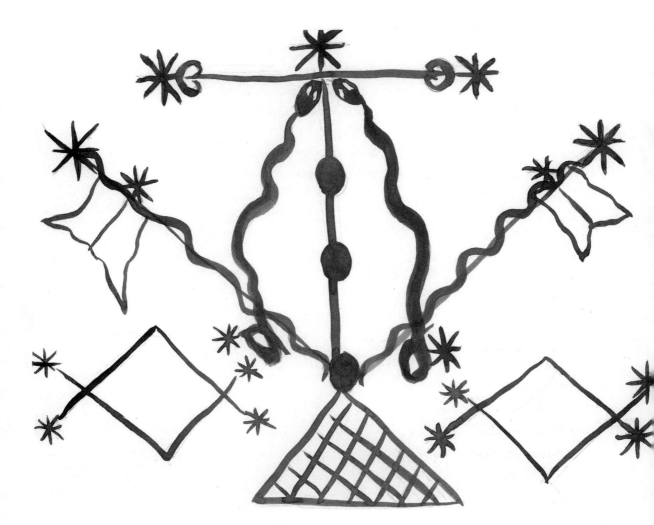

Damballah and Ayedo Hwedo with healing snakeroot plants

CHAPTER 5

Getting to the Root

ROOTS, BULBS, TUBERS, AND HEALTH

PLANTS IN FOCUS

- High John
- Little John
- Low John
- Wild yam
- African yam
- Cush-cush yam
- White Guinea yam
- Sweet potato
- Cassava
- White snakeroot
- Button snakeroot
- Virginia snakeroot
- Sampson's snakeroot
- Snakeweed
- Snakebite
- Beth root
- Angelica
- Dong quai
- Ginger
- Dogwood

Roots

Root is an important word in African culture. We celebrate our ancestral roots, as they are the source of culture, just as they are the basis from which plants grow. This has transformed with time and space. In Africa, people are rooted to their people, clan, or secret society, their village and spiritual practice. In the Caribbean and Americas, people have roots that tie them to a specific island, a part of the country, one coast or another, neighborhoods, or in some cases even specific counties. It has become very popular for us to try to find our roots in the Motherland and other cultures using genealogy. Meanwhile, a unifying element that holds us together culturally is our food and herbs, as well as specific ways of naming and preparing them. Within the naming and preparation of herbs and whole foods lie important keys to our roots.

Roots are important in parts of the United States in magical and spiritual practice. An herbalist is frequently called a *rootworker* since a great many formulas utilize the root of the plant above all other parts. *Rootwork* is also another name for *Hoodoo*. Rootwork consists of understanding the environment and herbalism and then incorporating indigenous wisdom. This includes the holistic approach that is the crux of African traditional medicine, African American folk medicine, and Jamaican bush medicine, as well as a myriad of practices whose base is in the ATRs of the Motherland.

Whereas once we were isolated from one another, dispersed on different islands and scattered across huge expanses of land in North and South America, today, increasingly, we are celebrating what we have in common. We see the commonalities within African culture whether the location is north, south, east, or west, not just in Africa, but also in the Black Atlantic. Though we have many different branches, languages, and appearances, there is that one strong root to our tree of life that unites us as a people and it is called Africa.

This chapter investigates the healing uses of some of our most celebrated roots, heralded for their multiple ways of making our lives more comfortable. Keep in mind that traditional African healing seeks to examine the core or root cause of a problem—this may be physical, metaphysical, environmental, or of the spirit realm. Whether used metaphorically—as amulets, charms, brews, or potions—or as a tasty side dish, roots are deeply embedded in African healing culture.

Roots: A Few Definitions

As I have mentioned, *root* is used to mean many different things in Hoodoo, including tubers and rhizomes, so I have done the same in this chapter. In the understanding of *roots* in herbalism, it is important to understand the differences. Here are definitions to keep in mind:

Root—the underground organ, lacking buds, leaves, or nodes that anchor the plant to the ground.

Tuber—a fleshy underground stem or root that serves as the reproductive food storage area of the plant.

Rhizome—a horizontal plant stem above the root.

Getting to Know Your Johns: High John, Little John, and Low John

There is a character that makes multiple appearances in African American folklore—his name is John. John is referred to as Big John, John Henry, High John, High John the Conqueror, Little John, and Low John. Sometimes John is the metaphor for a formidable man with superhuman strength and integrity, as in the story of John Henry. John can be naughty or unpredictable when connected to the story of the Eshu tricksters. In one story retold by Virginia Hamilton, "The Story of the Two Johns," one of the Johns is called the devil, and he performs brutal acts on animals. The other is the voice of reason. Other times, John becomes the symbol of courage and resilience, as in the stories of High John the Conqueror. High John the Conqueror is thought of as an enslaved African who could not be bound by his chains. He is the spirit of survival—a spirit that enables humans to survive disasters, atrocities, infractions, abuse, neglect, and diseases like cancer or heart disorders. High John is ultimately a radiant spirit of resilience that lies within the roots of all people.

High John the Conqueror (*Ipomoea jalapa*)

Naturally, we want to have an herb in our medicine bag that symbolizes the best qualities of John to help us confront difficult issues in our lives. In Hoodoo we have such a root: it is High John the Conqueror, a member of the morning glory family, related to our much-loved soul food, the sweet potato. High John the Conqueror is a natural amulet; as such, it is put inside a charm bag called a mojo bag. High John resembles a nut and indeed may be a stand-in symbolically for testicles. We all know the metaphors for *balls*; chief among them is the suggestion of courage. John represents the type of spirit energy we want to keep close, whether this sultry-smelling root is soaked in whiskey, dusted in magnetic sand for attraction, drenched in lucky oil like Van Van oil, or left as is to watch over us from a night table as we sleep. This natural amulet, which contains mild mind-altering constituents, plays an essential role in African American magico-spiritual magic as one of the strongest roots inside a mojo bag.

Little John Chew (*Alpinia galanga*)

Little John chew is a member of the ginger family. The general populace calls Little John galangal; it is a spice that tastes like a mild form of its cousin, ginger, which is discussed later in this chapter. Under the name *galangal*, you can find this root powdered at spice shops and specialty stores. With its connection to ginger, Little John chew is perfectly safe to consume. As an herb for the body, it is a stomachic carminative that soothes bellyache. It has found its way into our rootwork as a magical herb as well. Little John either chewed and spit or chewed and swallowed when doing court magic, or spells outside a courtroom, hence its nickname Little John chew. In traditional Central African and West African sculptures, spittle alone or combined with herbs is added to powerful figurative sculptures to imbue them further with that formidable energy known as ashe. Chewing the herb allows it to absorb the ashe of the practitioner, creating a forceful herb capable of doing the rootworker's bidding.

Low John (*Trillium grandiflorium*)

A third John, Low John is a relative of the lily. Low John is also called Beth root. As I mentioned earlier, there is the belief by the Yoruba people that there is great power in the naming of things. Power stems from the understanding of the name and the particular language of the plant when used for holistic health. High John the Conqueror, Little John chew, and Low John were so named by people of African descent with that particular thought and distinctive way of utilizing herbs in mind.

The Johns are important tools of rootwork whether used to help, protect, defend, attract, strengthen, or draw luck. These are not roots for dark work, hexing, or negativity. High John and Little John are used primarily in magical herbalism, whereas Low John is used medicinally.

Nurturing the Yam

When we harvest roots, inevitably we touch the earth—whether we dig the root or tuber up ourselves or handle it still touched by residual earth. This is a very important spiritual activity that author bell hooks expresses eloquently in her book *Sisters of the Yam: Black Women and Self-Recovery.*

"When we love the earth, we are able to love ourselves more fully. I believe this. The ancestors taught me it was so."[1] Hooks reminds us to remember our heritage as guardians of the earth, taking it as both an honor and our charge:

> *Living in modern society, without a sense of history, it has been easy for folks to forget that black people were first and foremost a people of the land, farmers.*[2]

Finally, there is a warning from this contemporary wisewoman that should be heeded:

> *If we think of urban life as a location where black folks learned to accept a mind/body split that made it possible to abuse the body, we can better understand the growth of nihilism and despair in the black psyche.*[3]

By convincing ourselves that we are an urban people, looking down upon all things rural as "country," we have lost an important part of our roots. We utilize roots like High John the Conqueror and Little John chew in magic and ritual. We would not consider a holiday joyous without consuming our favorite root called variously a sweet potato or a yam. The mind/body/spirit split was a malignant seed planted by others, nourished by us, or it could not have survived. In any case, it has yielded great harm. We must not embrace this concept

---

1   b. hooks, *Sisters of the Yam: Black Women and Self-Recovery* (Cambridge, MA: South End Press, 1993), 175.
2   hooks, *Sisters of the Yam,* 177.
3   hooks, *Sisters of the Yam,* 180.

but rather weed it out for the sake of spiritual enlightenment, which goes well beyond mere survival. Hold on to your yams, collards, watermelon, and roots; there is magic, mystery, connection, and healing stored up within them.

The Ubiquitous Yam

The word *yam* is derived from the Guinea word *nyami*, meaning "something to eat" because it is an important food. Portuguese slave traders could not pronounce *nyami*. It was called *igname* in French and, of course, *yam* in English. The family name of sweet potatoes is *Dioscoreaceae*, named for the Greek botanist thought to be the first physician in Europe. These starchy rhizomes can weigh as much as thirty pounds and are human and animal food. Using the words *yam* and *sweet potato* interchangeably to describe a beloved African tuber is not botanically correct. Sure, both tubers are an important part of African diets; they come from the earth and are celebrated in connection to culture and spirit. Wild yam, also called devil's bones or colic root, is a very important herb related to the African yams.

The next parts of this chapter will take you through the festivals on both sides of the Atlantic concerning yams, then discuss the differences between yam and sweet potato, followed by an in-depth discussion of wild yam.

Transatlantic Yam Festivals

The Igbo people of Nigeria believe in an almighty god named Chuku (Chineke). The affiliated gods are Ela, the earth mother; Anyanu, the sun; and Iwa, the sky. Ela is connected to the egun (the ancestors). Ndiche and Ajoku are associated with yams. The ancestors come to the animal festivals as marked dancers called Mmno.

The Igala, another group residing in Nigeria, have a main society formed around the ancestors called egun. The egun are remembered during yam harvest. No wonder sweet potatoes, also called yams in the United States, are so important to our annual harvest celebration of Thanksgiving.

The sweet potato (also called yam) is a very important crop for the region of Southwest Louisiana. Each year the yam is thanked for its goodness in a festival called Yambilee. The people in this area also cut roots, rhizomes, and tubers ritualistically to serve as natural amulets. This practice echoes the birthing ritual that follows.

Yam Birthing Ritual: Isu Egbegbe (The Mysterious Yam)

True yams contain diosgenin, which acts as a precursor to the hormone estrogen. This natural antioxidant has many beneficial effects on the body and is being used to improve lipids and the memory, among other things.

This African ritual is a part of the African practice of *agbo adoyun*, which translates as "liquefied herbs for pregnant women." I found this ritual of great interest because it unites the medicinal qualities of yam and its herbal uses for women with its earth symbolism.

African farmers have noticed the yam is near the top of the soil in the morning and it is located lower in the earth as dusk approaches. This is seen as mimicking the course of a woman's pregnancy—the child is higher earlier in the pregnancy, dropping lower and eventually traversing the birth canal during birth. Here is how the ritual goes:

- Healers put a yam cut into pieces into a bottle.
- The bottle is filled with water.
- A hole, perhaps suggesting the vagina, pierces the cover, which in turn suggests the round cervix cover.
- A feather of a beautiful bird is placed inside the hole (mucus plug).
- The bottle is hung; it cannot touch the ground (sacred view of the pregnant woman).
- The yam-infused water is consumed, ½ cup at a time once every three days. This causes vomiting, which is considered normal and may act out a desired course of action: the body's rejection of illness, toxins, and disease.[4]

This practice is believed to prevent convulsions in the newborn. Because of the purgative quality, this should only be done with the supervision of a traditional African medicine person.

Wild Yam (*Dioscorea villosa*)

Wild yam is kin to High John the Conqueror root and to the African yam. They are members of the trillium family. Wild yam is not, however, related to what we call a sweet potato

---

4   Makinde, *African Philosophy,* 110.

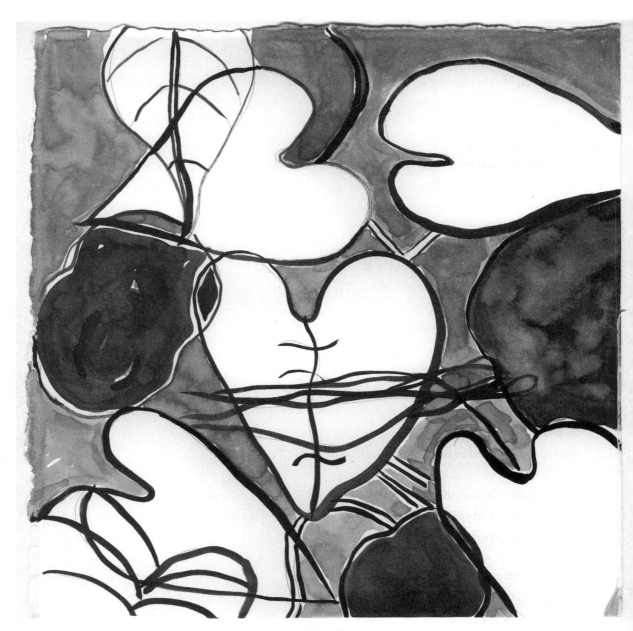

Wild yam

or yam in the United States. Neither of these are true yams. Yams grow well in Africa and the Caribbean. If you find African yams sold in the United States, they are usually sold in Latine neighborhood shops under the name *Africanos*.

Wild yam is a perennial climbing vine native to eastern North America: New England to Minnesota and Ontario, south to Florida and Texas. It grows well in damp woods, swamps, thickets, roadside fences, and hedges. It prefers a sandy to loamy medium-well-drained moist soil in partial shade. The prominently veined leaves rest on trailing vines.

Part used: rhizome.

How to use: tincture, capsules, or 8 ounces dried, cut, and sifted root decocted 25 minutes. Dose is ½ cup twice daily.

Constituents: steroidal saponins; dioscin, which yields diosgenin.

Wild yam is edible and medicinal. Ailments treated by Aztec and Mayans include a plethora of female reproductive organ complaints ranging from PMS, painful or absent periods, and childbirth pains to menopause. Diosgenin enabled the creation of the contraceptive pill. It contains high concentrations of dioscin, which is used to manufacture progesterone and other steroid drugs in contraceptives to treat reproductive organs. Steroids also help with asthma and arthritis. The phytosterols[5] (beta-sitosterol), alkaloids, and tannins make a powerful anti-inflammatory, antispasmodic, cholagogue, diaphoretic, diuretic, peripheral vasodilator, and relaxant.

Uses: As you can see, this plant is suitable for the maiden, mother, and crone—all stages of womanhood. Wild yam is used to relieve hot flashes, night sweats, mood changes, and vaginal dryness experienced by the crone. It has applications for males and females of all ages. Wild yam is used to treat irritable bowel syndrome (IBS), gastritis, gall bladder complaints, spasmodic cramps, and painful menstruation; it may help nausea experienced by pregnant women in small doses. The diuretic quality soothes the urinary tract and works well with any imbalances in the body, including the root cause to irritability. As a relaxant, it curbs stress and tension and shows promise at quelling the threat of miscarriage. As a food, wild yam contains twice the amount of potassium as bananas, one of our higher-potassium fruits.

---

5   *Phyto* meaning "plant" and *sterols* meaning "steroid constituents."

Sustainability: Perhaps with all these seemingly miraculous qualities, it is easy to understand that wild yam would become overused in modern society. United Plant Savers[6] has listed wild yam as an endangered plant. Care should be taken to seek substitutes and to grow this yourself rather than buying it in volume or wildcrafting[7] it to preserve the plant. Evolving research at Brigham Young University demonstrates that curing yams (letting them dry and age) increases their beneficial concentration of diosgenin. If that proves true, using cured wild yam will be optimal for efficacy and sustainability.

African Yam

There are a variety of African yams, including:

Cush-cush yam (*D. trifida*)—grown primarily in the Caribbean, this is one of the four most important food yams in the world. Surprisingly enough, it smells like bacon and eggs when cooking. The compact, ivory-fleshed tuber has a rosy underlayer beneath its skin. They turn dry and fluffy when cooked and taste like a fluffy, smoked potato.

White Guinea yam (*D. rotundata*)—originally from West Africa, this yam is used to make the popular dish fufu. It stores well and is tolerant of a long dry season. Wild Guinea yam might be a useful plant to grow in the United States because it does not require a lot of water and we have a tendency to overuse this precious resource.

Sweet Potato

Sweet potatoes are a soul food par excellence. They are loaded with goodness, and our ancestors chose very well in teaching us so many ways to use this nutritious starchy vegetable in a healthful diet.

Suggested amount: ½ cup daily.

Uses: preparation is roasted, boiled, baked, or mashed—go easy on the butter and salt. It

---

6   This is a sustainability organization.
7   *Wildcrafting* means harvesting a plant from the wild.

has a laxative effect due to high fiber content and is used medicinally to regulate bowels and to encourage a good complexion. Here are more highlights that make sweet potato a valuable contributor to our wellness:

- Sweet potatoes have some of the most disease-fighting antioxidants of all vegetables.
- Sweet potatoes' high beta-carotene quantity makes them apt to help the body boost its own natural immunity, which reduces the chances of cancers—even if you only eat a small amount every day. This suggestion carries over to lung cancer—one of the deadliest forms of cancer, for smokers or not—and even applies to those already diagnosed with cancer.
- Sweet potatoes help fight viral and bacterial infections.[8]
- They help deter cataract growth.

In short, sweet potatoes, that kindly comfort food we eat each Thanksgiving, Christmas, and New Year, and on other holy days, is a powerhouse root to tap for good health. For wholesome quality, reach for roasted sweet potato rather than candied sweet potatoes. Recipes follow in part III.

Cassava (Manihot esculenta), Also Called Manioc, Mandioca, Yucca, Sagu, and Tapioca

Cassava is second only to sweet potato in terms of importance as an African staple food and economic crop. It is the only member of the spurge family of plants to supply food. Cassava will grow where other things will not, and because of that, it is very valuable in areas without fertile soil and good growing conditions. Cassava is native to Central and South America. Cassava has been used since prehistoric times. Brazil is the principal growing country, along with Indonesia. The name *yucca,* pronounced *yoo-ka,* comes from the Arawak (indigenous) people of the Orinoco Basin who settled Greater and Lesser Antilles. The name refers to the roots, while *cacabi* refers to the bread made from it. The Portuguese took the crop to West Africa and it spread elsewhere from there. Cassava has been cultivated since

---

8   Research study by Ronald R. Watson, PhD, University of Arizona.

2500 BCE and contains a deadly poison inside that must be extracted from most types of cassava before it can be consumed.

- Cassava is prepared in many different ways around the world for food. The types imported into the United States come from Costa Rica and the Dominican Republic. They do not contain the toxins found in the African and Brazilian types, which are high in cyanide. Cassava is a low-protein, high-starch (energy) food.
- Flour called *farinha* is made from cassava in Brazil.
- The flour called *gari* in Africa is used to make flatbread.
- Cassava is eaten mashed or boiled as a vegetable or for dumplings and cakes, or mixed with coconut and sweetener to make biscuits.
- The West Indian dish pepper pot features cassava.
- Eighty-two million tons of cassava is produced mainly to make fufu.
- The cassava is washed, peeled, boiled, and pounded with mortar and pestle.
- In Brazil a superior variety called *mandiba* is ground extra fine and pressed to become the beginnings of tapioca—the dish that we are most familiar with in the United States. Tapioca is derived from another group of indigenous people, South American Tupi-Guarani people who call it *tipioca*.
- The sweet cassava is also widely used and does not require a detoxification process. It is eaten raw like melon, kiln-dried, or cooked.
- In Brazil a sustainable automobile fuel is being made from sugar, acetone, alcohol, and cassava.

The liquid of bitter cassava was used in earlier times, recorded in the activities of the enslaved Africans in the New World. The poisonous juices were used to cast worms out of meat and out of humans. Worms, snakes, and mythical serpents play a large role in African medicine, and so now we turn to them for the lessons they hold.

Snakes: Charming and Not

In my youth, a fear of snakes was quickly instilled when I happened upon a black water moccasin near our home by the lake. As children, we were fortunate because even though we saw snakes in the yard and wood and while swimming, most were harmless and none of us were ever bitten. Snakes still writhed around in my dreams for the longest time, harbingers of fear, symbols of misfortune, threats of impending betrayal.

Imagine my surprise when living with the Yolngu people on an island village on the top end of Australia, and Rainbow Snake was identified as my totemic animal. I wanted to shout to the elder who delivered the news, "You must be mistaken," but looking at his formidable appearance and huge mark of scarification on his belly, which looked as though he had hugged a cauldron to his stomach, I thought better of it. Clearly he had already made it through much more in his rites of passage during men's ceremony than I could hurl his way. Like a bad penny, snakes have been with me as long as I can remember, appearing in my paintings, my dreams, and my soul from here on out, as my totem.

In Haiti there is a snake that bears some resemblance to the all-powerful Australian Aboriginal Rainbow Snake of the Dreamtime, whom I had been linked to through my deep studies of my DNA ancestry—practitioners of Vodou know him as Damballah. The word is derived from the Dahomean word for reptile, *Dā*. Dā is the good serpent of the skies and is often linked with the Yoruba rainbow orisha Olumare. The good serpent of the sky, Dā, represents combined the male/female energy of the Mawa (female) moon that is cool and gentle and Liza (male) that is a tough, fiery representation of the sun. This balance of dualities strikes a chord with the Fon ideal personality—not too hot or too cold. Some people see Dā as being akin to kundalini[9] energy that exists in the earth and her children.

Damballah is the eldest and chief of the lwas, a primordial serpent deity who created the world and the god/desses who rule it. He is of such antiquity that he does not even need to speak to be heard; like DNA, he is at the core of our being.

Damballah Hwedo and his wife, Ayedo Hwedo, hold the entire earth in their coils. They set up the four pillars made from cast iron that support the four directions of the earth and hold up the sky. This was accomplished when the giant snake twisted around the columns, coloring them the multiple hues of the rainbow.

---

9   Kundalini is the electrical current of sensual or sexual energy that is at our core.

Earthquakes occur when these pillars are disturbed. The rainbow is the beautiful symbol of Dā Ayedo Hwedo, as is the color white. White represents the otherworld or the great beyond to the Dahomey people. People of African descent such as the Haitians understood the images of Saint Patrick quite easily when first presented with them. To them, Saint Patrick was Damballah Hwedo and Hwedo. Saint Patrick is seen as an elder wise man because of his white beard and the staff of power he holds. Standing upon the snakes he cast out of Ireland is seen more as an emblem of the unification of Damballah's power with that of the elder wise man and leader, than someone casting out serpents or devils from the land. Damballah Hwedo and his wife, Ayedo Hwedo, appreciate offerings of white things, especially eggs.[10]

The snake held power for us even in ancient Egypt. The rattlesnake's rattle is an emblem of ancient Egyptian goddesses Hathor and Isis. Isis used her sistrum, a rattlesnake-like instrument, to motivate the god/desses and humans to become active rather than passive. Isis, or Auset as she was called in Egyptian, brought the cobra into being. In our modern culture, snakeskin and rattlesnake rattles are used in various Hoodoo formulas for good or ill intent, including the infamous goofer dust, in which it is a key ingredient.

Dr. Buzzard, a renowned white Hoodoo from the Low Country, is remembered as someone who could implant snakes and other reptiles into his human victims with the power of his mind, a handshake, or a blow of dust. This is a well-documented practice that hails from Africa and has indeed continued in the New World. Anthropologists and authors Paul Stoller and Cheryl Olkes document snake venom sorcery in their book, *In Sorcery's Shadow*,[11] centered on the Republic of Niger. On whichever side of the Atlantic it is practiced, snakes and reptiles placed under the skin is a malignant act requiring a skillful healer familiar with the right roots for safe removal.

Snakes of various types have a prominent role in African myth, legend, and everyday life. The qualities of snake that are admired are its ability to survive on land and in the water; its ability to camouflage itself and blend quietly into its environment; its ability to hunt and eat much larger, more powerful prey than itself; and the potency of its venom, which demonstrates very strong ashe.

In the present-day United States, we have a huge mound outside Cincinnati, Ohio,

---

10 Thompson, *Flash of the Spirit*, 175–78.
11 Paul Stoller and Cheryl Olkes, *In Sorcery's Shadow* (Chicago: Univ. of Chicago Press, 1987).

called the Serpent Mound. It is the largest serpent effigy in the United States. People who honor snake energy go there to pay homage.

It is no wonder numerous roots are named for snakes and many magical formulas are dedicated to snake energy in one form or another. Snakes have a revered place in African culture; people who live in close proximity to wildlife seem to cultivate an awe for their power, mystery, and prowess.

The interpretation of snakes in Christianity is altogether different to that in ATRs. The snake is symbolic of treachery, deceit, and the devil in Christianity, and many people of African descent are now Christian—even those who practice other paths still incorporate elements of organized religion into much of their work.

To complicate matters further, serpents are a physical threat to small livestock, children, and rural people—perceived or real. We even need snake venom antidotes today, especially those living in rural areas, campers, and those who enjoy hiking.

IN AFRICAN AMERICAN FOLK MEDICINE, there are at least ten herbs named for snakes—all are called snakeroot of one kind or another. Below we examine a few of the prominent snakeroots. We will explore how they were, and in some cases continue to be, useful to the Gullah people of the Sea Coast Islands of Georgia and South Carolina as well as other African American rootworkers.

White Snakeroot (*Ageratina altissima*)
White snakeroot has leaves of three to six inches that are egg-shaped, connecting this plant to Damballah. They grow in the woods, thickets, and clearings and are used to kill worms.

Button Snakeroot (*Eryngium yuccifolium*)
Button snakeroot, taken as a tea with whiskey or cut with pine tar, life everlasting, and lemon is used to fight symptoms of the common cold.

Virginia Snakeroot (*Aristolochia serpentaria*)
Virginia snakeroot is a plant that grows in the woods, swamps, and wetlands with good shade, growing six to eighteen inches high. It is a slender, erect plant with heart-shaped leaves and pointed tips. Virginia snakeroot is used in traditional African American med-

icine to treat sprains by making a poultice of the leaves. A decoction of the root is used to treat infections and viruses similarly to penicillin. This plant is becoming scarce and is presented for its historical value and connection to Damballah more than as a suggestion for use.

Sampson's Snakeroot (Orbexilum pedunculatum)

Sampson's snakeroot is also called gentian root. It is a bitter digestive stimulant. It eases stomach pain and is especially useful for elders. It is a pronounced bitter gastric stimulant, cholagogue, tonic, antiemetic, anti-inflammatory, febrifuge, and refrigerant. It is also a treatment for anorexia nervosa, dyspepsia, and gastrointestinal upset. It is very useful in some malnourished individuals, especially the elderly who may become depressed and avoid food. Magically in Hoodoo, Sampson's snakeroot chips are placed in mojos and jack-balls because it is the symbol of power and strength, especially for men. They are useful in mojo bags that help men with love draw, fertility, and virility spells.

Snakeweed (Bistort) Root (Polygonum bistorta)

Snakeweed (bistort) root is a perennial growing in mountainous areas, damp soils, and wet meadows, as well as on stream banks.

Part used: root.

Dose and preparation: 2 teaspoons rootstock to 1 cup water. Simmered below the boil 5 to 10 minutes. One cup consumed per day.

Uses: alternative, astringent, diuretic, styptic. Snakeweed is an excellent remedy for diarrhea, mouthwash for gum disease, and treatment to stop hemorrhages. When directly applied to wounds, the powdered plant will stop bleeding quickly.

The chips of snakeweed (bistort) root are used magically in Hoodoo to draw luck and prosperity. The root serves as a natural amulet to repel snakes and protect against betrayal.

Snakebite (*Chenopodium album*)

Snakebite is more commonly referred to as lamb's-quarter.

Part used: root.

Habitat: snakebite is an herbaceous perennial plant found in rich soils and shady woods of central to western states of North America (grows as a weed in some locations).

Qualities: antiseptic, astringent, diaphoretic, emmenagogue, expectorant, tonic, soap substitute.

Uses: as a poultice or salve (for insect bites and stings), decoction, or tincture.

How to prepare: decoct 1 teaspoon root to 1 cup water or milk. Drink hot or cold one to two cups per day. Decoction would be used as an herbal component of salve.

Tincture: add chopped root to a sterilized bottle, cover with 100-proof alcohol, close, and steep for 4 to 6 weeks. Take ¼ to ½ teaspoon at a time.

Roots for Mothers and Children

Traditional African American and African Caribbean midwives and healers are called by a variety of titles, including one that is most fitting, which is used in parts of Africa and Jamaica—*mothers*. The *mothers* use these roots to address the mind, body, and spirit of moms-to-be and moms.

Beth Root or Birth Root (*Trillium erectum*)

Parts used: rhizome and root.

Qualities: steroidal saponins, volatile oils, diosgenin, fixed oil, gum astringent, antiseptic, uterine tonic, alternative, and expectorant.

Uses: contains the building blocks of female sex hormones; used for menstrual disorders and to lessen the pain of childbirth; stimulates uterine muscles to help labor proceed smoothly. Used to halt bleeding of the nose and mouth and internally. Used to stop diarrhea and dysentery. External uses include an antiseptic wash to treat vaginal infections, thrush, and trichomonads. Speeds healing and soothes skin ailments, hemorrhoids, and varicose veins in a sitz bath.

Warning: should not be used during pregnancy because it stimulates the uterus and could cause premature labor.

Angelica (*Angelica archangelica*)

Beloved by Hoodoo rootworkers, angelica, also called Holy Ghost root, is the preferred natural amulet that works as a charm to protect women and children. Angelica is a central feature of protective mojo bags, whole or powdered. Angelica is seen as an herb that possesses high spiritual powers. It smells extremely pungent. The root's metaphysical effects are believed to be as strong as its odor. Angelica root is used for beneficial purposes such as defensive and protective magic, and in that way it is a healing plant of the mind and spirit.

The Other Angelica (*Angelica sinensis*)

Angelica's cousin, also called dong quai, is an important preventative and treatment, particularly helpful to the well-being of women and children. Dong quai contains the antioxidant beta-carotene, known to deter cancers, as well as vitamins B and E; constituents include beta-sitosterol, angelic acid, myristic acid, and angeol. The root has antispasmodic, balancing, detoxification, tonic, analgesic, and emmenagogue qualities. It is also a nourishing root that can be eaten raw or taken as a tincture. When cooked, dong quai is warming and improves the circulation, reduces high blood pressure, and prevents blood clots. The main gift of dong quai is its ability to tone the reproductive and sex organs. Dong quai affects menstruation since the analgesic and antispasmodic actions relieve menstrual cramps and release suppressed periods. Dong quai is useful for the symptoms of menopause. Because it relaxes the uterus, it is not to be used during pregnancy. The tonic quality helps strengthen and revitalize women in any stage of their life. It is especially useful to the elder who suffers with arthritis or rheumatic pains, or those who are convalescing.

Ginger (*Zingiber officinale*)

Parts used: root and rhizome.

Constituents: volatile oils (borneol, cineole, phellandrene, zingiberol, zingiberene).

Uses: antiseptic, diaphoretic, expectorant, digestive, antioxidant, circulatory stimulant, hypotensive, decongestant, carminative, rubefacient, antithrombotic, anti-inflammatory, antibiotic (can kill salmonella and staph infections at specific concentrations), anti-ulcer in animals, antidepressant, antidiarrheal, and strong antioxidant. Ranks very high in anticancer activity.

Preparation: ginger is shredded and used as tea, taken in capsule form, used as a food additive/spice, used decoratively and magically, and used whole and dried in potpourri and mojo bags.

Gingerroot varies in size and is a warm yellowish-tan color with a paper-thin skin that is easily peeled. Ginger is pungent, warming, and valuable for its stimulating action that affects the circulation and heart, bringing warmth and well-being. Hot ginger tea promotes perspiration, brings down fever, helps clear catarrh, acts as an expectorant, aids digestion, stimulates appetite, relieves nausea, acts to reduce pain, promotes menstruation, treats delayed periods, and deters menstrual clotting, spasms, and painful ovulation. It is a blood thinner shown to reduce cholesterol and blood pressure.

Ginger is used to treat nausea, vomiting, aches, rheumatism, and nervousness. It is a proven antinausea, anti-motion-sickness remedy that matches or in some cases surpasses the drug Dramamine. Ginger thwarts and prevents migraines, headaches, and osteoarthritis, and relieves the symptoms of rheumatoid arthritis.

Ginger is not recommended for those who suffer from gastritis or peptic ulcers or those intolerant to heat. The types we use as a ground spice are grown primarily in Jamaica, Nigeria, and Sierra Leone, where it is used to flavor curries, stews, and baked goods and to make ginger beer.

Dogwood (*Cornus florida*)

On the East Coast of the United States, dogwood's perky blossoms are a harbinger of spring. The trees were often transplanted in African American yards from nearby forests, and my parents did this when we first built our home. The roots are decocted and used as tea. The tea has been traditionally used as a cleansing, strengthening tonic and to reduce inflammation. Dogwood is good for the mind and spirit, making a lovely addition to the garden with white, cream, or pastel blossoms in the spring and leaves that turn a deep red in the fall. Identified by Robert Westmacott in *African-American Gardens and Yards in the Rural South* as a plant recognized as part of Southern Black gardens, it adds a touch of tradition and nostalgia to the garden. Westmacott also recorded beautiful handmade dogwood branch brooms used to sweep yards.

Dogwoods are, however, susceptible to illness; care has to be taken with them. They will not grow in all zones, so check with your local garden center before trying to transplant a dogwood.

CHAPTER 6

Harvesting the Grasslands

THE PLAINS, SAVANNA, AND PRAIRIE

PLANTS IN FOCUS

- Wild bergamot
- Echinacea
- Speedwell
- Sunflower
- Sweetgrass
- Hemp
- Broomcorn
- Bermuda grass
- Couch grass

- Red clover
- Five-finger grass
- Palmarosa
- Vetiver
- Citronella
- Lemongrass
- Sugarcane
- Acacia
- Baobab

I HAVE A VERY INTERESTING relationship to the grasslands and prairie. I often speak about my upbringing near the New Jersey Pine Barrens within the wetlands. With the goddesses' grace, I have had the opportunity to make my life anew in other regions, for a time in the desert of Australia and in the arid lands of Southern California. Fortunately, I was there at a time before massive mall renovations and condo mayhem set in. In the 1980s there were

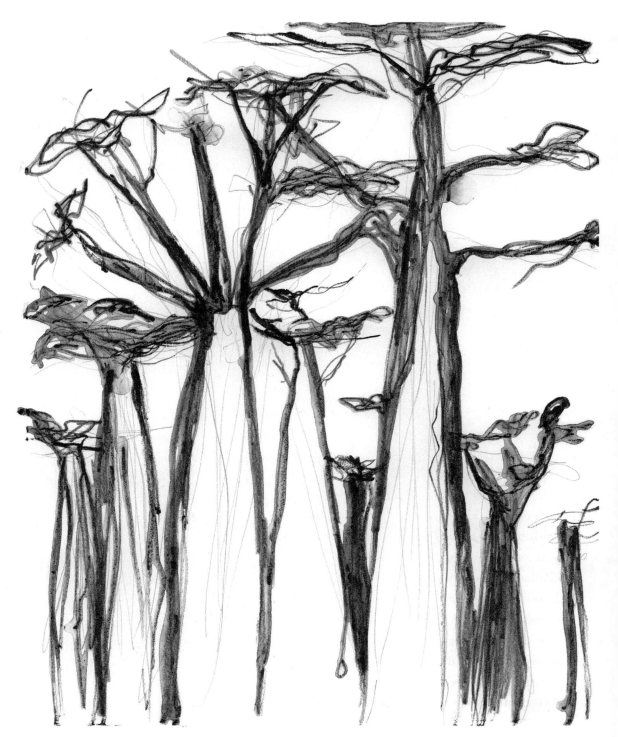

African savanna

still plenty of grassy mesas, eucalyptus groves, and wildflowers to discover. I have since left those arid lands, and now home is near the great tall grass prairies of the Midwest.

Often people comment on how dull and flat it is here. I'm sure when most people think of plains, the prairie, or even the savanna, they think boring. But there is a great deal of magic and wonder to be found in these unique places. I am proud of where I live and become moved spiritually when I take trips to the open prairie and ample fields of corn. These grasses bring life to the central and southern regions of our state and in many regards to the rest of the country and the world—as this is the breadbasket. On more recent journeys to my spirit home in Southern New Jersey, I see it with brand-new eyes. The Delaware Valley is indeed very diverse as well. Marshes, bogs, forests, swamps, and even savanna-like grasslands make that area a varied biome.

You may wonder, What exactly is a savanna? A savanna is rolling grassland scattered with shrubs and isolated trees. Generally there is not enough water to support large or numerous trees. There are some spectacular trees that grow amid the savanna, including one of the most curious you are likely to ever see, the baobab, as well as the acacia, which is imbued with an aura of the sacred—healer's bounty. Savannas are also known as tropical grasslands. African people have lived on the Serengeti plains of Tanzania, one of the world's most famous savannas, for centuries. People of African descent live in Brazil and Venezuela's grasslands. We are also populating the plains states; some even walked the Trail of Tears with the Cherokee and settled out west. We also have a rich history in Indiana, Missouri, and here in Illinois—all states with rich biodiversity and seemingly endless fields of grain. There are plenty of open prairies to fill the heart with wonder and the medicine bag with the jewels amid the grasses. Moreover, you can recreate a miniature prairie on quite a small patch of land. I know because I have done so myself. Having your own prairie wildflower plants allows you to help the environment and nurture wildlife while avoiding the endangerment of overharvested plants such as echinacea.

Similar to people of African descent, plants of the savanna, grasslands, and prairie have long taproots and are highly adaptable. These types of plants know how to make do with very little; they do not need the best conditions to grow—some actually flourish best on rugged terrain. They also can go a long time without water. Often the tree trunks of savanna trees are virtual warehouses storing massive amounts of water in their trunks and healing medicine in their nuts, barks, and leaves. People who live in arid regions, the

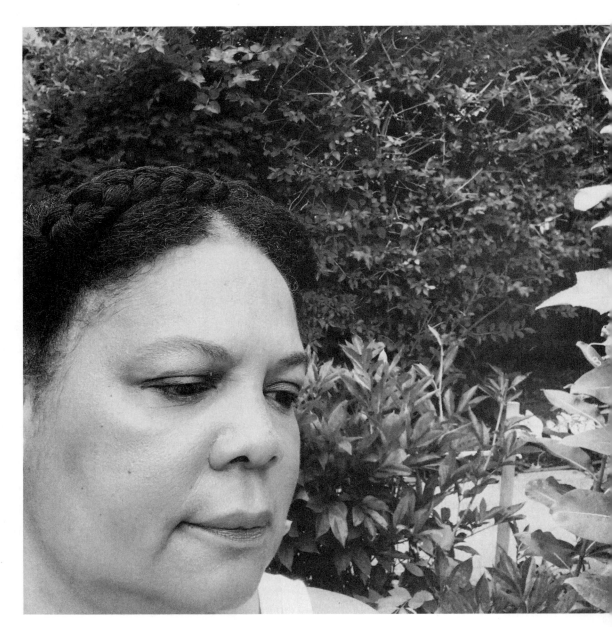

Priestess Bird in her summer garden

prairie, or what used to be the prairie, can help sustain biodiversity and conserve natural resources by growing drought-resistant plants such as:

- The family Echinacea
- Black-eyed Susan
- Sunflowers
- Wild bergamot

Finding the Prairie Through Ritual

I vividly remember when it finally dawned on me that for now I am a woman of the prairie. For years I almost delighted in saying, "I am not from here; this is not my place." Finally, I found a group of spiritual women, who taught me to appreciate the sacred nature of the prairie. I was humbled by the spiritual power of my elders in the Limina Society as they led us through this ceremony in a grassy field in suburban Illinois:

> The gathering
> Maidens, mothers, and crones
> We women of the prairie
> Nicneven casts the circle 'round the flaming bonfire
> Fire, stoked with collective energy, anxiety, and prayers
> Multi-colored fingers wave inscribed leaves
> To the feather-filled autumn sky
> Jubilant chanting ensued:
> Fire, fire, burning bright
> Illuminate, purify, this sacred night
> We women o' the prairie
> We who are lit by your amber glow have a request:
> Cleanse us
> Brighten us

Help us heal
May we reflect your light
Fire, fire, ever so bright
Reach into our hearts
Warm our souls
'Till the return of spring
Protective shawl of the winter crone
Shroud us with silver light
This chilly Autumn Solstice night
With Nicneven's order, there was a hush
Leaves were offered
To feed the fire
In honor of Goddess Ix Chebel Yax
Sure 'nuff, as the New Moon rose
We were refreshed, cleansed, ready to begin anew
Resilient, hearty
Brimming with sunny souls
We, women of the prairie.

Essential Prairie Medicines

Bergamot (*Monarda didyma*)

Bergamot is an unusual plant with scarlet-red frilly petals that are quite thin. Birds and bees absolutely love it, hence the nickname of its near relative, bee balm (*Monarda punctata*). Bergamot is one of those comforting plants, at once a source of wonder and a total delight, with a dash of humor thrown in for good measure. Wild bergamot has some of the scent of bergamot orange, from which the essential oil is created. Bergamot is a member of the mint family. It is a perennial that produces cheerful flowers that are charming and lift the spirits. The domesticated *M. punctata* requires lots of moisture, whereas the wild variety, like most meadow plants, does not. The dried flowers make fragrant additions to potpourri, wreaths, swags, and wall hangings. All in all, bergamot is a very worthwhile garden plant.

Coneflower Echinacea (*Echinacea angustifolia, E. pallida, E. purpurea*)

There are several varieties of echinacea:

- *Angustifolia,* also called black sampson coneflower, has eight-inch leaves, large soft violet flowers, and a dark cone-shaped center. Called Missouri snakeroot because the root is used to treat snakebites, it detoxifies the body and treats rabies.
- *Pallida,* also called pale purple coneflower, has rosy purple blossoms with drooping flower petals. It boosts immunity by stimulating white blood cells and regulating red blood cells. It is considered antitumor and antiallergenic.
- *Purpurea,* also called purple coneflower, grows up to five feet tall and has large red or purple flowers four inches in diameter. Purple coneflower stimulates the immune system and is used to treat colds and deter the flu.

Parts used: root, rhizome, leaves, flower petals.

Constituents: vitamins A, B complex, B_3, C, E, iron, calcium, magnesium, manganese, potassium, selenium, silicon, sodium, essential oils, polyacetylenes, polysaccharide, glycoside, resin, betaine, inulin, and sesquiterpene.

Qualities: alternative, antiallergenic, antiviral, antifungal, antimicrobial, anti-inflammatory, immunity booster, diaphoretic.

Uses: echinacea tea is standard for infections; it is used at the onset to stimulate immunity and speed recovery from colds, influenza, viruses, glandular swelling, lymphatic congestion, boils, abscesses, and inflammatory conditions.

Echinacea Tips

Decocted root is commonly used, but leaves and even flowers offer some of the same medicinal qualities. Using varied parts of the plant helps sustain them and protect the family Echinacea from facing extinction. To decoct the root, dig up part of the root, wash it, and chop it into small pieces. Put the pieces in a pot of water, bring the water almost to boil over medium heat, cover, and simmer for 25 minutes. Do not boil any herbs.

It is very easy to propagate echinacea. My local gardening neighbors and I cut down the plants late in the autumn (before a killing frost), shake out the seeds where we want more plants, and then lay the flowers down as mulch. Inevitably during the next growing season, there are lovely new echinacea plants. This practice is good ecologically and economic to boot.

Echinacea does not appreciate being transplanted; you may well lose your plant in the process or at the very least stunt its growing season. It is worthwhile to make a plan for where you will plant them and try to stick to it.

Other than providing stability, you do not need a green thumb to grow echinacea. Like many prairie plants, echinacea is quite happy if there is simply adequate sunlight and rainwater, though it does tolerate drought.

One month is the maximum time to use echinacea treatments, after which time you need to take a break for at least one month to let your system work on its own.

Speedwell (*Veronica officinalis*)

You already know I love this gorgeous plant, as it is mentioned as one of the foundation plants in my garden in chapter 2. The plant with the tall, elegant habit (shape and form) and deep purple blossoms grows in the prairie here, but it also grows in West Africa and on the Sea Coast Islands where the Gullah have made good use of it. In Francis Porcher's "Report on the Indigenous Medicinal Plants of South Carolina" more than one hundred years ago, Porcher reports the leaves and flowers were used as a tonic, expectorant, and to treat asthma as well as coughs. Infusions of the leaves were employed on the West Coast of Africa medicinally. They contain tannin. The official uses are as a diaphoretic, diuretic, and expectorant.[1] I recommend speedwell as a magical, spiritual, healing plant. The purple color of the flowers is a color of serenity and grace; the upright growth of the plant reminds us to hold our heads high no matter what the obstacles. This is a nice plant to give to someone who is feeling blue or ill or who is in recovery.

Sunflowers (*Helianthus annuus*)

As a sun-loving culture, the ancient Egyptians would have loved this plant. The plant's name tells why; it is the Greek *helios,* meaning "sun," and *anthos,* meaning "flower." The French word for it is *tournesol,* or "turn with the sun," which is precisely what it does. The plant is called phototropic, meaning that it follows the sun.

---

1   Francis P. Porcher, "Report on the Indigenous Medicinal Plants of South Carolina," *Transactions of the American Medical Association* 2 (1849): 815.

Native American people of various groups make great use of sunflowers, using them for healing poultices and skin washes as well as eating the seeds and working with the stalks to make life-preserving floats. Spiritually, some groups leave bowls of the seeds on the graves of loved ones.

Today, sunflowers are being grown in the sunny climate of South Africa as well, where they are utilized to create healing oil from the seeds. South African sunflowers are known to be rich in unsaturated fatty acids, especially oleic (monounsaturated) and linoleic, which is diunsaturated. Polyunsaturated fatty acids are found in sunflower. Sunflower oil is inexpensive; it provides vitamins A, D, and E and helps boost the immune system. Sunflower oil is an unsung hero in this market so saturated with oils. It has many healing applications, including herbal infusions used in massage, hot oil treatments, nail soaks, cooking, salad dressings, marinades, and homemade cosmetics. A cup of unshelled sunflower seeds contains:

- 162 calories
- 10.5 g protein
- 8.6 g carbohydrate
- 22.8 g fat (unsaturated)
- 4.8 g fiber
- a good source of zinc with 2.3 mg

Sunflowers are a special flower in the Midwest and they are the state flower of Kansas. They grow quite freely alongside the highways, beautify waste dumps, add color to fields, and of course grace our gardens. Basically wherever their seeds blow, sunflowers take root unless they are disturbed. Called an annual, they reseed themselves, making them a perennial in many a garden.

Each year, I almost look out at them in chagrin. Treelike in their massive ten-to-twelve-foot splendor, they threaten to overtake my garden and choke out the light from other less-aggressive or small-stature plants year after year. But then each year the ones I allow to grow share their metaphysical gifts. I can peer out my front window to the most gorgeous sight. Green finches, the tiniest little critters, sing cheerfully as they eat the sunflower seeds. There are plenty to go around as well. In the autumn I cut the mature plants and take the seeds inside for my family and our bird—all of whom absolutely love them.

Holistic Healing with Sunflowers

- The flower is aesthetically pleasing, hence the wide variety of artists who have dedicated canvases to them. Try painting, drawing, or pressing the leaves to use in collage.
- The seeds invite wildlife that in turn share their magic and mystery with those who will take time to enjoy.
- The seeds are inexpensive, plentiful, and nutritious.
- You can make a mildly antibacterial infusion from the leaves and use it to treat scratches or minor irritations.
- If you are truly industrious, you can utilize the stalks to make a very strong textured handmade paper, sprinkling in the bright-yellow petals for visual interest.
- Cut a bunch of flowers and cheer up a sick room, dining room, or anywhere you please.
- Last but not least, you can follow the example of our nation's First People: put a bowl of the seeds on a grave, or adapt this rite by putting a bowl of them on your ancestral altar.

Opening the Way with Sweet Grass

Wherever you live, it is wonderful to engage the spirit of the prairie in your healing work. Sweetgrasses and corn afford a wealth of opportunity to perform healing or nurturing work with grass.

The Sweetgrass Goddess

Sweetgrass (*Hierochloe odorata*) is often used at the beginning of rituals and ceremonies, as it is an invitation to positive nature spirits and the ancestors. A fragrant herb, reminiscent of warmed vanilla, sweetgrass is in fact sometimes called vanilla grass. It is beloved by various First Nations peoples, particularly the Sioux and Aniyunwiya, or Tsalagi (commonly called Cherokee in English). The Lakota people connect this scented rush with the compassionate creation goddess Wohpe.

Wohpe is a striking, well-balanced, spiritual goddess associated with the mysterious seventh direction. She is thought to appear at the moment a puff of smoke appears. According to Lakota stories, the braided grasses symbolize the beautiful plaited hair of Wohpe, though other nations associate sweetgrass with various other mothers of creation.

Sweetgrass herb creates quiet, seductive incense that assists during the process of spiritual cleansings, clearings, rituals, and blessings.

Like many beloved plants, sweetgrass is becoming endangered in certain states, especially along the East Coast and in New England. It is being grown by dedicated organic farmers and by Native American groups in Upstate New York. Sweetgrass grows well both in North America and in Europe around the Arctic Circle. In fact, the sacred nature of sweetgrass is shared among Native Americans and European groups who have utilized it as a strewing herb on church stairs during Saint Days. Sweetgrass has been cultivated for at least ten thousand years. Thirty species have been identified. Since the species *Hierochloe odorata* is disappearing rapidly, it is worth considering using the slightly less fragrant *H. alpina*, *H. hirta*, *H. occidentalis*, or *H. pauciflora*. Sweetgrass can also be cultivated, and some even grow it as an indoor houseplant under the right conditions.

Sweetgrass: The Welcome Basket

Sweetgrass and other types of woven baskets are an earth-embracing way to coddle your child. Our brothers and sisters, the Gullah people of the Sea Coast Islands, continue the basketmaking traditions their ancestors learned in Africa. I kept every one of my babies in a small handwoven grass basket that could easily be carried from place to place. The baskets have the sweet smell of the sea grasses and they embody the spirits of the earth. The grasses called *sweetgrass* by the Gullah are frequently harvested on James Island and in Mount Pleasant in the Low Country. One of the grasses is the very tall, thin *Muhlenbergia filipes*, and it smells of newly mown hay. Some weavers add bulrush, which makes the baskets sturdier and more colorful. Saw palmetto leaves are split until they are very thin and then used as a thread to hold together the sweetgrass. See page 254 for more on saw palmetto. The woven strands of grass and rush hold ancestral energy. Today, many of the Gullah basketmakers display and sell their crafts in the open-air marketplace of Charleston, South Carolina.

The way of the Gullah people is to not give away their secrets by talking. The Gullah keep a great deal inside, which may be a key to how they held on to so much West African culture. Owning one of these baskets is a way of supporting a valuable though waning traditional craft and a way of keeping their story, which is also a part of our story, alive—this is good spiritual medicine.

If you want to use a basket of the right shape and size as a baby basket, the blanket placed inside should be made of soft organic cotton, hemp, or flannel. Pillows are not desired within the basket, but a dream pillow containing rose petals, lavender, and chamomile can be placed in the bedroom to assist the child's sleep. Alum can be sewn into the outside of the sleep basket, blanket, or hat and used as an amulet of protection.

Broomcorn (*Cytisus scoparius*)

Broomcorn is a grass; it is also called sorghum. Sorghum is used in the production of molasses—a significant ingredient in African American magic—and as the sacrificial offering to goddess Oya and god Shango. Molasses also plays a key role in African American soul food cooking, most notably in the preparation of baked beans and gingerbread.

Broomcorn is a stiff grass, related to raffia, another highly valued material and commodity used in West African ceremony, ritual, and art. Palm is another relative to broom—it is used for myriad purposes: food, wine, oil, soap, housing, basketry, crafts, ceremony, and ritual. Raffia and palm fibers or fronds are not only related to broomcorn; they are also symbolically interchangeable in magico-religious practice. Finally, dragon's blood, a resin from palm trees, is used in Hoodoo as a potent incense, filled with powerful intent, capable of serious juju.

To the African mind, natural grasses in all their incarnations are representatives of the wild, untamed nature of the forest. As such, they are denizens of power, for grasses embody and contain the living spirits of the forest. Along with nature's ability to comfort and provide comes an awesome helping of unpredictability. There is not much of the concern that we have in the United States for taming or controlling nature. *Nature* isn't really a word found in the primary traditional languages of West Africa; instead the word *wilderness* prevails as both a place and a concept.

Folklore, Brooms, and Africans in the Americas

I remember when I was a girl, my family respected broomstraw for its curative powers. My aunt pierced my ears using a needle and thread. The thread was knotted and left in my ear for six weeks of healing. Then a tiny piece of broomstraw was singed and inserted into my ear for another six to eight weeks. The broomstraw was believed to form a core, sealing off the hole, so that the pierced ear would never close. This special process of piercing, knotting, and inserting broomstraw was used to fight infection and scarring.

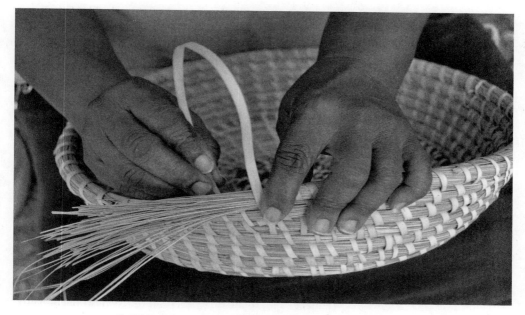

Gullah with a sweetgrass basket in Charleston, South Carolina

The book *Folklore from Adams County, Illinois* presents several other ways that broomstraw is used for healing. Primarily, broomstraw is cited as a potent herb that can be used for lancing warts and then placed on top of the lanced wart in the shape of a cross to encourage complete healing.

Folklore from Adams County, Illinois is but one volume in Dr. Harry Middleton Hyatt's exhaustive research on Hoodoo. He devotes an entire chapter to brooms and sweeping. A few of the entries are quite telling in their connection back to West African beliefs, and in particular Mande beliefs surrounding the wild, unpredictable quality of brooms. The Mande language survived slavery in a creolized form with the Gullah people of the Carolina Lowlands, so it is no wonder that Mande beliefs regarding brooms have flourished in Hoodoo and the African American community at large. Georgia and the Carolina Lowlands hold a vital link to African Americans' connection with tribal West Africa and it is one of the major bases for Hoodoo.

Several of Hyatt's informants warn that resting a broom improperly invites injury, pain, or loss. In particular, resting a broom on the bed is believed to cause the sleeping person to die. How a broom is approached is also a subject of much lore—if you step over a broom or if it falls as you start to leave, you may expect death to follow. Carrying a broom inside the house is a sign that death is coming to descend on the family. However, proper handling of the broom brings luck, happiness, and prosperity. If you go to look at a home for rent or purchase, informants advise you to carry your broom (under your arm) or even to throw it into a window so it enters before you do. Holding your personal broom under the arm is also a shield against arguments and domestic unrest. If arguments or fights occur, go outside with the broom tucked under the arm and throw it inside the door. The first thing to enter a new home should be your broom. Brooms should be treated with respect and broomstraws should be stored facing upward.

Broom: As Symbol, Tool, and Cleanser

The idea of a swept yard discussed in chapter 2 may have come as a surprise, but the humble broom holds an elevated position in African and African American folklore, magico-religious beliefs, and spiritual practices. The rustic dogwood and bulrush brooms created by Southern Black folks and Cayman Islanders to pattern the sandy soil of their yards attest to a reverence for brooms and a trust in them to serve us well.

Most folks are aware of our reverence for the broom because of its role in the Jumping the Broom ceremony. As we look into the elaborate broom etiquette and customs of early African Americans, we gain partial understanding about the broom's multiple purposes. For an in-depth understanding of the relationship between brooms and Black folks, we must journey much further back in time. Tracing the broom's usage back across the Atlantic sheds the brightest light on its complex articulation in African and African American culture.

Beyond the utilitarian, brooms are often thought of in terms of European witchcraft—the wild rides under the full moon and highly sexually charged sabbat rituals. While Europeans have an intriguing history of broom magic and broom making that goes all the way back to the Middle Ages, broomcorn itself originated in Central Africa. The following paints a picture of how the broom is perceived in the Motherland.

Spirits Who Lurk: The Frightening Spirits of the Grass

The negotiators who deftly mediate between the wilderness spirits and civilized society are hunters and metalsmiths, and to some extent healers, diviners, and warriors. Since so many groups of Africans live in or near the wilderness (forest, bush, and savanna), a strict separation between what is considered *wild* and *civilized* is observed. The hunter, metalsmith, healer, diviner, and warrior regularly cross the boundaries that separate the distinct worlds, helping their communities integrate the power of nature into their daily lives. Generally these arbitrators recognize and honor the subgroups of beings that reside in the wilderness. These beings are somewhat akin to fairies or pixies of Northern Europe, yet they are more grotesquely misshapen inversions of humans (even walking and doing things backward). The forest folk who grass-clad masqueraders either invoke or repel during annual purification ceremonies include:

Bori—a densely populated species living among the Hausa people. Bori bear resemblance to humans but have hooves. These tricksters readily shape-shift and are known to be fond of taking the form of snakes.

Eloko—a people-eating dwarf that lives among the Nkundo people of Democratic Republic of Congo. Eloko live in the hollows of trees in densely forested areas. Eloko blend in well with their environment, since they are covered in grass and their clothing is made from leaves. These little people are minute, green, and easily mistaken for grass—pity the fool who does! If you mistake an eloko for grass, they become infuriated. Only a hunter's metaphysical prowess can dispel an angered eloko, which is why it pays to be acutely aware of the environment.

Abatwa—much smaller than a common fairy, abatwa hide under a blade of grass and sleep inside anthills. Typically, the entire species rides into a village on a single horse. These grass-loving spirits murder victims with poisoned arrows.

It is only on rare occasions and for specific reasons that these types of spirits of the wilderness are invited to be a part of civilized society. These occasions include: annual performances, harvest festivals, fertility rites, and purification and sweeping activities.

Common people often fear mysterious and unpredictable forces of nature. Spirits of the savanna and bush are believed to cower around the doors of humans' homes, waiting for discarded food, drinks, or clothing to bring to their own villages and families. It is frowned upon to sweep dirt out the front door or even to throw wash water there. To repel or dispel tiny spirits who hang about doorways and stoops, both are meticulously cleansed on a daily basis, using spiritually charged herbs and special waters. The spiritual cleansing of doorways and front stairs is important in many parts of West Africa, as well as to practitioners of Vodou and Hoodoo in the diaspora.

Judicious Grasses

Grasses are also used to cast judgment in certain villages. The Go Society has a mask and costume called a *Ga Wree Wree*. The Ga Wree Wree is a fierce symbol of the powers that lurk within the forest. The mask contains leopard teeth and raffia and is primarily red—the essential color of life force (blood). The huge bell-shaped skirt of the costume is made entirely of raffia. A Ga Wree Wree performer walks or sits immersed in the grassy folds of the skirt. Ga Wree Wree is a creature that oversees and then passes judgment on the activities of the community, according to unwritten law.

The Dan people of Côte d'Ivoire have their own masks and costumes, which almost always feature grass such as raffia to indicate the power of the wilderness. Wo Puh Gle is a talking entertainer, while Yeh To Gle is an authority figure. The Boma clan of Ijo village in Rivers State, Nigeria, has a time of the year when costumed performers wear a mask of natural raffia and other wildcrafted materials. The lead performer moves from one end of the town to another, like a gigantic broom, sweeping the community clean of its annual buildup of spiritual and physical clutter. These groups and many others throughout West Africa have a vital tradition of wearing costumes constructed of natural grasses and straw to enhance their spiritual duties.

Grass and Deities

These examples highlight a strong appreciation for broom, grass, straw, and raffia as a part of African ritual. Ritualistic use of natural materials allows us to see them as extraordinary, distinct from mundane life. A fear of brooms remained intact well after enslavement; respect for the broom was a remarkable characteristic of early African American life. A peek into the Yoruba orisha Obaluaiye brings greater understanding of the fear and foreboding that brooms incite.

Obaluaiye is a fierce god who has the power to either create epidemics like smallpox or heal them as he sees fit. Obaluaiye's scarlet-clad followers are feared and dreaded. It is believed that devotees of Obaluaiye can strike down people who walk around at high noon under the bright sun. Epidemic-causing diseases like smallpox are dispensed by Obaluaiye when he feels the need to raise the consciousness of society. When the fierce god is angered or appalled by society, he uses his special broom to spread *yamoti* (sesame seeds) on the earth. The seeds spread by an ever-widening concentric sweeping motion. As his broom touches the dirt, dust rises into the air. The seeds ride on the sweeping winds, hitting people hard, causing horrible pockmarks to be left in their wake. The horrific tool of Obaluaiye is a magical broom called a *shashara*.

In Benin, worship of Obaluaiye is called *Sakpata*. Sakpata worshippers are also in Cuba and Brazil. The *shashara* (brooms) of Cuba are extraordinarily beautiful. Reflecting their Dahomean style, the brooms have a special handle of blood-red cloth imbued with medicinal power and heavily embroidered with intricate cowrie shell patterns that hold significance and power. In Bahia, Brazil, the broom is called *ja,* whereas in the Dahomean language it is *ha*. The *ja* is exalted to the level of nobility. The whisk broom transcends utilitarian function, becoming instead an elaborately decorated power object approaching the beauty of finely crafted jewelry.

When Obaluaiye appears in Bahian temples, he doesn't carry a club, arrow, or spear for protection—his single weapon is his *ja* (broom). Obaluaiye's broom is paraded about with flowing movements by his followers; this weapon is at once beautiful and terrifying. The motions can suggest both the dispersal of disease-causing sesame seeds and the sweeping away of them. The Bahian *shashara* (broom) is an unusual yet potent royal scepter. The fierceness of forest energy is further enhanced by the *ade iko* (all-raffia crown) and the complementary *ewu iko* (all-raffia gown) worn by devotees, since they are filled with the dual powers of Obaluaiye and the spirits of the forest.

Nana Baku, whose followers live north of Fon in Benin, is Obaluaiye's mother. Her symbolic image sits on a baobab tree shrine, represented by a conical piece of earth, wearing the clothing of the spirits—raffia. She appears to be a large, benevolent whisk broom. The duality of the broom's uses and the gods and goddesses who imbue them with powers make it an object that can generate luck, domestic bless, purification, destruction, disease, despair, and sadly, even death.

Island Green: Bermuda Grass (*Cynodon dactylon*)

Bermuda grass is a bit of a paradox; it is an invasive, competitive weed and it is also a low-maintenance medicinal plant. Bermuda grass is from the Cynodon family, originally from Africa. There are two East African species. Now found in many warm climates, Bermuda grass was introduced to the United States from Bermuda. Like most savanna/prairie plants, it has deep taproots and grows well in poor soil.

Couch Grass, Also Called Witch Grass, Quack Grass, or Dog Grass (*Agropyron repens*)

Couch grass is a relative of Bermuda grass with the same negative qualities—it's a creeping, tenacious weed—yet it has useful medicinal qualities. This grass grows in Europe, Russia, North Africa, and North America.

Constituents: contains carbohydrates, mucilage, saponins, a variety of mineral salts, silicic acid, iron, and vitamins A and B.

Medicinal and spiritual uses: the tea is used as a blood cleanser and the high carbs help stimulate the metabolism and the elimination of waste. Couch grass is a diuretic that is used to clear the skin. Cleansing and detox qualities lend it to be used in the treatment of bronchial complaints, rheumatism, gout, and lower urinary tract or upper airway obstructions. In the past, it was used as incense to disinfect and purify the home or sacred spaces and was thought to chase away demons.

Magical Grasses

Clover (*Trifolium pratense*)

Time-honored herbalists like Jethro Kloss, author of *Back to Eden*, touted red clover blossoms as a panacea. At one time, red clover was heavily used to fight cancer. Today many of us add it in small quantities to herbal tea blends and tonics for its more traditional uses—coughs, bronchitis, skin issues, eye infections, and as an emollient—and as sweet flavor for herbal teas and desserts like clover blossom honey.

Magical and Spiritual Uses of Clover

It is always nice to find healing uses for weeds and invasive wildflowers such as clover, which you can find growing almost anywhere. Rabbits love to eat them. They are also a highly sought-after good luck charm used magically as a natural amulet—especially the less-common four-leaf clover. If you find a four-leaf clover, clip it, bring it home, press it with a warm iron between two pieces of waxed paper, and you'll have a preserved charm. You can cut this down to the parameters of the clover and put it inside a large locket or add it to a mojo bag. Four-leaf clovers are used for luck, fertility, and prosperity.

Five-finger grass (*Potentilla erecta Rosaceae*)—the Latin name says a lot: *Potentilla* means "little powerful one" and also refers to the Native Americans who developed some of potentilla's medicinal uses after it was brought over from Europe. In *Pow-Wows, Or, Long-Lost Friend: A Collection of Mysterious and Invaluable Arts and Remedies,* it is suggested that you can get anything you want when you carry five-finger grass with you.[2] Five-finger grass—also called cinquefoil, five-leaf grass, and septfoil—is an erect, hairy plant with sparse though attractive flat-topped clusters of pale-yellow flowers. *Cinquefoil* is Old French for "five leaf." Flower stalks are long and slender, lending it an upright bearing. There are usually five petals and five sepals, along with numerous stamens and pistils. The leaves are palmately compound and divided into five to seven rounded, toothed leaflets that range from one to three inches long. The lower leaves are alternate and short-stalked.

Five-finger grass is an astringent like many herbs; it is also a febrifuge and a tonic.

Part used: The rhizome, which is an underground plant stem that extends shoots and roots into the soil, is collected in the spring. Leaves may be collected anytime up until frost.

Habitat: Grows wild as a weed along roads and in fields from Ontario to Nova Scotia; south from New England to Virginia; west to Tennessee, Arkansas, and Kansas.

Medicinal uses: used to treat stubborn skin conditions such as seborrhea.

It is a bitter gargle for sore throats, sore mouths, and bleeding gums. It is used as a tea to treat irritable bowel syndrome (IBS), colitis, diarrhea, and rectal bleeding.

The external portion of the roots is decocted and the brew is used to soften corns and

---

2 Hoffman, *Pow-Wows,* 13.

calluses. A salve is made to treat hemorrhoids and wounds and to help heal burns. Five-finger grass is also used in facial treatments and baths, as a tisane added to the water.

Magical uses: five-finger grass is a greatly sought-after natural amulet used to help gain luck with all manner of things that require manual dexterity. With its petals and leaves symbolically suggesting the human hand, it fits well into the African idea that healing plants reveal themselves to the observant. Five-finger grass is used for all situations in which luck is sought, including relationships, empowerment, health, and prosperity.

Palmarosa (*Cymbopogon martinii stapf.* var. *motia*)—palmarosa essential oil is an old favorite of Hoodoos and soapmakers alike. It is a pleasant-smelling essential oil that can be used to suggest rose, though it is much less expensive. Palmarosa is a steam-distilled or water-distilled oil from the wildcrafted, fresh, or dried grass of palmarosa. While the grasses grow well in India, Nepal, and to some extent, Pakistan, they have been enjoyed around the world for a very long time. Palmarosa oil is versatile and blends well with other ingredients to scent or mask odoriferous herbal blends used for homemade cosmetics or topically.

Van Van or khuskhus—another popular name for Hoodoo blends, it refers to the inclusion of vetiver. To make matters even more confusing, you will discover a variety of spellings for *vetiver*, including *vertivert* and *vertiver*. To be certain of the authenticity of the vetiver used in recipes for khuskhus, look for the botanical name *Chrysopogon zizanioides (L.) Roberty*. It is no longer called *Vetiveria zizanioides (L.) Nash* (1903–1999) or the even older name *Andropogon muricatus Retz.* (1783–1903). Khuskhus is so named because of one of its chemical components, khusinol. Vetiver is called khus in older books. In present-day India, oil from the wild vetiver grass is used to make a perfume called ruh khus or "oil of tranquility." Vetiver has a deep, earthy, relaxing aroma; chemically, it acts as a fixative; spiritually, it strengthens and adds sensuality.

Blended Grasses
The Lively Grass Blend: Van Van

Van Van is a popular name for various Hoodoo formulas. Palmarosa, citronella, lemongrass, or ginger, and grasses of the *Cymbopogon* (*Spreng.*) genus and the *Poaceae* family are the sources of Van Van's scent and power. These aromatic grasses flourish on lands where our people have traditionally thrived. These grasses, used alone or in combination, form the herbal base of Van Van and Chinese Wash. Van Van oil is quite lemony, and original formulas contain bits of magnetic sand (magnetite) to accelerate its luck-drawing qualities. Van Van oil can be used to feed mojo bags and dress candles, for anointments, or as an additive to baths, or can be worn on the charkas. Chinese Wash is considered to be a spiritual floor wash to bring well-being and abundance to the household. It also has a lemony scent that speaks of the inclusion of lemongrass.

Sugarcane (*Saccharum officinarum L.*)

Whether we like it or not, sugarcane is a deeply embedded part of African history, particularly in the Americas and Caribbean. The grass came from Asia and was cultivated in New Guinea, Indonesia, and India. It was introduced to the West Indies by Columbus and was already being cultivated in Brazil. Sugarcane is a labor-intensive crop, requiring long, dedicated work. This sparked the desire to enslave Africans and bring them to various locations in the Caribbean—to process sugarcane. At one point, so many enslaved people were working the sugarcane fields of the Caribbean that some of the islands were simply referred to as the Sugar Islands. Often the slash-and-burn method of cultivation is used, which requires hand-cutting with machetes. This is not the most ecologically sound way of farming, but it is a tradition that was brought to the New World by African people nevertheless. My neighbor, who was born and raised in Jamaica, still uses the method of slashing weeds, trees, and undesirable plants in her yard with her machete; believe me, I stay on her good side! It always brightens her spirits if I can find her a ripe piece of sugarcane in our local shops. To be sure, we have a love/hate relationship with sugar.

In the early-nineteenth-century literature on African Caribbean cures and treatments, it is reported that "Negro" children prone to worms, starvation, or wasting diseases were treated with sugarcane, sucking directly from the grass until they regained their health and strength.[3]

Botanically, sugarcane belongs to the *Poaceae* family of grasses. It is one of the most important species of food-producing grasses and for economic botany in the world. Sugarcane is a perennial grass, and that is a rare occurrence in terms of crop grasses. It has the highest growth rate of any plant. When the flowers form, it means the stalk, which resembles green bamboo, is loaded with sugar.

---

3   Descourtilz, *Flore pittoresque et médicale des Antilles.*

In the United States, we eat far too much sugar, mostly as an additive to processed foods. Eating high quantities of sugar and sugared foods contributes to cavities and gum disease, raises insulin levels, and adds "empty" calories to the diet. It is likely that if one consumes excessive amounts of sugar they will gain weight, since it not only adds to one's caloric count but also reduces the motivation to exercise because of its tranquilizing effect.

Medicinally, sugar is very high in antibacterial, antimicrobial qualities and is used to treat wounds. While there is a buzz about sugar being the culprit of hyperactivity in children, sugar is cited by recognized nutrition writer Jean Carper as being a relaxant with a tranquilizing effect that can diminish insomnia.

Sugar and sweets play an important role to this day in our celebrations and in traditional ATR ritual. Mother healers in Jamaica each have symbols; one of those is sugarcane. Mother of the orishas, Yemaya, enjoys an offering of sugarcane. Sugar and sweetness are associated with the orisha of love and sensuality, Oshun. Sweets or plain sugar are offered to her spirit across the Caribbean and in the United States as well as Brazil, where different types of ATR are still practiced. Moreover, two of the chief sugar by-products, rum and molasses, are also intricately woven into the fabric of magical and spiritual practice.

An interesting new development with sugar and its checkered past is that in Brazil it is being used to create a renewable source of ethanol-based automobile fuel.

Acacia (*Acacia nilotica*): Medicine Tree of the Savanna

The acacia is a much-loved tree, especially by the ancient Egyptians, who linked it to divinity, birth, death, the afterlife, and immortality. Some believe gods were born underneath Goddess Saosis's acacia tree, north of Heliopolis. Horus is said to have emerged from within the acacia tree. With its association to figures held as sacred in the Egyptian/ Khemetian cosmology, it is no wonder the tree is considered healthy and magical and is linked to divinity. Today acacia trees continue to grow abundantly in Egypt.

Gum acacia consists primarily of arabin, a compound of arabic acid, with calcium and varying amounts of magnesium and potassium salts along with a trace of sugar.

Medicinal qualities and other uses: gum acacia is a demulcent that sheathes inflamed interior surfaces. Used to treat respiratory, digestive, and urinary tract ailments, it is useful in the treatment of diarrhea and dysentery. It has been known to combat low stages of typhoid fever. It is administered as mucilage (meaning it is soaked and dissolved) called *mucilago acaciae.* Artists use gum acacia as a medium, particularly with watercolors.

Dosage: 1 to 4 drams gum.

Types of acacia are:

- **Mucilage of acacia**—is nearly transparent, colorless, viscid, with a faint though pleasant taste.
- **Senegal gum**—refers to acacias gathered from the Sudan, Egypt, or Kordofan. Senegal gum possesses properties that make it superior and always preferred to other gums. *A. Senegal (Willd.)* is different and comes from Senegambia in West Africa and the Upper Nile region of Eastern Africa.
- **Acacia resin**—is added to "sacred blend" incense and lends it a high frequency.

Anchor of the Savanna: Baobab

Baobab (*Adansonia digitata*) is also called muuyu, lemonade tree, or cream of tartar tree.

The baobab tree is such a rich reservoir of mythology, folklore, and medicines that it has become emblematic of the Motherland. One story by the Khoisan people states that when all the animals were given a special tree during the creation time, hyena was given the baobab. Disgusted by the odd appearance of the baobab, the angry hyena threw the baobab tree down to earth, where it landed upside down. This explains some of its lofty position in their society, as well as offering an explanation for its strange appearance. Baobabs are frequently called upside-down tree because their branches are spindly and gnarled, suggestive of roots rather than branches. The tree is also called lemonade tree because of the beverage made from it and cream of tartar or tartar tree because it contains tartaric acid.

These fascinating trees are one of the only trees that grow on the savanna, accentuating their reputation as being bizarre, as they seem out of place in their homeland. Baobabs grow in arid, semiarid, and subhumid tropical climates.[4] Extremely long-lived, a baobab's life span is between one thousand and three thousand years. The seeds contain pulp with numerous uses. The vitamin C[5] content of the fruit averages 300 milligrams per 100 grams, nearly six times as high as an orange.[6] Baobab is also rich in vitamins B_1 and B_2, phosphorous, iron, trace minerals, and protein. It contains essential fatty acids (EFAs) and polyunsaturated fatty acids (PFAs), lending medicinal and food value. Baobab oil is useful in cooking and cosmetics. The nutritious oil has a faint aroma, making it suitable for massage and natural products. Baobab has a long shelf life, meaning it is suitable for international shipping and storage.[7] I have found it to be a comforting, useful oil for skin treatments; to deter the appearance of wrinkles; and to condition the nails and soften the heels, elbows, and hands.

4   International Centre for Underutilized Crops, "Baobab Fact Sheet," 2003; see also https://www.namibian
-naturals.de/media/factsheets/fact_sheet_Baobab.pdf.
5   Vitamin C is an antioxidant that helps renew cell growth.
6   PhytoTrade Africa, 2003.
7   International Centre for Underutilized Crops, "Baobab Fact Sheet."

CHAPTER 7

Where There Is a Will, There Is a Way

PLANT LIFE ON ARID LAND

PLANTS IN FOCUS

- Aloe vera
- Frankincense
- Myrrh
- Balanites
- Tamarind

- Dom palm
- Moringa
- Jatropha / physic nut
- Henna

I LOVE IT WHEN THE character Dr. Malcolm in the movie *Jurassic Park* says with foreboding, "Life will find a way," when considering the proliferation of offspring from supposedly sterilized dinosaurs at the fictional theme park. Dinosaurs aside, the sentiment certainly holds true for people and plants. They do indeed find a way to survive tough situations, variable conditions, and change. The insertion of chaos theory through Malcolm's character is also interesting—the assertion that making a ripple across the oceans will slowly but surely be felt by the entire ecosystem.

The Caribbean is a good example. The people, landscape, and plants are beautiful, maybe because of or perhaps despite their rugged history. Whenever you see advertisements for travel to "the islands," there is always the promise that the "natives" are friendly, happy people. I could not help but wonder what is held beneath the picture-postcard palms, sandy beaches, and smiling faces.

Barbados has a fascinating history to follow when you are considering survival. Sure enough, behind the sunny picture is a brutal history for both the land and the people.

- Around 1623 BCE a group of indigenous people from Venezuela arrived on the island and settled it. They became known as the Arawaks. The Arawaks are recorded as being a small-stature people with tan skin. They bound the heads of their children so they would grow pointed. They painted themselves with charcoal and chalk so that they appeared black and white—clearly a creative people. The Arawaks grew cotton, cassava, corn, peanuts, guava, and pawpaws, also called papaya. The cotton was woven into various small textiles. The cassava was ground and grated to make serviceable flour.
- Circa 1200 CE, a stronger, more warrior-like people called the Caribs (hence the name Caribbean) conquered the Arawaks. They were allegedly cannibals.
- Around 1492, the Spanish colonists arrived. They enslaved the Caribs and eventually wiped the entire race out through a combination of brutality and the smallpox and tuberculosis they introduced.
- British colonists arrived between 1625 and 1644. When the colonists felled most of the trees, the island became arid. They aimed to wipe the space clean of the natural forests to make way for tobacco and cotton fields.
- The British colonists took a shine to the idea of having other people raise and process sugar crops for them, so they enticed lower-class white people from Europe to come work on the island as indentured servants. They also began a massive scheme to bring thousands of Africans to work as slaves.
- Between 1644 and 1700, sugar and other plantations flourished; in fact, the island came to be known as Sugar Island because of the superior product grown and processed on Barbados.
- From 1700 to the 1830s, Mother Nature interceded. There were a series of natural

disasters—hurricanes, drought followed by massive rains—and some of the island approached desertification.

- Slavery was abolished in 1834.

Today Barbados is known as a spectacular island where pleasant people called Bajans live and extend open arms to visitors. There is a spirited annual festival that lasts an entire month. The Crop Over festival began in the 1800s at the end of sugar growing/processing season. Beginning in July and ending the first Monday in August with a closing ceremony, the festival remembers African culture and celebrates the harvest with song, dance, showy costumes, and a parade. The terrain holds the history in its rugged and craggy landscape.

Before we move along, a bit of island hopping is in order. It is worthwhile to visit the not-so-typical island of Aruba. I say not typical because the island is not what you would think of as a "tropical island"; parts of it resemble a desert and it is filled with dozens of species of cacti. Not to get tedious, suffice it to say this island also became a sugar island with its attendant disregard for native people, local flora, and the underclass. Under British colonists, thousands of Africans were stolen from Sierra Leone, Guinea, Ghana, Côte d'Ivoire, Nigeria, and Cameroon and were forced to work the crops. Aruba was in the throes of sugar and slavery from 1644 to 1807.

Aloe was brought to the island of Aruba between 1840 and 1850, and ever since then it has been grown there on a large scale. Aruba has an ideal climate to support aloe. This member of the Kingdom of the Netherlands has an average rainfall of less than twenty inches per year, and the temperature remains rather stable in the low to middle 80s year-round. Soon enough, thousands of acres of aloe were grown and many Aruban families lived from the harvest, export, trade, and raw materials, which are used primarily as laxatives. Aruba aloes were deemed to be of very high quality; at the beginning of the century they were the largest exporter of aloe in the world. The island went from a sugar island to the Island of Aloe. Today, tourism is a much bigger industry, but the jaunty aloe plant remains in the Aruban coat of arms. The official name of the laxative derived from aloe is curacao, after the harbor from which Aruba aloes were shipped.

We ended the last chapter speaking of grasses and other plants that thrive in less than perfect conditions. We continue to explore that theme, now traveling to even harsher conditions of arid and semiarid lands. This chapter begins with the story of aloe because it affords the opportunity to understand will, survival, and healing; it ends with a personal story of how henna helped lift my spirits from an incredible depth.

Aloe (Aloe vera L.), Modern Egyptian Arabic

Aloe is a succulent plant with clusters of long, bayonet-like leaves, prickly at the edges and tips. It can produce a woody stem up to fifteen meters tall. It has spikes of flowers of various colors including yellow, orange, and red.

The aloe plant has a lengthy history in Africa and the Middle East. Prospero Alpini reported that Egyptian women perfumed their genitals with aloe. Aloe was used in remedies to treat fever and plague. The plants are reported as growing in Somalia in the times of Alexander's conquests. In the Holy Bible, aloe is referred to as ahaloth and is recorded as a perfumery herb. The Copts used aloe with other ingredients to treat eye disease, swelling, and other disorders.[1]

In our recent history, people felt they could gain health benefits from orally consuming aloe juice and sometimes even the gel. Aloe does contain volatile oils and aloins that are very purgative. Because of its purgative quality, it is definitely contraindicated for pregnancy and hemorrhoids. Consumption of aloe in large quantities could prove very painful. As it stands, there is no thorough scientific test evidence to indicate health benefits from internal treatments with aloe but the people speak up for it, particularly those from the Caribbean. It is widely available at grocery shops and online.

Uses: the Jamaican people have a great adoration for aloe, which they call sinkle bible. In Jamaica it is used to cut the sweetness in the blood. It is also used to purify the blood in the following ways:

- For its constituents actions:
  - Glucomannan, an antidiabetic
  - Rhein, an antiviral and antibacterial

---

1   Lise Manniche, *An Ancient Egyptian Herbal* (Austin: Univ. of Texas Press, 1989), 72.

- Emodin, an antiviral and viricide
- Aloin, a viricide
- For tuberculosis:
  - Barbaloin, an antitubular
- For cleansing, called "washout":
  - Lignin, a laxative
  - Barbaloin, a laxative and purgative
  - Rhein, a purgative
- For the nervous system, "nerves":
  - Coumarin, a sedative[2]

Today, aloe is mostly used in skin care, and it makes an excellent hair gel, especially for locs (also called dreadlocks). Aloe gel can be easily accessed with this method:

- Thank the aloe for sharing her medicine with you.
- Cut off just enough of the leaf as is needed.
- Slit it open using your penknife or sharp kitchen knife.
- Scrap the gel into a plastic bag, plate, or container.
- Apply to the area to be treated.
- Thank and nurture your plant so she will continue to grow and share her medicine.

Aloe is widely available in health food stores and even in mainstream shops and pharmacies. I recommend purchasing the product pure and organic if possible rather than an adulterated product whose benefits are questionable.

Frankincense and Myrrh

Both of these resins are mildly sedative and uplifting. They are natural resins sacred to the Khemetians. The rich scent of the natural form is related to Anubis, Osiris, and Ra. When the resins are used as essential oil, they take on the feminine form, suggestive of Isis. Since

---

2   Payne-Jackson and Alleyne, *Jamaican Folk Medicine*, 165–68.

Isis's attributes center around her protective abilities, she is thanked for security and abundance. Frankincense and myrrh are important for observing holy days and creating sacred space and are used as a sacred invitation to Ra, Isis, Osiris, and Anubis. The two are ground with a mortar and pestle to create incense. There should be two parts frankincense, which is light and airy, to one part myrrh, which is the deep base note. This combination helps you create a highly charged bright spiritual vibration. Here is a breakdown of each resin:

Frankincense (*Boswellia sacra, B. carterii*)

Frank means "free," and *incense* means "lightning." The Arabic word for frankincense, *luban*, means "milk of the Arabs." Information about the earliest-known use was inscribed on the tomb of Queen Hatshepsut in the fifteenth century BCE.[3] Somalia's commercial history began with incense, and Northern Somalia gained significance through its incense trade. Beyo, also referred to as olibanum, is the classical frankincense distilled into essential oil. Beyo is used locally as a fire starter, to deter snakes and scorpions, for purification, to perfume hair and clothing, and in incense, holy ointments, and even a cola soft drink. Beyo is still imported primarily from Somalia (ancient Punt) in East Africa.[4] It also grows around the Horn of Africa and the Hadhramaut region of Yemen and Oman.[5]

Maydi is the top-grade medicinal frankincense. Used as a chewing product in Saudi Arabia, maydi comes in seven grades. The highest two are preferred: mushaad and mujaarwal, numbers one and two respectively, are close to transparent and are sold as quite large, unbroken pieces. The maydi that survives shipment abroad is usually the smaller, opaque, lower-grade types.

Swahili speakers use frankincense as a diuretic. The bark of the resin is used as a tonic in East Africa.[6] Frankincense is enjoyed in the African diaspora, particularly in the USA, as incense and anointment oil. British herbalist Anne McIntyre suggests frankincense to heal many conditions, including respiratory infections, catarrh, laryngitis, asthma, fevers, scars, sores, and wounds.[7]

---

3   Celestial Tides, 2003; the original www.scents-of-earth.com.
4   James A. Duke, *Herbs of the Bible: 2,000 Years of Plant Medicine* (Atlanta, GA: Whitman, 2007).
5   Celestial Tides, 2003; the original www.scents-of-earth.com.
6   Duke, *Herbs of the Bible.*
7   Anne McIntyre, *The Complete Woman's Herbal: A Manual of Healing Herbs and Nutrition for Personal Well-Being and Family Care,* 1st edition (New York, NY: Holt McDougal/Holt Paperbacks,1995).

Myrrh (*Commiphora myrrha*)

There are 135 species of myrrh growing in Africa and the Middle East. Just as with frank-incense, the highest grades still come from Somalia. Heliopolis myrrh was burned at noon as incense to invoke and praise the ancient Egyptian sun god, Ra. Myrrh is also burned to honor the Egyptian moon goddess, Isis.[8]

Practitioners of many paths and religions use myrrh spiritually. Anne McIntyre recommends it medicinally in her *Woman's Herbal*, citing it as a stimulant, carminative, vulnerary, expectorant, antiseptic, antiviral, and detoxifier that is useful for bronchitis, asthma, colds, indigestion, and inflammation.[9] It is an excellent dentifrice; a mouthwash is made from it to help topical ulcers, gingivitis, periodontal disease, and toothache. The versatile resin is added to lotions, potpourri, perfumery, soap, baths, and food (approved by the FDA) as a preservative of scents. Ghanaians fumigate clothing with the fragrant smoke of burning myrrh wood.

Balanites—Balanites Oil (*Balanites aegyptiaca*)

Called *heglig* in modern Egyptian Arabic, balanites are heavily thorned trees, a protection from attacks. They are found in most arid and semiarid to subhumid tropical savannas, in hot dry areas, along waterways, and in forests.[10] The tree is native to the Sudano-Sahelian zone, Israeli, Palestine, and Jordan.[11] Balanites trees are flexible but they cannot tolerate prolonged flooding.[12] Thirty to forty percent of the balanites seed is oil. The plant is useful as a soap substitute since it has a high saponin content. Locally, balanites is useful in treating sore throat, colic, mental diseases, epilepsy, and toothache and it serves as a laxative.[13] Balanites may be useful to those with overprocessed hair. Analgesic qualities lend balanites oil the ability to reduce the sensation of pain, making the oil useful when warmed in massage. An astringent oil, balanites should be combined with other emollient ingredients like avocado, jojoba, or castor oil when used on dry skin or hair.

8   Judika Illes, *Earth Mother Magic* (New York: HarperCollins Publishers, 2001), 38.
9   McIntyre, *The Complete Woman's Herbal*, 1995.
10   McIntyre, *The Complete Woman's Herbal*, 1955.
11   EROS Data Center, 2003; https://www.usgs.gov/centers/eros.
12   EROS Data Center, 2003; https://www.usgs.gov/centers/eros.
13   EROS Data Center, 2003; https://www.usgs.gov/centers/eros.

Moringa Oil (*Moringa stenopetala,*
M. oleifera, M. pterygosperma, M. aptera)

The moringa is also called the drumstick tree, and in modern Egyptian Arabic, it is *ban* or *jasar.*

Moringa oil comes from Egypt, the Sudan, and the Arabian Peninsula. *M. pterygosperma* is indigenous to Egypt and still grows there. It is favored for cosmetics and cooking.[14] Moringa has a long history recorded in Egyptian medical papyri as a woman's pregnant belly rub called *ben.* The pharaohs also used it medicinally, for example a treatment for gum disease included moringa, gum acacia, figs, water, ochre, and four ancient plants.[15] Moringa contains 73 percent oleic acid and other nutrients. Today, Moringa continues to be used medicinally in skin care, cosmetically in perfume and soap, and as lamp fuel. This oil also makes a delightful vehicle for essential oils.

Parts used: roots, seeds, and leaves.

- **Roots**—acrid, digestive, anthelmintic, constipating, anodyne, bitter, alexipharmic, stimulating, and vesicant. Moringa is useful in inflammation, fever, cough, cold, bronchitis, pectoral diseases, epilepsy, and hysteria.
- **Seeds**—an acrid bitter used as an anti-inflammatory and a purgative, useful in neuralgia, inflammation, and intermittent fevers.
- **Leaves**—used to treat scurvy and vitiated conditions.

Jatropha (*Jatropha curcas* L.),
Family Euphorbiaceae

Jatropha was introduced to Africa and does very well there. It grows on Cape Verde Islands and has been naturalized in the West Indies and South America; it also grows in Jamaica and Brazil. It is well suited to arid and semiarid conditions. Most Jatropha thrive in areas that have seasons of dry weather such as the grassland and savanna previously discussed, as well as thorny forests. It is a tenacious, drought-resistant perennial, growing quickly and well

---

14 Manniche, *Ancient Egyptian Herbal,* 122–23.
15 Manniche, *Ancient Egyptian Herbal,* 122–23.

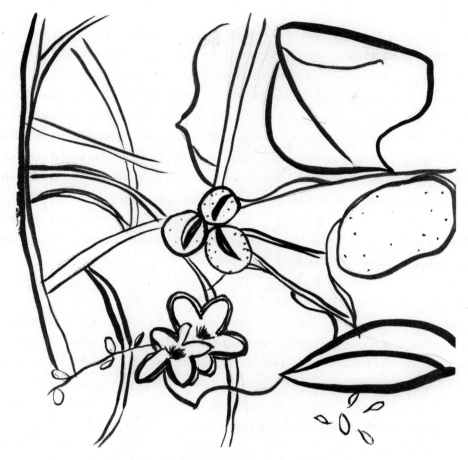

Jatropha (also called policeman's nut, Barbados nut, and physic nut)

in poor soil and producing seeds for fifty years. Jatropha is considered a small tree that can grow from eight to fifteen feet. It has large simple soft green leaves with three to five lobes and spiral phyllotaxis. The oil is rich in glycerin, making it useful in various hair, scalp, and skin treatments. In 1999, the Alternative Resources Income (ARI) project successfully mobilized women to produce handmade soaps from Jatropha oil to fight skin ailments such as eczema, acne, rashes, psoriasis, and fungus.[16] In Surinamese traditional medicine the leaves are used as a treatment for bellyache in children; the boiled leaves are used as a dentifrice for gingivitis

---

16 *Arusha Times*, September 9, 2002; Global Facilitation Unit for Underutilized Species, (*Jatropha curcas L.*), in Africa. http://apirs.plants.ifas.ufl.edu.

and throat ailments. Leaves are also used to treat urinary blockages, constipation, and backache as well as other areas that become inflamed. Rubefacient properties are contained within the leaves, making them suitable for poultice, salve, balm, or soak treatments for rheumatism, eruptions like boils, and piles. The seeds are emetic, causing drastic cathartic effects accompanied by burning feces, as well as stomach and other serious symptoms. Their use should be avoided. Jatropha contains constituents capable of attacking infections of the scalp that normally deter hair growth. It is considered an invasive weed but obviously it is useful for multiple purposes. Seeds are 50 percent oil. This oil is being used for an eco-friendly fuel that burns smoke-free, powers simple diesel engines, and does not need to be refined.

Tamarind (*Tamarindus indica*), Caesalpiniaceae Family

Tamarind is a flexible tree. It grows in semiarid or monsoon climates. The trees produce up to fifty kilograms of fruit in West Africa, where rainfall totals less than five hundred millimeters annually. It manages through six-to-eight-month-long droughts that are common where it has established itself. The tamarind actually produces more fruit when there is less rainfall. It is, however, not tolerant of lengthy cold temperatures or even a brief frost.

Tamarind originated in the East African country of Madagascar. Arab people spread the seeds, establishing it elsewhere. Tamarind fruit makes a wonderful bittersweet sauce for curries, syrups, and processed foods. The pulp is also added to chutneys, preserves, pickles, sherbets, and beverages. Most people come across it frequently, whether they realize it or not, as tamarind is an important ingredient in steak sauce and Worcestershire sauce.

The pharmaceutical industry in the United States processes one hundred tons of tamarind pulp annually. The fruit is used to reduce fever and cure intestinal ailments and it is well documented against scurvy. It is a common ingredient in cardiac and blood-sugar-reducing medicines.[17] The pulp is being used more frequently in commercial botanically based skin care products. The wood is hard and dense and burns well as charcoal. Tamarind wood also takes a brilliant polish and is used for furniture.[18]

---

17 Von Maydell, 1986.
18 O. N. Allen and E. K. Allen, *The Leguminosae: A Source Book of Characteristics, Uses, and Nodulation* (Madison: Univ. of Wisconsin Press, 1981).

Dom palm (Hyphaene thebaica L.)

The dom palm has a characteristic bifurcate trunk and grows in Upper Egypt. The fruits are about the size of an orange and have little pulp. A sweet juice is contained inside. Dom palm is used in basketmaking and woodworking as it is capable of achieving a high shine. White nuts are used as a vegetable ivory substitute to make jewelry and buttons.

Dom palm was well appreciated by the ancient Egyptians as well. Egyptian tombs from prehistoric times contain art or artifacts of the palm. Ramesses III offered 449 and 500 measures of dom fruit to Amun-Re at Thebes.

Bread of dom fruit is used by the Saharan people to cure stomach complaints and treat fevers.[19]

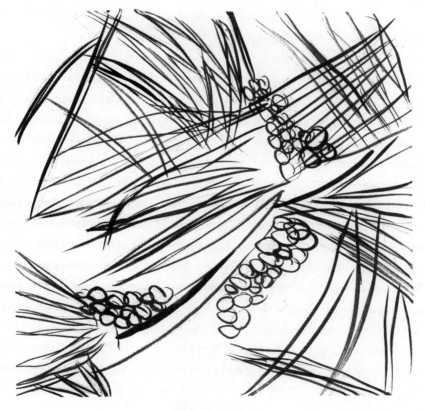

Egyptian dom palm

19 Manniche, *Ancient Egyptian Herbal*, 108–9.

Cool Medicine for the Beauty Way

While many people know henna as a gorgeous hair colorant of varying tones, the cosmetic use of the plant barely scratches the surface of the plant's dynamic story. Once we begin to explore henna from the perspective of the people who have been growing and using it for thousands of years, we find that it is truly a miraculous plant. Henna possesses a complex array of healing possibilities. More than simply a beautiful dye for the hair, henna is symbolic of blood, the essence of life itself. I hope you will find the ways it is most meaningful for you to use as you walk the way of inner and outer beauty.

History of Henna

Henna is an herbaceous shrub called *Lawsonia inermis* in botanical Latin, named after the British explorer John Lawson in the early 1700s. The plant thrives in the hot dry climates that are the focus of this chapter. The use of the herb for health and beauty is far older than the British discovery; it is carbon-dated back to 3500 BCE and has had a continuing presence in human civilization recorded in the arts for seven thousand years.

Henna is a Persian word for the plant that has many names. In Arabic it is called *khanna*. In India, henna is called by many names depending on the dialect—*menhadi, mehendi, mehedi, mendi, hina*—and in Sanskrit it is *mendika*. Ancient hieroglyphs in tombs in the Valley of the Nile refer to it using the Egyptian name, *pouquer. Pouquer* refers to the dye created from the plant used to color the fingernails of mummies. A lovely perfume created from the henna plant is referred to as *camphire* in the Koran. Since the Hindus of India call it *mehndi*, a name synonymous internationally with the henna plant used for temporary tattoos, I will use it here alternately with *henna*.

The reddened hands created by henna applied in patterns are preserved in the early civilization of Catal Huyuk from around 7000 BCE. The Ugaritics, Canaanites, Cycladics, Minoans, Mycenaeans, and Egyptians all created other early artifacts showing henna patterns.

In early India, henna was applied by dipping palms and soles into a thick paste of crushed fresh leaves, creating a solid red stain without pattern. Middle Eastern henna was done by mixing dried powdered leaves into a paste and applying it with a stick. Henna is still in use in parts of Asia, especially India, as well as in the Middle East and North African countries, where it flourishes; it is also catching on in Australia, North America, and Europe.

Table 1: A Rough Timeline of Henna Use*

Catal Huyuk	7000 BCE
Turkey	5000 BCE
Syria	3000 BCE
Cycladic Islands	3000 BCE
Israel/Palestine, Jordan, Lebanon	2100 BCE
Crete, Cypress, Greece, Libya, Nubia	1700 BCE
Iraq, Iran	1300 BCE
Tunisia, Kuwait, Morocco, Algeria, Mali, Sudan, Yemen	1200 BCE
Jewish culture	1000 BCE
Muslim culture	550 BCE
Pakistan, India	400 BCE
Christian (Coptic, Armenian)	1–100 CE
Asia (Sri Lanka, Turkmenistan, Uzbekistan, China, Tibet, Myanmar, Thailand)	700–800 CE
Ethiopia, Nigeria	800 CE
Indonesia	1200 CE
South Africa	1800 CE

---

*   Research according to henna historian Catherine Cartwright-Jones.

Uses of Henna: Cool Medicine for Health and Beauty

To move beyond the concept that henna is solely a cosmetic for the hair and skin, we can explore its health benefits. Here are some of the medicinal uses of henna:

- It is antipyretic (a natural coolant), hence its popularity in hot climates.
- Henna is antispasmodic (soothing), antiseptic, astringent (drying), antibacterial, and antifungal.
- It contains natural sun-screening chemicals and is effective for soothing sunburn when applied topically as a paste.
- Henna is a natural deodorant and antiperspirant, especially for the feet.
- Dyeing the sole of the feet is called a step-in design. This insulates the foot from hot desert sands, making the alluring adornment a painted substitute for sandals.
- In Ayurvedic medicine henna tea is a beverage used to treat headaches and soothe fevers and stomach pains.
- A paste is applied to the skin for soothing dermatitis (skin ailments).[20]
- Folk remedies from around the world feature henna as a curative for rheumatism, nervousness, and certain types of tumors, cancer, and sexually transmitted diseases—and even for leprosy.[21]
- In aromatherapy, the scent of the fragrant henna flower is used to make *hina* perfume. Gul hina or hina perfume is purchased in small bottles (drams) of thick oil from health food stores and specialty Asian suppliers. The oil can be applied neat (straight) by dabbing it onto the pulse points, temples, or crown of the head. The oil-based perfume called hina mehndi attar or gulhina has a spicy, floral, musky scent. Gulhina and hina are calming and balancing scents used by both men and women.
- While henna can be applied anywhere and even taken internally (if prepared by an Ayurvedic practitioner or herbalist), it is best known and most widely used as an application to the hair, hands, and feet.

---

20 Duke, *Herbs of the Bible,* 144–48.
21 Duke, *Herbs of the Bible.*

Henna Tattoos
in Africa

While some folks do not associate henna tattoos with Africa, it has a lengthy history on the continent, as table 1 demonstrates. It is believed that the seafaring Canaanites spread the tradition of using henna across the Mediterranean to North Africa between 1700 and 600 BCE. Nefertiti was a famous redhead whose name translates to "the beautiful one comes." It is thought that her hair was made red with henna. Cleopatra used henna and rosewater to create an alluring dip for the sails of her boat when she was approaching Mark Antony; henna/rose scent paved her path.

The Imazighen/Amazigh and Tuareg people have a distinctive way of ornamenting with henna that incorporates pre-Islamic mythology, folklore, and symbols. The Imazighen/Amazigh and Tuareg formulate a deep, almost black color of henna paste, which is then applied in large, bold geometric patterns.

Henna was incorporated into the customs of Muslim peoples in the sixth century BCE. Henna traditions were long established in Arabia and it was used by Muhammad's wives to color his beard. The henna flower is considered the favorite of Muhammad. Muslims use the henna plant in various ways. Some of the most complex and elegant henna designs ever created were done between 900 and 1700 CE in the Islamic countries of Africa and the Middle East.

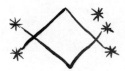

DIRECTIONS FOR HENNA USE[22]

In the Middle East and Northern Africa, particularly Morocco, henna is incorporated into everyday life. Typically, a tattoo specialist is consulted to carry out a design. If you would like to try it on yourself, follow these instructions.

- Bring a cup of water to a boil. Add 2 rose hip (or hibiscus) tea bags and 1 black tea bag. Cover and steep overnight.

- Pour approximately 1 cup of green henna powder into a nonreactive (stainless-steel or Pyrex) bowl.

- Add the tea to the powder.

- Stir to form a thick paste. (Add liquid slowly so that the mix doesn't become watery.)

- Add a few drops of eucalyptus essential oil or oil of clove to enhance the staining power of henna; this is called a mordant. (Use sparingly as these oils are skin irritants; avoid them altogether if you have allergies.) Let the mixture sit for one hour so the color can mature.

- While maturing the henna batch, create a lemon sugar glaze: Squeeze and strain the juice of a ripe lemon. Add 3 tablespoons white sugar. Stir and set aside.

- Dip fingers or soles of the feet, or create a pattern (see following pages). When the henna begins to dry, apply the lemon sugar with a cotton swab. Reapply lemon sugar every twenty minutes until a protective glaze forms.

- You can also use a porcupine quill (easily purchased from a beading supply shop or craft store) or bamboo skewer to draw more intricate designs. Most henna artisans prefer pastry-decorating tubes with very narrow tips to spread henna.

- When the glaze forms on the hennaed design, gently wrap the area in gauze or toilet paper to protect the designs.

- Be sure to keep the area warm. Hold it near a lit fireplace or over a candle flame (far enough away so that you do not burn yourself) or drink hot tea.

- Keep henna on your hands or feet as long as possible—at the minimum, four hours; overnight is preferred. Your dreams will be informative.

- Flake off henna.

- Massage with sesame or olive oil.

---

22 Powdered henna leaves can be easily purchased in pure form from reliable herbal shops or health food stores or suppliers.

Hennaed Feet

Another simple form of *mehndi* is to henna the feet. Henna can be applied individually to the toes, to the tops or bottoms of the feet, or as a simple step-in design, similar to the fingertip dip. Just as it sounds, with the step-in design, you simply step into a bowl or plate of henna, smooth it out, and follow the directions on page 134.

Patterns

Once the henna bug takes hold, you will find that you are quickly ready to move from dots and dips to exquisite patterns. Begin with a simple pattern like diamonds, patterned dots, or stars. Explore traditional patterns from the powerful centers of the *negasset*, Fez, Marrakech, and Casablanca in Morocco. In these cities, intricate lacelike patterns abound, similar to the Islamic architecture that flourishes there.

The patterns are generally abstract and geometric since the Islamic faith that inspired them forbids the use of realistic imagery. Abstract, stylized patterns are commonly shaped into symbols. One of the most important is *elain*. *Elain* is a defensive eye shape that appears in ritual and crafts, including *mehndi*. Triangles, diamonds, circles, dots, lozenges, and crosses are also popular. Other Moroccan symbols include magic numbers, magic squares, verses of the Koran, Arabic script, geometric figures (such as triangles, squares, crosses, eight-point stars), spirals, circles, diamonds, floral and vegetable shapes, and abstract human hands and eyes.

Images of fierce animals are utilized for protective, defensive magic. These include the snake, a prominent image whose symbolism was discussed in the previous chapter. The snake appears realistic or abstract. It is a symbol of male sexuality, virility, and fertility. The dangerous scorpion is used in imagery in Morocco as a protective symbol. Fish are associated with rain, which assures good crops, sustenance, and fertility. Turtles are associated with the highest character, for example saints and protective energy, as well as fertility. Birds are considered messengers in the Koran, emblems of heaven and earth. The eagle is a symbol of power. Lizards and salamanders soak up the sun and thus are symbols of the individual's search for spiritual enlightenment.

Henna Medicine for the Mind, Body, and Spirit

One of the most revered qualities of henna is its ability to cool. It is a good idea to reflect on the cooling qualities of henna herb:

- Henna is a cooling plant that aids with numerous medical disorders.
- The soothing patterns of *mehndi* tattoos are considered to be a calming influence that uplifts depression.
- *Mehndi* requires patience; cultivating patience quells anxiety and alleviates stress.
- Henna invites communal activity, as it is difficult to accomplish alone.

Personal Reflections on Mehndi: Walking the Beauty Way

Hands help us express our being; they help us shape and define our way of being in this world and beyond. We use our hands in greeting, farewell, to identify things (pointing), in invocation and worship (hands pressed together or outstretched), and as a sign of goodwill (the peace sign); in weddings and handfastings, hands come together sensuously. Raising our hand in the air is our way of saying, "I am here; I exist."

When my mother died, I reflected on her hands, placed neatly on her belly, in the coffin. I had always looked at Ma's hands. When I sat on her lap as a toddler and she stroked my head, I looked to her tender hands; when she and I made meatballs together, I marveled at her crafty hands; when they were polished, I noticed the beauty in the shape of her oval fingernails; and when she smoothed her skirt, I saw the finesse in the movement of her fingers.

My head is full of images of both my parents' hands.

When my father lay in the intensive care unit (ICU) on life supports, his eyes were clamped shut as he was in a medically induced coma. Deprived of his hazel eyes, the routes to his soul, I was left to reflect on his hands. He had strong hands, the hands of a carver, sculptor, fisherman, and laborer. Sadly, these hands that I had come to identify with Dad were swollen almost beyond recognition. Still, each day I would massage his hands with cooling essential oils in hopes that somehow I was calming his spirit, and connecting to our past together as father and daughter, through the touching of our hands.

This was one of the darkest times of my life. I could not shake the feeling of coldness. When I was ready for warmth, I huddled near my hearth, finding things to cook just so I could be near it. I looked above it to the calendar. It said March, a cold month where I live. On this "Women of the African Ark" calendar,[23] a mother and daughter huddled together wearing the black *buibui* that is the dress of orthodox Islamic faith in Kenya. Below the days of the month was a small inset of hands being treated to black henna in Lamu, Kenya; I was intrigued.

My heart began to swell with hope; perhaps the healing traditions of my sisters in Kenya could help me pass through this dark passage—help, once again, was in the palm of my hand through the grace of my friends from nature. I began to focus on the art created from henna, which I had heard people call *mehndi*. I did some research and found the best *mehndi* artist, typically called a *negasseh*, available in my area to have my palms, hands, and wrists tattooed in memory of my parents.

I reached to *mehndi* because it honors the beauty of our hands. *Mehndi* would allow further reflection on how my parents' hands shaped my life. Full recognition of ancestry reminds us that we are but mere vessels, pots shaped neatly by the DNA of our ancestors. My hands are a living testament to the lives of my parents and their parents before them who have now passed on the wings of birds to the great beyond.

Our hands are sensual instruments, leading us forward in this journey toward the divine. We want our experiences to transcend the present; we want to see the past and divine the future. In short, we have an endless quest to grasp spirit. Hands are a type of conduit that leads to and from the soul. The hands are also our tools for touching one another, thus they have the potential to heal, acknowledge, and protect and to express love.

Our palms hold magical potentiality. Interesting enough, of all the parts of the body, the palm takes henna the best, staining the deepest color. As a very flat surface, palms are loaded with design possibilities. Traditionally, palms are decorated with mandalas or paisley or spiral shapes. Palms are ideal surfaces because of their even temperature, their thickness, lightness of color, the fact that they are hairless, and because of the dazzling effects that can be produced as a combination of these factors. The wrists are also promising

---

23 *Women of the African Ark: Photographs by Carol Beckwith and Angela Fisher* (Pomegranate Press) contains images of a Swahili mother and child with henna hands and a Tuareg woman in Niger with a henna-patterned face.

palettes. An important joint and home to important veins, wrists are typically decorated with vines as symbols of growth and renewal.

The *negasseh* I was fortunate enough to find covered my palms, wrists, and fingers, as well as the backs of my hands, with an intricate, lacy pattern, Moroccan style. He chose specific designs to brighten my dimmed spirit. I'm happy to say he accomplished this task using the shrub we call henna. Soon after painting up my palms, hands, and wrists with elaborate patterns in *mehndi*, I was back dancing with my sisters, doing American Tribal Style (ATS) belly dance.[24] Belly dancing is a joyful way to express with the hands what henna can do for the soul. You have probably already seen many dancers with hennaed hands and feet.

Henna can imbue your life with health and happiness, fill your heart and home with joy, and most definitely lift the spirits. Life is short. Henna forces us to slow down. Take some time with family or friends while enjoying the supreme desert healing medicine called henna.

---

24 For more on henna and ATS, see K. Djoumahna, *The Tribal Bible: Exploring the Phenomenon That Is American Tribal Style Bellydance* (Black Sheep BellyDance, 2003), 6, 139–46, 221, and 226.

CHAPTER 8

The Healer's Heart

MATTERS OF HEART AND BLOOD

NATURAL MEDICINES IN FOCUS

- Beets
- Rose hips
- Rooibos
- Rose madder
- Camwood
- Nettle
- Raspberry
- Black cohosh
- Motherwort
- Garlic
- Bloodwort
- Hawthorn
- Yarrow
- Adam and Eve root

- Dragon's blood
- Mandrake root
- Hyssop
- Life everlasting
- Licorice root
- Rosemary
- Astragalus
- Lavender
- Calendula
- Shea butter
- Red roses
- Red wine
- Chocolate

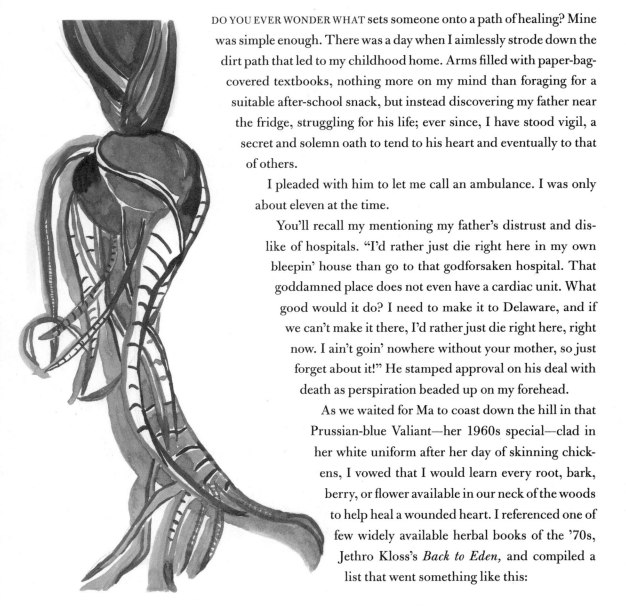

DO YOU EVER WONDER WHAT sets someone onto a path of healing? Mine was simple enough. There was a day when I aimlessly strode down the dirt path that led to my childhood home. Arms filled with paper-bag-covered textbooks, nothing more on my mind than foraging for a suitable after-school snack, but instead discovering my father near the fridge, struggling for his life; ever since, I have stood vigil, a secret and solemn oath to tend to his heart and eventually to that of others.

I pleaded with him to let me call an ambulance. I was only about eleven at the time.

You'll recall my mentioning my father's distrust and dislike of hospitals. "I'd rather just die right here in my own bleepin' house than go to that godforsaken hospital. That goddamned place does not even have a cardiac unit. What good would it do? I need to make it to Delaware, and if we can't make it there, I'd rather just die right here, right now. I ain't goin' nowhere without your mother, so just forget about it!" He stamped approval on his deal with death as perspiration beaded up on my forehead.

As we waited for Ma to coast down the hill in that Prussian-blue Valiant—her 1960s special—clad in her white uniform after her day of skinning chickens, I vowed that I would learn every root, bark, berry, or flower available in our neck of the woods to help heal a wounded heart. I referenced one of few widely available herbal books of the '70s, Jethro Kloss's *Back to Eden,* and compiled a list that went something like this:

Mandrake root, garlic amulet, and Adam and Eve root charms

- Angelica
- Arnica
- Balm
- Barberry
- Bear's foot
- Bear's garlic
- Bennet
- Betony
- Bistort
- Black hellebore
- Bloodroot
- Blue cohosh
- Blue vervain
- Borage
- Buttercup
- Calendula
- Cayenne
- Cowslip
- Cucumber
- European mistletoe
- Foxglove
- Fragrant valerian
- Garden violet
- Garlic
- Green hellebore
- Hawthorn
- Horse chestnut
- Kolar tree
- Lady's mantle
- Lily of the valley
- Mexican tea
- Milfoil
- Mistletoe
- Motherwort
- Mugwort
- Oat
- Onion
- Pasqueflower
- Primrose
- Rosemary
- Rue
- Saint-John's-wort
- Shepherd's purse
- Silverweed
- Strawberry bush
- Virginia snakeroot
- Wahoo
- Wormseed

The idea of a wide array of herbs that could be wildcrafted or cultivated was comforting. It was what I now call my first Spiritual Heart Healer's medicine kit. This was the beginning of my passion for tending to the heart—there was no choice, apparently; it was in my blood. As a child I listened with wide-eyed wonder to stories of the healers that came before me, my maternal grandmother, in particular, who used old-time Southern remedies combined with spirituality. My paternal grandmother had the seer's gift and dreamer's way. Her mother, my great-grandmother, was also well versed with spirit; she could speak in tongues. I heard it for myself.

I am not alone on this path—blessed be. In fact, a huge portion of healing treatments and concerns in African healing is dedicated to matters of the heart. Treatments for the heart in a spiritual, mental, or physical way, as well as an array of equally idiosyncratic blood treatments, are perhaps the most distinctive elements of African healing found throughout the diaspora. This can be the love magic practiced by Hoodoos—drawing love and keepin' it close. Love or drawing magic is an eclectic group of practices that combines herbs, minerals, incantation, and sometimes prayer. It is also an evident preoccupation within the work of the mother healers of Jamaica, whose very name shows their work is imbued with love; they are healers with heart and they employ spirit heavily to accomplish their work. The Jamaican traditional forms of medicine are diverse. The vein that runs through them is how to treat the blood: strengthen it; balance it, so it is not too sweet or too bitter; build it up; and cool it down.

Tonics and purifiers are taken to keep the blood strong, thick, and circulating properly in Jamaican medicine. In Trinidad, Puerto Rico, and Guadeloupe there is more concentration on cooling the blood so it is not too hot, whereas in Jamaica the focus is on reducing sweetness.[1] Rastafarians avoid foods that are not organic. Inorganic foods, treated with pesticides and fertilizers, are deemed too hot. Since chemicals can actually burn plants, it is thought that those plants will also heat up the blood.[2]

In *Walkin' Over Medicine,* Loudell Snow dedicates an entire chapter to African American heart healers and another to our conceptions of ailments of the blood. The healing practiced by African American heart healers and the mother healers of Jamaica is not surprisingly quite similar. They synchronize the Greek Four Humors, which we learned of from the ancient Egyptians (and presumably from the nearby early African civilizations like Nubia, Kush, and Axum that served as cultural crossroads) who inform all of Africa's cultures. There is influence also from the colonists whose medicine is informed by the ancient Greeks and (although it is seldom discussed) by the Egyptians who influenced them. The aspect of greatest focus within the Hippocratic humoral theory is the focus of the blood as a primary health concern. This complements the African belief based on Egyptian philosophy that the blood is an organ.

In Egyptian medicine, heart was *ab,* or the heart-soul. It was considered the most important of the seven souls of the seven birth goddesses called the hathors. The hathors were also called the holy midwives and are associated with the seven heavenly spheres. Judicious goddess Ma'at weighed the *ab* against her feather of truth to see if it was too heavy with sin. Osiris's mummy received an *ab* in the form of an amulet made from a red stone to assure vitality. Eventually *ab* came to mean both "offering" and "heart." The hieroglyph for *ab* was a dancing figure, so it also became associated with the mystical dance of life going on inside the body—the heartbeat.

1   Payne-Jackson and Alleyne, *Jamaican Folk Medicine,* 89.
2   Payne-Jackson and Alleyne, *Jamaican Folk Medicine.*

The hathors gave each Egyptian seven souls at birth, one of which is the heart-soul.[3] Bantu witches remember the Egyptian way. They cast a death spell by symbolically eating the heart of an intended victim to consume their "heart-life." Egyptian ideas of the heart, passed down into African diasporic healing, consider the heart the seat of the self. This is where the terms *heavy-* or *lighthearted*—as a reflection of one's mental state, heartache, or heartbreak—stem from for describing longing for a loved one.[4]

Linda Camino found this Egyptian-inspired heart health practice in a very odd place—the fundamentalist, "holiness" Pentecostal church in a Piedmont city of Virginia. In her work, *The Cultural Epidemiology of Spiritual Heart Trouble,* Camino reveals the intriguing condition her studies unearthed. Spiritual heart trouble is a very specific type of mind/body/spirit illness that presents itself almost like depression. There is apathy and loss of joy and spiritual desire. People in this faith believe the self is split in three:

1. Heart/blood is the body.
2. Truth/knowledge is the mind.
3. Joy/desire is the spirit.[5]

The blood and heart are full of metaphor; that is, they go way beyond the physical into the metaphysical. The culprit in *spiritual heart trouble* is a heart that could not pass Ma'at's feather test; it is too heavy with sin, remorse, and regret. In the case of this unique heart ailment, redemption is through the cleansing blood of Jesus Christ.

3   Barbara Walker, *The Woman's Encyclopedia of Myths and Secrets* (Edison, NJ: Castle Books, 1991), 375.
4   Walker, *Woman's Encyclopedia,* 376.
5   Linda A. Camino, "The Cultural Epidemiology of Spiritual Heart Trouble," in *Herbal and Magical Medicine: Traditional Healing Today,* eds. James Kirkland, Holly F. Mathews, C.W. Sullivan III, and Karen Baldwin (Durham, NC: Duke Univ. Press, 1997), 118–36.

Red Blood Herbs: Rich and Strong

In many indigenous cultures as well as ATRs, animals are sacrificed, and the blood, a most precious gift, is submitted to the spirits to ask for their blessings and show appreciation. The mystical quality of blood is a unifying element in our stories about health and what it means to be whole and sound. In the four quarters of the African diaspora, there are vegetables, fruits, and herbs that, when prepared, resemble blood. These are utilized medicinally, sometimes even as cure-alls. This is because of an underlying belief in the mystery, strength, and power of blood and the special symbolism of the color red. After all, as long as our blood flows, we are alive. When it stops, we have passed over into the great beyond. This carries over to rituals of life and death and also impacts health. In the Yoruba cosmos, red, called *pupa*, includes the colors yellow, brown, and red. Red is the color of the earth, and the sky is white.[6]

Beets

Parents and caregivers have many ways of trying to encourage their children to eat a wholesome diet. I remember my mother could wax on for hours on end about beets. She would say things like, "Beets give you strength, vitality, and strong blood," and then later, "Beets are sexy." I ate beets; though they did not taste terribly good in my young opinion, I was sparked on by her unending enthusiasm for them. As an artist, I did a painting that combined word with image. It was a rendering of a bunch of beets, roots resembling dripping blood and healthy greens springing from the tops; scrawled underneath on the white paper was the word *heart*. At that point, I was not heavily involved with herbalism, nutrition, or folklore—at least not consciously. There was just a seed, planted by my mother, whose seed was probably planted by her mother, and so it has gone. Somehow for us there was a connection between beets, blood, and the heart.

Researchers have investigated the red in beets to see whether they contain any phytonutrients. Phytonutrients are plant constituents that are thought to be beneficial to our health and they are employed to prevent disease. The betacyanins that give beets their red color also lend the color to the lovely bougainvillea flower. In a clinical trial of the antioxidants present in fruits and vegetables capable of reducing the damage caused by oxygen

---

6   Anthony D. Buckley, *Yoruba Medicine* (Brooklyn, NY: Athelia Henrietta Press, 1997), 55.

radicals, Ronald Prior and Guohua Cao found beets to contain 840 of the 3,500 ORAC units needed per day.[7] Beets are among the top ten antioxidant vegetables and legumes. The other red ones are red bell pepper and kidney beans;[8] in terms of fruits, watermelon is ranked high, as are red grapes, strawberries, raspberries, and cranberries. Beets contain betaine, found in only a few other foods. It is a colorless crystal that plays a role in detoxifying homocysteine, a troublesome amino acid implicated in heart disease. Beets contain salicylic acid, a close relative of aspirin (acetylsalicylic acid) and have some of the anti-inflammatory qualities of aspirin, so perhaps the mothers were not off track with their "color equals good health" theory after all.[9]

In the 1950s, a Hungarian doctor treated inoperable cancer patients with beets. They ate a diet high in organic beet juice and raw beets. Twenty-two of the twenty-three patients had some degree of improvement. Alexander Ferenczi saw tumor regression and weight gain. Dr. Govind Kapadia, professor of biomedicine chemistry at the historically Black college Howard University, has also conducted experiments that found beet extract profoundly inhibits skin, lung, and liver tumors in mice.[10]

Beet greens are also used to fight addiction to cigarettes.[11] To be sure, chomping down on fruits or vegetables dramatically reduces the chances of developing cardiovascular disease.[12] The *pupa* medicines, as the Yoruba call them (those fruits, vegetables, and herbs that are red, yellow, or orange), have particularly strong medicine from both a traditional African medical standpoint and a Western biomedical one.

Henna (*Lawsonia inermis*) was discussed at length in the previous chapter. It also belongs in this conversation because its renowned red dye plays an important role in West African healing. Henna is used to stop bleeding.[13] The leaves and fruit are used to bring on absent periods (amenorrhea).[14] Hina, the plant oil, combined with sandalwood is used as an aphrodisiac, particularly by men in North and East Africa.

---

7   Ronald Prior and Guohua Cao, USDA-Agricultural Research Service, https://www.ars.usda.gov/news-events/news/research-news/1999/antioxidant-power-of-natural-product-supplements-highly-variable/.
8   Joseph, Nadeau, and Underwood, *Color Code*, 30.
9   Joseph, Nadeau, and Underwood, *Color Code*, 54–55.
10 Joseph, Nadeau, and Underwood, *Color Code*.
11 Carper, *Food—Your Miracle Medicine*, 449.
12 Carper, *Food—Your Miracle Medicine*, 32.
13 Abbiw, *Useful Plants of Ghana*, 190.
14 Abbiw, *Useful Plants of Ghana*, 173.

Rose Hips (*Rosa canina, R. rugosa, R. centifolia*)

Roses were first grown in the Middle East in Persia and spread through Saudi Arabia, North Africa, and then to Europe. *Rosa damascena*, one of the most fragrant types, is used to make perfumes and rosewater. It grows well in Morocco and is cultivated in North Africa. In North Africa, rose is used to calm irritability and anxiety; these are considered matters of the heart spiritually. The petals create a hemostatic powder when mixed with oil, which is used to treat nasal, auricular, and blennorrhagial infections. In temperate zones, rose hips provide a vibrant red color in the otherwise drab-colored winter landscape. When infused in very hot water, rose hips release a deep burgundy tea. The tea of rose hips is high in vitamins C, A, D, and B complex, as well as bioflavonoids. The bioflavonoids allow our bodies to more readily absorb the vitamin C. Rose hip also contains minerals: calcium, iron, silicon, selenium, manganese, magnesium, phosphorus, potassium, and zinc. It is used as a tea served hot or cold for building immunity, strength, and vitality. Rose hips contain antioxidants and act as an antidepressant. Rose helps scavenge free radicals; it is a tension tamer, soothing the nerves; and it helps regulate the circulation. Also, it is considered a recovery tonic, spring tonic, and system cleanser.

Rooibos, the Cure-All of South Africa

Annemarie Fillmore-Nava hails from Cape Town, South Africa, and is a descendant of the Zulu people. In this interview, she fondly recalls what the tea meant to her growing up and why she now gives it to her young son as a preferred beverage:

Annmarie: First a pronunciation key: in South Africa we spell the name of this herb *rooibos* or *rooibosch*, but it is more commonly called *bossie*. Bossie is pronounced as if "o" were an "oa" sound, as in "coat." Bossie tea has been a staple in my life ever since I was a young child. It is a common drink in South Africa not only because it is native to our land but also because of the health properties. The Adventist Church, of which I was a member growing up, follows a very regimented diet, abstaining from pork, shellfish, alcohol, and caffeine, among other foods and ingredients. Bossie is the preferred hot beverage for most Seventh-Day Adventists because it fits into our beliefs about health and spirituality. It contains no tannin or caffeine and is renowned for immune-boosting properties. It is a very versatile herbal tea in that you can drink it with or without milk. You can buy it in loose leaves or already in tea bags, either way is fine, although we found the bags to be more convenient. It has a very clean, naturally sweet taste to it and such a beautiful red color.

Whenever we had a cold, my mother would say, "I know what you need, you need some bossie tea with lemon and honey. That will get you better in no time." And that is exactly what she would give us. Because this tea is so pure, you can give it to babies who have colic, in which case you simply give it to them plain. Plain means no milk or sugar (older children through adults usually drink it with milk and sugar, also called "English style.") Bossie really doesn't require sugar because it has a naturally sweet taste. Infants will gladly accept this tea because of its mild natural sweetness.

We also use it for children or adults who have diarrhea as it settles the stomach. Again, it would be served plain. This tea is also used as an appetite stimulant; during recovery from an illness when you need to eat but just can't seem to, a cup of plain bossie tea will do the job. Needless to say, it is not a dieter's tea. However, this drink is great for those nights when you just can't seem to relax. The best way to serve it for this purpose is to brew the bags with milk on the stove. When you use only milk with it, it has a very creamy texture and really warms the insides, much like the effects of hot chocolate on a cold day.

Many a day in the winter during my childhood, we would play in the rain and come inside to a warm milk and bossie drink. There were five of us coming at different times to make our tea, so my mother would often be very irritated with us children because, as you well know, what happens to milk when it comes to boil? It boils over. I can still hear her saying, "I just cleaned the stove. Who made bossie tea and did not clean the stove?" I remember standing in front of the stove, waiting for that boiling point so that I would not have to clean the stove. My brother never learned that trick, so he was always stuck cleaning the stove.

Besides the medicinal purposes, this is just a great all-around drinking tea. One does not need any specific reason other than that you would like a hot beverage to drink. In South Africa, we drink our tea typically with milk and sugar. Even though we drink a lot of English tea for enjoyment, I continue to use this tea for my son who is six years old. He has been drinking this tea since he was born for all the reasons and purposes I spoke about. He absolutely loves it and usually drinks it with milk. Bossie tea is a wonderful replacement for teatime with kids because of the absence of caffeine and the clean, sweet taste. If you are looking for a tea with excellent health properties to enjoy, this is the one.

We also use this tea as a first aid for wounds and cuts. In this case, we use loose leaves and make a paste with water, which is applied directly to the wound. It draws out any infection. So as you can see, it is our cure-all. Thanks to the Khoisan people who discovered it and its many uses ages ago.[15]

Rooibos (*Aspalathus linearis*) grows exclusively in the Clanwilliam district of the Western Cape of South Africa,[16] where the age-old tradition of wildcrafting the organic herb continues. It is truly a remarkable red medicine. Rooibos contains fifty times more antioxidants than green tea. It contains a free radical damage scavenger, superoxide dismutase (SOD). SOD helps keep fat from turning into harmful lipid peroxide. Quercetin, a flavanol, brings the greatest gift to our blood, lending the tea the ability to prevent hemorrhaging, increase circulation, build capillary strength, and fight infections.[17] Rooibos mineral counts, per 200 milliliters tea, are:

- Calcium: 1.09 mg
- Copper: 0.07 mg
- Fluoride: 0.22 mg
- Iron: 0.07 mg
- Magnesium: 1.57 mg
- Manganese: 0.04 mg
- Sodium: 6.16 mg
- Zinc: 0.04[18]

15 Annemarie Fillmore-Nava interview.
16 Eve Palmer, *The South African Herbal* (Cape Town, South Africa: Tafelberg Publishers, 1985).
17 D. J. Cobb, "Red Bush Blessings," in *2005 Herbal Almanac,* ed. Llewellyn et al. (Woodbury, MN: Llewellyn Worldwide, 2005), 266–67.
18 Cobb, "Red Bush Blessings," 267.

Rose Madder (*Rubia tinctorum L.*)

The root of rose madder, or madder, as it is also called, makes an exquisite dye used in fine arts and crafts. The dye is also very useful for hair; when used in an infusion, it stains the hair a deep claret red.

Madder root is cultivated in Africa from Libya to Morocco. The roots are boiled as an emmenagogue. The stems and leaves are used to treat hypertension. The powdered plant is used to create a tonic or an emmenagogue, or for dressing contusions and wounds. Madder is used to treat all blood diseases, and it is also used as an aphrodisiac.[19]

Rites of Passage

Women see their blood vividly from menarche through menopause. Each month, we see evidence of the power and mystery of creation flowing from between our legs. To the Yoruba medicine people, this is the hidden secret of red manifest. Menstrual blood is examined for its health and used in ritual. It is not considered a dead or useless substance, as it tends to be from a Western biomedical view. In Yoruba medicine, ideal menstruation—in terms of color, duration, texture, and scent—is called *pupa daadaa*.[20] Not surprisingly, we have a cache of herbs to address various elements of our blood passage.

Camwood (*Baphia nitida*)

In West Africa, impending weddings are a time of celebrations of a new, productive stage in a woman's life. The color red figures prominently. During her prenuptial period, the bride-to-be is elevated to the position of royalty. While our bridal showers are a one-day event, young West African "queens" are lavished with gifts and treated to indulgent natural beautification recipes over an extended period.

In West Africa, betrothal is reminiscent of the limbo between life and death. There is a dread of what the woman may suffer filled with unpredictability. The bride-to-be is encouraged to gain weight, so she appears capable of bearing many children, quite unlike the American tendency to diet and shed pounds. While most folks shy away from intentionally

19 Loutfy Boulos, *Medicinal Plants of North Africa* (Algonac, MI: Reference Publications, 1983), 155.
20 Buckley, *Yoruba Medicine*, 225.

packing on additional pounds, the idea of taking time out to be spoiled should be required medicine. The entire village gathers to sing praise and blessings for the marriage that is about to take place. The bride-to-be is taken to a small hut and stays there until her husband joins her. Her husband gives gifts to the community. The marriage is consummated. The next morning a goat is sacrificed and its blood is poured as a libation on the threshold of the hut. If the bride reports to her mother that she is pleased with her husband, dancing and celebration ensue. People are invited to offer money to either visit with the bride or rub her body with camwood, which creates a red dye. Camwood is a traditional symbol of good fortune because it is red medicine. When camwood is rubbed on the skin, it acts as an exfoliant, removing dead skin and bringing a healthy glow. Considered a restorative, camwood brings a healthy complexion to all ages. The color balances so there is not too much bitterness held within.[21] The blood libation is designed as an offering to bring good fortune and fertility to the couple.[22]

Nettle (Urtica dioica, U. urens L.)

Nettle is a mineral-rich all-around body strengthener, blood cleanser, and detoxicant. Where *U. urens L.* grows in Egypt to Morocco, it is used as an aphrodisiac and antihemorrhagic, and for dysmenorrhea, nosebleeds, and eczema.

Several types of nettle also grow and are used medicinally in South Africa, including bush stinging nettle, also called *bosbrandnetel*. The powdered leaves are stuffed in the nose to stem nosebleed and also used for blood disorders. River nettle (*riviernetel*; *Laportea peduncularis*) is a South African native nettle used much the same way.

Raspberry (Rubus idaeus)

I recommend young girls begin drinking this as a part of their woman ritual near the onset of their first period and continue throughout life. In the wisewoman way, raspberry leaf is considered one of the most important plants to a woman's reproductive development. Raspberry, a member of the rose family, contains fragarine, an alkaloid that strengthens the uterus, helps produce effective contractions during labor, tones the womb, and expels the

---

21 Buckley, *Yoruba Medicine,* 225.
22 Buckley, *Yoruba Medicine,* 209.

afterbirth. With miscarriage or abortion, raspberry leaf is used to help regain the strength, vitality, and tone of the uterus.

For good health, vitality, and strength, the fruit of the raspberry is also recommended for its super antioxidant status and abundant red medicines. Seasonal organic strawberries, cherries, red grapes, and cranberries are also highly recommended for the same reasons.

Black Cohosh (*Cimicifuga racemosa*)

Black cohosh is also called *rattleroot* and *black snakeroot*. This herb is a traditional women's healing herb appreciated for its ability to assist with PMS, menstrual discomfort, and menopause. Black cohosh is native to eastern North America, where it is found in rich shady forests from Maine to Ontario and Wisconsin, and south to Georgia and Missouri. Black cohosh, as its folk names of rattleroot and black snakeroot indicate, carries snake energy. Black cohosh is a top-selling herbal supplement.[23] According to the Expanded Commission E of the American Botanical Council, it influences the endocrine and regulatory systems, affecting them in a way similar to estriol, one of the milder endogenous estrogens. It binds weakly with estrogen. As a popular herb, black cohosh has gone through numerous scientific tests for its efficacy. The Commission E approves the use of black cohosh root for PMS, dysmenorrhea, and menopause. One of its constituents, actina, is being evaluated for the treatment of peripheral arterial disease. One side effect is occasional gas. It is not recommended during pregnancy or lactation.

How to use: 40 milligrams per day: cut the rhizome and root and decoct in simmering water.

Motherwort (*Leonurus cardiaca*)

A native of Europe, motherwort, meaning "mother herb," is known to be an herb of the blood. The stem shoots straight up; it is strong and thick. There are three large three-lobed leaves. Motherwort helps maintain heart health and is beneficial to women's reproductive systems. It is calming and soothing to the nerves. This mothering tea helps the woman's reproductive system by assisting with some of the discomforts that may arise with menses and menopause. Motherwort is also used for heart palpitations. The word *cardiaca* in the

---

23 Michelle Cora, "Black Cohosh Herbal Extract and Hematologic Alterations in B6C3F1/N Mice," *Toxicologic Pathology* 50, no. 7 (October 2022).

Latin name demonstrates that it has a long history as a heart tonic herb. The herb contains calcium chloride, which calms the heart and eases palpitations. Motherwort is a great stabilizing herb that stops internal tremors. Apparently a good herb for the nerves, motherwort is recommended by the Commission E for heart palpitations that result from anxiety attacks or other nervous complaints. Historically, motherwort has been a medicine to treat heart weakness, absence of periods, and any cardiac symptoms associated with nerves.

Uses: as a cardiac tonic, antispasmodic, nervine, diaphoretic, uterine stimulant, sedative, emmenagogue, and carminative.

Contains: vitamin A, alkaloids, bitter glycosides, bufanolide, and tannins.

Recommendations: utilize the stem, leaves, and flower; gather these during the plant's blooming season.

Warrior Herbs

Blood red is associated with life, yet it is also connected to violence and death. In the Yoruba cosmology, Ogun is the orisha of war, weaponry, metals, and strength. He is also orisha of the heart region. His herbs include motherwort, which we just discussed, garlic, bloodwort, and hawthorn, which will be explored in this section. In addition, we will look at other herbs that are useful for the wounds, cuts, bleeding, and other ailments that a warrior might come up against.

Garlic (*Allium sativum*)

The health warrior of all warriors, no wonder it is the ewe (herb) that traditionally represents Ogun. Garlic is a broad-spectrum antibiotic that combats bacteria, intestinal parasites, and viruses. It contains more than two hundred compounds, including at least twenty germ killers, antioxidants, and a dozen anti-inflammatories. It has cured encephalitis in high doses. Garlic lowers the blood pressure and blood cholesterol while discouraging blood clots. Two to three cloves per day are recommended to reduce subsequent heart attacks. Garlic contains anticancer compounds that act as antioxidants; in fact, garlic tops the National Cancer Institute's list of cancer preventatives. It is particularly useful for stomach cancer. Garlic is known to boost immunity, making the body stronger overall. It is an antidiarrheal, estrogenic, and diuretic that lifts the mood and has a mildly tranquilizing effect.

Garlic Growth

Garlic is a bulb, with multiple wedge-shaped cloves and a papery white or sometimes purplish skin, beloved in African stews and curries as well as dishes from North Africa and the Caribbean. The pungent garlic is used as a spice to balance the sweet fruits used in cooking as well as honey.[24] In South Africa, wild garlic (*Tulbaghia violacea*) grows on the Eastern Cape and Natal. Its leaves are eaten to strengthen the body and it is rubbed on the forehead for sinus pain. *T. alliacea*, another African wild garlic, grows from Cape Province northward to Natal and the Transvaal and west to Botswana. The roots are boiled and used in a bath to treat rheumatism and cure paralysis.[25] In North Africa garlic is called *thoum* or *toum* in Arabic. It is used as an antidote for many different kinds of poisons and as an antibacterial, stimulant, tonic, and antiseptic. Garlic is inserted as a suppository to treat hemorrhoids and it is also used as an animal medicine.[26] Shallots are grown in the savanna area of West Africa. The Awuna people of the Volta region in Ghana are the traditional African shallot growers. Shallots are eaten in Ghana raw, prepared with hot pepper to make kenkey. They are used this way to disinfect and to purify the blood.[27]

Magically, four thieves vinegar is a popular potion used in Hoodoo and similar practices to ward off evil. Garlic hangs over doors to ward off burglars, malintent, and illness. Garlic amulets are worn in specially knotted strings made by *treaters* (healers from parts of the Caribbean).

Bloodwort

Also called bistort, this is used to stop hemorrhaging. Bloodwort is an alternative, astringent, diuretic, and styptic. It is directly applied to a wound as a powder and is said to stop bleeding. The recipe is 2 teaspoons rootstock to 1 cup water. Boil 5 to 10 minutes, and drink 1 cup per day.

24 Tami Hultman (ed.), *The Africa News Cookbook: African Cooking for Western Kitchens* (New York: Penguin Books, 1985).
25 Palmer, *South African Herbal*, 157.
26 Boulos, *Medicinal Plants of North Africa*, 25.
27 Abbiw, *Useful Plants of Ghana*, 38.

Hawthorn (*Crataegus oxyacantha, C. monogyna*), a Sacred Herb

Hawthorn is a powerhouse—no wonder it too is associated with the warrior orisha Ogun. Hawthorn is common in Asia, Europe, and North Africa. It is a heart tonic that enhances blood circulation and improves the uptake of oxygen; it also helps regulate the heart rate, stabilize blood pressure, increase relaxation, and reduce stress on the nerves.

Contrary to popular belief, the Commission E, who studies herbs intensely and verifies their efficacy with evidence-based studies, recommends the leaves and flowers rather than the berries for maximum health-producing benefits.[28] The Commission E report includes hawthorn as a support for cardiovascular health and states that it is frequently used in conjunction with cardiovascular medications like digitalis and ouabain to increase recovery time from cardiovascular disease as well as to help patients tolerate biomedicines used in the treatment.[29]

Hawthorn contains vitamin A, B complex, and C, as well as sodium, silicon, iron, manganese, potassium, phosphorus, selenium, saponins, glycosides, flavonoids, tannin, and procyanidins. It is a cardiovascular tonic, hypertensive, vasodilator, relaxant, astringent, antispasmodic, and diuretic.

Yarrow (*Achillea millefolium*)

Yarrow has a traditional reputation as a warrior's herb. Women of the world involved in Goddess Spirituality and other types of earth medicine utilize it as an overall toner and systemic strengthener. Yarrow is used as a gargle to stop bleeding gums. It is used to tone the pelvic muscles, for uterine disorders and to relieve tension or pressure on the lower body. Yarrow is used to regulate the menstrual cycle and reduce heavy periods or the feeling of uterine fullness. Yarrow works with the veins as an anti-inflammatory to reduce vascular appearance. It is an antiseptic and is used as a poultice on varicose veins. For hemorrhoids, yarrow sitz baths are recommended. Wounds are cleaned and the cuts sealed quickly with yarrow tea or poultice. Yarrow is used to treat burns, ulcers, and inflamed skin. The silica in yarrow repairs damaged skin. My favorite yarrow poultice is simple: chew fresh clean yarrow; moisten it with saliva; and apply it to a nosebleed, cut, or wound. Yarrow is traditionally used to treat high blood pressure.

---

28 This refers to physical health, not the spiritual or mental benefits that have been traditionally associated with hawthorn berry as a charm and natural amulet for a variety of magical purposes.
29 American Botanical Council, *Expanded Commission E report*.

Parts used: plant and flowers.

Contains: vitamins A, B complex, C, and E, bioflavonoids, minerals, amino acids, sterols, coumarins, saponins, salicylic acid, and more.[30]

Hoodoo's Magical Love Herbs

One of the most frequent requests of a Hoodoo or conjurer is to work love magic. There are several herbs used in love magic. Here are three prominent ones, apart from rose, which is discussed elsewhere in this chapter (page 163):

Adam and Eve Root (*Aplectrum hyemale*)

A talisman of an orchid root—one being more rounded and suggesting the female (Eve) whereas the other is more phallic and pointed, suggestive of the male (Adam). The two are natural charms used to cultivate love and strengthen relationships. They are featured inside love draw mojo bags, which would consist of a red (flannel) drawstring bag; a pair of matched lodestones (magnetite stones also in male and female shapes); powdered herbs such as rose, orris root, and cinnamon; and a sprinkling of magnetic sand or Van Van oil. Sweet fragrances are preferred for love draw magic like neroli, orange, Queen of Sheba, palmarosa, geranium, lemon verbena, lavender, or the ubiquitous rose. Most Hoodoos create their own unique blend using precisely measured amounts of these and sometimes a few other ingredients.

Dragon's Blood (*Dracaena draco*)

To form agreements and pacts or write love letters, people often use dragon's blood ink from the resin of an African tree in the palm family. Dragon's blood is also associated with passion, strength, vitality, and motivation, symbolized by the color red. Some people simply buy a normal red ink and add a few small chunks of dragon's blood to imbue the ink with the dragon's power. Dragon's blood is sold as an incense, powder, and ink. In West Africa, dragon's blood is consumed as an aphrodisiac.

---

30 Victoria Zak, *20,000 Secrets of Tea: The Most Effective Ways to Benefit from Nature's Healing Herbs* (New York: Random House, 2009).

Mandrake Root (*Mandragora officinarum L.*)

Since it is shaped like a man, mandrake root is one of the preferred herbs for attracting one. Mandrake roots are also used to create a poppet, which is a stand-in for a human; as such, it is utilized for sympathetic magic. The person's initials are carved into the root; it is cajoled, talked to, and played with. Sometimes the infatuated person even sprays their own perfume on the man-root in hopes that their intended will become taken with them. Mandrake root contains a deadly poison. It should only be handled by adept herbalists and kept out of reach of animals and children.

Disease Through Tainted Blood: HIV/AIDS

The fact remains that the combination of heart disease and AIDS threatens the very existence of our people, and it hits any healer directly in the heart. For instance, HIV and AIDS have made significant incursions into the lives of the Kalahari Kung. Working in the mines of Johannesburg, one way or another, the Kung men got infected, brought that infection back to the women, and now it is in the children as well.

There has been a buzz in the Black community for almost as long as HIV and AIDS have existed that it is a conspiracy, a planted illness to wipe out our race. Folks point to the Tuskegee syphilis experiment for proof. A recent scientific test by sociologists indicates that over 50 percent of African-descended people believe the AIDS virus is planted.

Whether or not it is true remains to be seen. The fact of the matter is that it is a very real and very deadly disease that does not care what culture, age, lifestyle, or sex it infects—take the Kalahari Kung for example. In Africa, and elsewhere for that matter, there has been strong resistance to treatment, suggestions about prevention, and education on the topic. To our culture, there is nothing—and I do mean *nothing*—worse than the notion of bad blood. Diagnosing, treating, and flushing out bad blood are at the very crux of our healing ways.

HIV/AIDS Therapy

The worry by some, which I also share, is that belief in the conspiracy theory will make people feel hopeless and encourage them to lose their fighting spirit—the will to survive that is the spark that has been our cultural glue. If there was the possibility of creating a virus that would weaken the mind, body, and spirit of people of African descent, it would most certainly be a virus that created "bad blood." We know that, but we must get over theory and dwell in fact to prevent the spread and to treat those already infected. There is no cure.

A variety of complementary therapies offer support to people with HIV/AIDS. Many African and indigenous healers in general seek to comfort and support the person so that they have the will or spirit to heal. As I have stressed throughout this book, within African medicine there are spiritual, mental, and physical aspects. Biomedicine is fixated on the physical.

Many of "my people" in an ethnic sense—my family of artists of all sorts and my extended family of relatives—were wiped out by AIDS, especially when it first struck and there was little awareness of its cause. As I mentioned earlier, my uncle who had HIV for many years managed his life with the help of spirit. He practiced divination, became heavily involved with djembe drumming, and would sing praise songs, chants, and blues and jazz songs from time to time. Divination helps us to know what the future holds and helps us understand alternate realms of possibility. Djembe is a way of activating those realms of possibility. Sometimes drumming can induce a state that is meditative or trancelike; this is enhanced by controlling the breathing. My uncle was strong of heart and spirit until shortly before he passed over, but this is not true for everyone. It does not mean, however, that music cannot still offer spiritual support. If the person who is suffering knows a drummer or drumming circle, he can ask that they come in to play for him. If there are drumming circles in the community, perhaps they can make an effort to go to a local community center and play with spirit for people with HIV, AIDS, or other serious illnesses. Play with spirit. Play from the heart. The beating of the drum can help one cross over so that the idea of death is not as scary.

Singing brings joy to the self and to the spiritual entities around us. It is a way of expressing joy and sorrow. It is no mistake that Negro spirituals sprouted up in the fields alongside cotton and tobacco plants. Negro spirituals are a call to nature, to the ancestors, the spiritual guardians, and angelic beings for help, release, and grace. Prisoners who were forced to work down South created beautiful and haunting chants and songs. They are touching.

Prisoner field songs and chants speak of all kinds of suffering, regrets, and remorse, and some are concerned with forgiveness. The African people have always found release from misery through making joyful noises as well as movement and the arts.

When singing, drumming, movement, or art take too much energy, there are more passive forms of lightening the heavy heart, including comedy. Comedy, jokes, poking fun, laughing—these are all incredibly important in African culture. Laughter is one of the heart medicines that cannot be bottled, sold, or made into a cocktail; nevertheless, its efficacy cannot be argued. I would find that even my healer's heart, my daughter heart, and my niece heart would become heavy with the imminent possibility of loss. During these times I felt my heart would break into a million pieces, I was advised by my uncle, Babalawo of Shango, "Girl, you just too serious. Why don't you watch a funny movie? Rent a video of your favorite comedian; laugh your ass off, girl." I followed this advice. Laughter is great medicine, and for the most part it is free.

In turn, I found some of the African herbal healing ways to offer comfort and, yes, to alleviate the pain of terminal illness. One of these is to gift—to give, to share self. This can be accomplished by writing emails and letters, making phone calls, stopping in to visit, and even giving a tender hug. There is nothing more painful than feeling as though you are dying and doing it all alone. Gifts of herbs like lavender, chamomile, and rose dream pillows seem to offer huge comfort. These herbs have a time-honored tradition of being soothing and calming and helping to induce sleep. Jasmine makes another nice addition.

HIV/AIDS Medicine Bag

There are widespread discussions of traditional medicine people in Africa and the African diaspora using their oral traditions to perform miraculous healings based on holistic principles. There is not too much clinical evidence of HIV/AIDS cures, though a number of herbs have piqued the interest of researchers, including:

Hyssop (*Hyssopus officinalis*)—used in moderation, hyssop is a good herb to treat dry throat, coughing, and upper respiratory ailments that may result from AIDS.

Life everlasting (*Gnaphalium polycephalum*)—a traditional curative in Gullah medicine and in Hoodoo, where it is used as a tea and as a charm held within a mojo bag. As its name indicates, life everlasting is one of those herbs thought to be imbued with such high vibration that it can bring about a long life. The bright-yellow flowers bring cheer to the weary spirit.

Licorice Root (*Glycyrrhiza glabra*)

A perennial native to the Mediterranean, central to southern Russia, and Asia Minor to Iran, licorice is now cultivated through Europe, the Middle East, and Asia. Most of what is sold comes from semiwild plants from Turkey, Greece, Iran, China, India, Pakistan, Afghanistan, Syria, Italy, and Spain. Licorice has been extensively researched. The roots contain glycyrrhizin, a compound that is very sweet. Many people come into contact with licorice root as a flavoring in teas, liquors, and food. Its use is documented in Assyrian tablets and Egyptian papyri. It was used in ancient Arabia to treat colds, cough, and sore

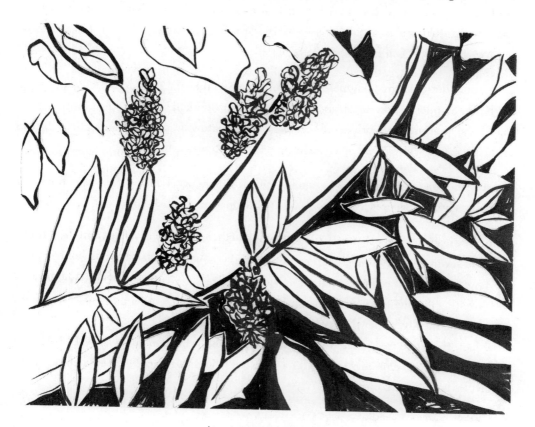

Licorice plant and root

throat and as a stomachic. From ancient times to the current day, licorice root is considered a broad-spectrum healer.

Most often an herb will arouse interest because of the effects it has on those around us. We have heard the stories of freshly enslaved Africans chewing roots similar to licorice root during the terrifying ship rides of the Middle Passage. These were used to settle the stomach. When my grandmother was stricken with cancer, she frequently requested licorice to soothe her symptoms. Observing this made an indelible impression that it was an herb with potential to be a great healer.

I have noticed there has been a battery of tests to explore the medicinal quality of licorice root. It has undergone clinical trials as a treatment for hepatitis C, hemophilia with HIV-1 infection, and the inhibition of HIV replication in patients with AIDS. It has also been studied for its use in treating anxiety and as a stress reducer. The constituent glycyrrhizin has been studied as a controlled dosage for therapy for patients with HIV. Patients showed improvement with their clinical symptoms.

Recommendations: the Commission E has approved internal use of licorice root for catarrh of the upper respiratory tract and for gastric or duodenal ulcers. The German Standard License approves licorice root infusions for loosening mucus, alleviating discharge in bronchitis, and helping with spasmodic pains of chronic gastritis.

Uses: decoction or infusion 1 to 4 grams in 150 milliliters water, after meals three times per day unless otherwise prescribed by an ND (naturopathic doctor).

Contraindications: liver disorder (including cirrhosis of the liver), hypertonia, hypokalemia, and severe kidney ailment. Not recommended during pregnancy or lactation.

May cause sodium and water retention with prolonged use. Potassium could result along with swelling (edema), hypokalemia, and hypertension, among other ailments.[31] Use with care therapeutically, under the care of an herbalist or ND.

In fact, there are many herbs useful in treating the symptoms of HIV/AIDS because these are symptoms not only thirsty for a cure but also in dire need of treatment to calm, soothe, invigorate, and protect.

---

31 American Botanical Council, *Expanded Commission E report.*

Rosemary (*Rosmarinus officinalis*)

Rosemary is grown in the Middle East and Africa, from Libya to Morocco and in Egypt. Rosemary is used in these areas for aromatic baths, as a carminative and antispasmodic, and to treat wounds and eczema. Leaves are added to the bath for strength. Powdered leaves are used to treat wounds due to their antiseptic properties, which appear to have anti-HIV potency in vitro. Studies conducted in France indicate that rosemary compounds suppressed HIV replication without damaging cells studied in the laboratory.

The first of the two herbs I feel most confident about for treating the broad spectrum of symptoms of HIV is pau d'arco, also called divine bark. Divine bark will be discussed in chapter 10, "The Sacred Wood," because it deserves a place of high honor among the sacred trees of the world. The second is astragalus, which we will explore next.

Astragalus (*Astragalus membranaceus*)

I have the highest respect for this native of China and Mongolia. Astragalus is a member of the native perennial legume family. It has pea-shaped leaves on the middle stem, from which rows of pea-shaped flowers hang like bells.

I respect astragalus because it is a single herb that holds a wealth of holistic health benefits. It helps balance body fluids, detox, invigorate, and stimulate immunity. It is useful after chemotherapy, radiation, and surgery or during the course of an exhausting illness. Astragalus is recommended for the recovery and replenishment of the mind, body, and spirit. This herb revitalizes white blood cells, stimulates the production of natural antibodies, is a natural interferon, improves antiviral resistance, and fights fatigue from colds and flu. In Chinese medicine it is considered to have protective energy. Moreover, it increases the ability of other herbs to heal when it is brewed along with them. Andrew Weil, a renowned healer who helped bring greater attention to the benefits of holism, recommends astragalus to his HIV and AIDS patients.[32]

Qualities: tonic, energizer, immunity stimulator, cardiac toning, and antimicrobial.

Properties: amino acids, polysaccharides, linoleic acid, betaine, and choline glycosides.

---

32 Andrew Weil, *Spontaneous Healing: How to Discover and Embrace Your Body's Natural Ability to Maintain and Heal Itself* (New York: Ballantine Books, 1995), 78.

Preparation: as a tough root, astragalus needs to be decocted. Decoct 2 teaspoons per cup of water for 20 minutes.

Lavender (*Lavandula officinalis*, *L. angustifolia*, *L. stoechas L.*; North African Variety)

Lavender is called *khuzama* in Arabic. In Africa, lavender is used as a stimulant, an antiseptic, a tonic, and a cure for irritability.[33]

Calendula Skin Wash, Ointment, or Bath

Calendula, those perky flowers also called marigold, release an effective healing medicine for the skin when prepared as a skin cream or oil infusion or included in soaps or a water infusion added to the bath. I have seen wonderful results with itching, lesions, and eruptions using calendula in all these forms.

Shea Butter

Explored in depth in chapter 10, shea butter makes an excellent simple (one-ingredient) healing skin balm for skin lesions that can form due to the lowered natural immunity experience by people with HIV/AIDS. Shea butter often brings relief to dry skin and makes a soothing addition to the bath.

---

33 Boulos, *Medicinal Plants of North Africa*, 101.

Love: Mind, Body, Spirit

All the concerns in this chapter are matters of the heart. In ATR we do not just look at the end result—for example, an illness or disease, but also at environment and spirit. I find it of great interest that the emblems of our love day, Saint Valentine's Day—roses, red wine, and chocolate—are all good for the heart medicinally; we already knew they were good for the spirit.

Red Roses (*Rosa rubiginosa*)

Roses are flowers that stimulate the senses—in the akashic sense of our extrasensory perception, as well as smell, sight, taste, and touch. The rose's gift to the akashic realm is that it stimulates the storehouse we hold of ancient memories of past lives; ancestors, angels, and deities around us seem to enjoy their presence as well. The smell is fresh and sweet, reminding us of the gentle qualities of life. Often they are given as a token of love and for healing; thus they are intimately tied to the heartstrings. Roses are available to us in many forms that lend them to aromatic applications, including attar or otto, a pure rose oil used as a natural perfume. Attar of roses is thought of as an aphrodisiac; it also increases energy and desire for action of all sorts. Rosewater is a hydrosol that can be sprayed on the body, sheets, and clothing, as well as in the air, to bring a positive loving presence. Dried roses are used to give vitality and a softly romantic scent to potpourris. This is all in addition to the abundance of cosmetic products like body sprays, bath scrubs, powders, bubble baths, salts, and soaps containing pure rose oil. Rose petal paper makes a nice stationery for love letters, and rose oil can be added to ink to scent the paper. Rose petals make a nice addition to salads and honey. You can also give a delicate flavor to sugar by adding rose petals to the sugar jar. In Africa and the Middle East, rosewater is added to cakes, beverages, and delicate dishes.

By far the preferred gift exchange between lovers is a dozen red roses. The feel of the delicate flowers paired with the delightful scent makes the heart swell, the face blush, and warmth prevail between friends, relatives, and lovers.

Red Wine

Usually writing about red wine extols its virtues first and its detractions afterward. Seeing as how alcoholism has depleted the energy of many indigenous people after its introduction, and how it has decimated many Black neighborhoods, I decided to put the warnings up front. While there are many researchers reporting the virtues of red wine and its benefits to the cardiovascular system, I know all too well from personal experience the heartbreak that results from alcoholism. In fact, if you have a tendency toward addiction, it is best to skip the next two items—red wine and chocolate—because their use will harm, not heal. I say that because, with addictive personality disorder that can lead to alcoholism or over-eating, the "off" button that says to use with discretion or only eat a one-inch square of chocolate is permanently malfunctioning. If you are unable to know when to stop, do not be seduced by the virtues of red wine or chocolate. They can only benefit those able and will-ing to take in very small amounts (1 glass red wine a day or 1 to 2 ounces dark chocolate). Moreover, if you have issues in your family history or ancestry that include alcoholism, it is best to avoid red wine.

One additional note: the type of wine recommended for health benefits—Bordeaux, cabernet sauvignon, and claret, desired for their anticoagulant properties that counter-act fat during meals[34]—are dry red wines. Traditionally people of African descent drink sweeter wines, although that is changing. There are sweet fruity wines like a rosé, or those made from strawberries, peaches, apples, or other harvested fruits have been used in the United States to make wine in the Black community. Palm wine is the preferred wine in many countries in Africa. These types of wines are not mentioned in most of the current studies; when white wines are mentioned frequently, it is to say they do not offer the same health benefits as red.

For those abstaining from wine who desire some of the same health benefits, try adding grapeseed oil to your salad dressing as it raises good cholesterol, or eat more red grapes since they contain antioxidants. Resveratrol belongs to a family of compounds called poly-phenols that combat damaging free radicals in the body. This is the polyphenol that lends red grapes, grapeseed oil, and red wine many of their benefits.

It seems as though drinking in moderation with meals has greater benefits than drink-ing alone.[35] According to the popular South Beach Diet author, Dr. Agatston, drinking with the meal fills the stomach, decreasing the amount of food consumed at the meal. Dr.

34 Carper, *Food—Your Miracle Medicine*, 38.
35 Alice Lichtenstein and Eric Rimm, in Kathleen Zelman, "How Much Wine Is Good For You?" WebMD, January 26, 2005, https://www.cbsnews.com/news/how-much-wine-is-good-for-you/.

Agatston recommends red wine because of the antioxidant resveratrol.[36] Another doctor from WebMD, Dr. Rimm, reports that although red wine has the antioxidant, not everyone can readily absorb it. Dr. Rimm suggests eating raw vegetables (salad) to get antioxidants rather than imbibing. Alcohol has very powerful effects on the increase of good cholesterol (HDL), improving it as much as 20 percent if used moderately and combined with regular exercise. Recently the *New England Journal of Medicine* evaluated more than twelve thousand elder women (ages seventy to eighty-one) and found the moderate drinkers scored well in mental function tests.[37] The 2005 Dietary Guidelines by the US Department of Health and Human Services recommend one drink a day for women and two a day for men.

Chocolate

Chocolate contains flavonoids called catechins that also give antioxidant strength. Dark chocolate, which has hardly any sugar, is preferred and recommended in very small amounts. Dark chocolate has 35 percent more of the brown paste of ground cocoa beans than other chocolate. Milk reduces the health benefit in chocolate, thus milk chocolates are to be avoided when eating chocolate for health benefits.

Dr. David Katz, nutrition expert at Yale School of Medicine, reports that chocolate offers some important health benefits. He also states that the right kind has to be consumed and eaten moderately—and even then, it is not as wholesome as fresh fruit and vegetables. The benefits according to Dr. Katz are derived from the fact that cocoa has more flavonoids than green tea, for example. It may well have the highest source of flavonoids of any food in our diet. The problem is that eating lots of chocolate, as we well know, means we are also consuming large amounts of fat. Couple that with lack of activity, and you may well gain weight, which has all sorts of negative health implications.

Nutrients in chocolate include protein, calcium, riboflavin, iron, vitamin A, and thiamine. Remember: half the calories in chocolate come from fat, and white chocolate is chocolate in name only.[38]

There are a wide variety of botanical products containing cocoa butter and chocolate scent. One that I'm very fond of is the powdered form of cacao. I add it to hot cereals instead

---

36 Arthur Agatston, in "How Much Wine Is Good for You?"
37 Agatston, in "How Much Wine Is Good for You?"
38 "Does Chocolate Qualify as a Health Food?," ABC News, December 12, 2004.

of sugars or fats and it provides a big blast of satisfying flavor. Cacao powder is enjoyable with coffee and with mushroom hot chocolate. Enjoy it for its health benefits to the skin without any guilt.

I suggest purchasing your cacao powder organic, gluten-free, and non-GMO. Here are a few of its nutrient facts:

- 0% sugar
- 1% daily value of fat
- 2% daily value of potassium
- 7% daily value of fiber
- 10% daily value of iron
- And 100% good taste!

One last tip is to freeze a banana, chop it up, and put it in a food processor with two teaspoons of cacao powder for a yummy, fat-free chocolate banana freeze, similar to ice cream.

Because the heart crosses so many boundaries and means so many different things to different people, there are numerous ways of practicing heart healing. Scents provided from essential oils, particularly sandalwood, also help the heart of the person stricken by illness, saddened by mourning, or drained from healing.

CHAPTER 9

Funfun Health

MEDICINES OF THE SWAMPS, MANGROVES, LAKES, AND SEAS

NATURAL MEDICINES IN FOCUS

- Sandalwood
- Holy basil
- Transvaal basil
- Zulu basil
- Basil
- White willow
- Bentonite
- Rhassoul
- Lotuses
- Papyrus
- Various salts
- Kelp
- Wakame
- Kombu
- Dulse
- Irish moss
- Spirulina
- Libations

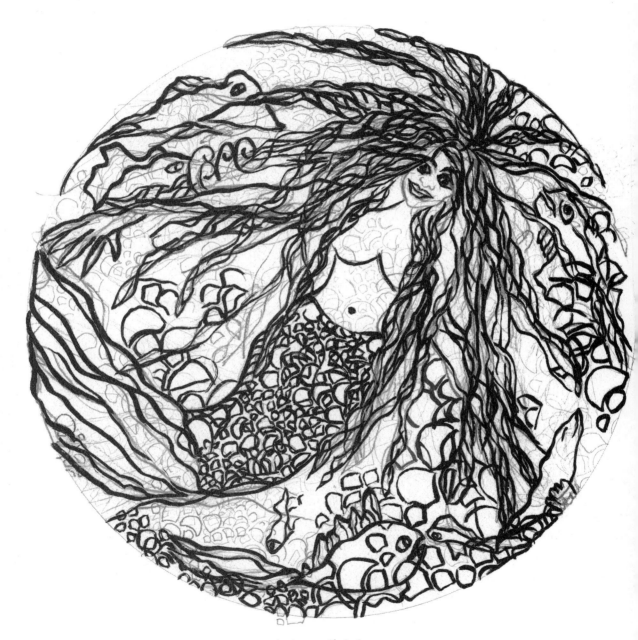

Lasiren and Labalen

Funfun

"The Healer's Heart" discussed the heart in its myriad interpretations, including a discussion of the blood in relation to well-being. This chapter delves into the mysterious world of *funfun*. *Funfun* is a Yoruba word for the white or colorless realm of the water—a realm that, though crystal clear, remains mysterious. In the previous chapter we began to understand heart through the color red, called *pupa* by the Yoruba people. They call the white realm *funfun*, and it's another important color signifying a distinctive worldview.

Funfun realm is concerned with the ways Africans view the clarity of water in a metaphysical sense. *Funfun* is not only populated by fish and sea plants, but also by the ancestors, spirits, and beings that cross between human, fish, and serpent. The essences of bodies of water, clay, seaweed, and salt also play a role because they contain the spirit of *funfun*. This area is seen as mysterious, benevolent, foreign, and full of unimaginable treasures. Some African groups believe there are fully intact underwater worlds, similar to Atlantis, inhabited by not only the ancestors but also entire societies of water spirits.

In Western health, we are admonished against white foods as being dull and lifeless. These foods are interpreted literally as white in color: the potato, white sugar, denatured and bleached white flour, and so forth. To avoid confusion, I utilize the Yoruba word *funfun* because it allows us to explore white in conjunction with healing medicines of the water spirit without the other implications. Whereas red is the color of earth, white is the color of sky in Yoruba cosmology; color-wise it includes white, blue, green, and clear. *Funfun,* then, is the world of spirit, air, and water.

The water is considered a place where spirits who carry healing medicine abide. Our passport to this mysterious world are deities: Obatala, orisha of the immaculate white realm; Isis, creation water goddess and mother of the ancient Egyptian floods; Yemaya-Olokun, mother and father of the sea; Oshun, sweet orisha of fresh water; and of course those mysterious lwas, Agwe and the simbi, who weave magic as they slither through water. There are also the fascinating engineers of ashe medicine who serve as conduits for transformation; they are called the masa. Other Haitian spirit beings of interest include Lasiren the mermaid and Labalen the whale. In North Africa there are the *djinn*, but for now we shall leave them rest, as they are dubious. White mountain man, deities, mermaids, sea mammals, orishas, and sea serpent spirits will act as our trusty guides. We will navigate the turbulent waters aided by this group in an effort to understand the potential of water medicine.

Mangrove Medicine: Sandalwood

In Africa and the diaspora, water spirits are often exotic, foreign, and not of the soil. Some are represented as foreigners with long straight hair and fair skin like Mami Wata, while others are, well, extraordinary and not of the earth in any way. Our first stop is a visit with one of the great spiritual trees of that world; interestingly it grows on the precipice between earth and water. In the mangroves we find the sandal tree. It is coveted for its fragrant wood called sandalwood, and it is an esoteric herb of the orisha Oshun.

Oshun is the orisha of many desirable things, like many of her riverain friends. She brings prosperity, fertility, refinement, sensuality, beauty, and protection, especially for women and children. Oshun is a freshwater and sweetwater orisha. Her domain, then, is rivers, streams, lakes, and ponds as freshwater orisha. Her love of sweetwater means she has a predilection for cologne and heavenly scented aromatic botanicals like sandalwood. Exploring Oshun's sandalwood allows us to visit a neighboring non-Western system called Ayurveda.

Most of the water spirits and their attendant cosmology developed along African trade routes. Frequently, water spirits embody elements of cultures of interest to Africans. East Indians have lived in Africa for hundreds of years, and they also live in the African diaspora, often in or near Black communities. There have been wonderful crossovers, sometimes even resulting in a shared spirituality. Ayurveda may sound different, but it shares the African concern for holistic health. It has exerted significant influence on Jamaican healing ways. The professors Payne-Jackson and Alleyne, who did several comprehensive studies of Jamaican healing medicine, report Hindu spirituality influenced Jamaican beliefs including Rastafarianism. Unani, a faith of Islamic origin, plays a role, and Ayurveda, Buddhism, and Yoga figure quite prominently as well.[1] Perhaps now it is time for these non-Western paths to influence the rest of us farther afield. Buddhism, Yoga, and Ayurveda in particular have certainly been influential personally.

---

1   Payne-Jackson and Alleyne, *Jamaican Folk Medicine*, 52–53.

The Mystical Sandal Tree: Shelter for the Spirit

I knew for several years that my father had been deemed "terminally" ill; still, when I got the phone call we all dread, my blood ran cold. "Dad is in the hospital—in a coma . . . they cannot bring him out of it," my brother said solemnly. When I spoke with the doctor, and he said they would *keep him going* until I got there, I knew the outlook was grim.

On that snowy February day, I went through a predictable range of emotions, from hopefulness to sinking dread, and finally deep sorrow, in a matter of hours. I knew that within twenty-four hours I would take the cross-country flight to be at his bedside, February snowstorm or not.

It is difficult to pack for such a trip. I remember rummaging through my medicine cabinet. Bach Rescue Remedy, the buffer for sudden shocks, was a definite item to take. In terms of essential oils, the choice was equally simple: sandalwood was the first to be gingerly packed. Just as the mangroves are mysterious, the wood of the sacred tree would accompany me on the trip into spiritually unknown territory, the death of my last surviving parent. I packed it because it is a spiritual panacea. Just as I provided space for my precious oil during the trip, I want to devote ample space to the psychological and spiritual applications of sandalwood here as my chief herbal savior on the journey through grief and mourning. Knowing this tree is in the domain of Oshun helped because she is all that is lovely. I also looked to the ancient Buddhist and Hindu traditions of healing to shape my understanding of sandalwood, so they are utilized here as well. Before exploring the sandal tree in depth, let's explore Ayurveda.

Ayurveda and Sandalwood

The word *Ayurveda* is derived from the Sanskrit words *Ayu* ("life") and *Veda* ("science"). Ayurveda is rooted in cherished scriptures called Vedas that date back to 1500 BCE. The Vedas are sacred literature, including the Rig-Veda, which contains one thousand hymns and was written between 1700 and 800 BCE. The Rig-Veda asserts considerable influence over Indian healing traditions. While ancient, the Vedas still influence the contemporary interest in holistic healing, since they stress care of the entire being. The ancient concepts of Ayurveda continue to influence and direct the use of healing herbs and aromatic treatments.

According to Ayurvedic practice, the mind exerts profound influence on the body. A well-balanced, tranquil mind can free the body from illness. Sandalwood cultivates acute awareness central to achieving the balance sought after in Ayurvedic healing.

Sandalwood (*Santalum album*): An East Indian Perspective

> *Maillaagar bereh hai bhuyiangaa. Bikh amrit basahi ik sangaa.*
> The snakes encircle the sandalwood trees. Poison and nectar dwell there together.
> —*Sri Guru Granth Sahib,* The Divine Teachings of Gurbani (SGGS 525)

Wood from the sandal tree has been used for at least four thousand years, and it is mentioned in the oldest Vedic scripture, the Nirukta. Sandalwood is called *chandan* in Hindi. It is believed that *chandan* imparts a sweet scent to all of nature. The aroma of *chandan* blesses every tree near it and even the axe that cuts it. To the Hindu people, *chandan* symbolizes mystery, sanctity, and devotion. Lovely sandalwood-based incense exported internationally from India is called *chandan.*

In India, the heartwood of sandal trees has divine status; sandalwood is a manifestation of divinity and holiness. The oil is used to anoint images of sacred deities, as it is considered pleasing to the gods. Sandalwood is used in the last rites of Hindus; the wood is used on funeral pyres to carry the soul to its eternal abode.

Sandalwood is beloved in numerous cultures as a spiritual aid to meditation and devotion. Medicinally, it is cooling, aphrodisiac, emollient, anti-inflammatory, and mildly astringent. Sandalwood is also admired for its ability to break insomnia. The psychological (aromachology) applications of sandalwood include easing inhibitions, boosting self-confidence, inducing a calm, sedate mood, and releasing emotions. These are all qualities I knew I would be drawing on when I visited with my father, potentially for the last time.

✳

Sandalwood and the Elements

Air

Sandalwood essential oil is the concentrated extract of the heartwood of the sandal tree. The oil is considered an aphrodisiac that builds self-confidence and generates wellness in the workplace or living environment. Sandalwood essential oil is widely available and works well dispersed by air.

- Add an appropriate amount to an aromatherapy-vaporizing unit. Light a votive candle beneath the unit. (Never leave this unattended.)
- Add oil to a scent ring that works with a regular light bulb. Follow manufacturer's directions.

Water

Hydrosol is a term coined by aromatherapist Jeanne Rose for what were once referred to as flower waters. According to Rose's website for the Aromatic Plant Project, the word *hydrosol* is made up of *hydro* ("water") and *sol* ("solution"). Hydrosols are the fragrant waters collected through the steam distillation of plants, thus they contain essential oils in a water base. To release sandalwood energy in water try the following:

- Add pure sandalwood hydrosol to a spray-top bottle; spray the face and hair for conditioning, spiritual benefits, and balancing of moods.
- During rinsing of hand-washables, add ½ cup sandalwood hydrosol to the washbasin. Swirl fine linens, lingerie, or scarves in this water; complete the process appropriate for the fabric, using clothing manufacturer's directions.
- Purchase ready-made unscented bubble bath, shampoo, conditioner, or lotion. Add the suggested amount of sandalwood hydrosol for the quantity of product and its directions. Mix thoroughly before use.
- Create, melt, and pour (handmade) soap. Scent with sandalwood essential oil using product directions.

Earth and Fire

- Apply neat (straight sandalwood essential oil) to the charkas or pulse points; body heat will disperse the scent. The oil is gentle enough to use on humans or animal companions.
- Sandalwood oil is used as a base for many fine herbal perfume oils from India called attars (*attar* means "of the air and wind"), including gulhinas from the henna plant (*Lawsonia inermis* and from kewda (*Pandanus odoratissimus*), motia (*Jasminum officinale*), and rose (*Rosa damascena*). These are also applied neat to temples, pulse points, or charkas.
- Sandalwood oil and the attars above can be used in massage when diluted with sweet almond oil or jojoba oil. Add ½ teaspoon to 8 ounces oil; swirl to mix.
- Light a candle for a few minutes. When there is a pool of melted wax, extinguish the candle. Add a couple drops of sandalwood essential oil to the candle and relight it.
- One of the most satisfying ways of combining sandalwood with fire is the age-old practice of enjoying smoldering incense. Next we explore the allure of loose sandalwood incense.

The Sweet Breath of Buddha

According to various Buddhist texts, the red sandalwood tree is sacred, a sage among people. Buddha's words are perceived as being scented, thus fragrance is central to Buddhist faith. There are many beautiful scents associated with Buddhism; the five most important are:

1. **Buddha family (Vairocana) aloeswood**—transmutation of ignorance
2. **Vajra family (Akshobhya) clove**—transmutation of aversion
3. **Ratna family (Ratnasambhava) borneol**—transmutation of pride
4. **Padma family (Amitabha) lotus/sandalwood**—transmutation of desire
5. **Karma family (Amoghasiddhi) turmeric**—transmutation of envy

Baieido creates traditional Japanese incense from the five families of scents listed above. Established in 1657, Baieido is the oldest incense company still in existence. The "fine" and "connoisseur" grades of sandalwood incense are Byakudan and Byakudan Kokoh, respectively.

Byakudan (Japanese for "Old Mountain") is suitable for mixing with other incense ingredients or burning on a charcoal block alone. As you will see below, sandalwood blends well with many herbs and resins. The Byakudan incenses are used in initiation rites and during meditation. Baieido incense blends are renowned, and they were one of the earliest suppliers to the head temple of each Buddhist sect. Here are some age-old Japanese incense blends:

Zuikun Jirushi chips—sandalwood, clove, cassia, and Chinese herbs; used for ceremony and meditation.

Tokko Jirushi chips—sandalwood and star anise; used to invigorate the mind, lead to clarity, and calm body and spirit.

Sutoko Jirushi chips—aloeswood and sandalwood; a gentle, calming blend that restores the mind after hectic activities and stress.

Sandalwood incense enjoys a central role in various Asian faiths. According to Hindu religious writing, worship must include burning fires of fragrant woods at the four cardinal points, where consecrated oils are placed.

Sandalwood for Letting Go, Grief, and Mourning

Understanding the history of sandalwood in Asia and its connection to Oshun in Africa, as well as being familiar with its practical applications, enabled me to harvest its healing energy in a dire time of need, and it may hold that gift for you as well. Each morning before I went to the hospital, I not only dabbed the essential oil on my pulse points and temple but also packed it into my purse so that I could share it with my father. I knew that, as a determined fighter, my father would continue to hold on to life on earth. Once I understood from my dreams, intuition, and talking to his team of doctors and nurses, as well as reviewing his X-rays and test results, that there was little hope for him to continue to exist on our spiritual plane, I wanted to do what I could to help him pass over to the next dimension. Sandalwood is believed to help us break ties with the past.

I wanted him to feel relaxed, loved, and fearless; sandalwood reduces anxiety and balances mood. I utilized sandalwood alone and sometimes in concert with neroli and attar of roses applied neat to his temples to help him not only let go but also anticipate a new life after passing over to the great beyond. As a healer and a loving daughter, I found this to be one of the most difficult tasks in my life. I realized with more than a little remorse that his passing on was the way things had to be.

For months after his passing, I continued to utilize the gentle gifts of sandalwood. The oil helped me sleep and relax, and it gradually eased my depression. I used sandalwood oil neat, added six to eight drops to my bath, burned sandalwood candles, and did the type of outdoor sandalwood ritual that follows.

Sandalwood for Closure

Following is a ritual and altar suggestions so that, when the time comes, you have additional tools in your healing arsenal. This ritual involves a circle, symbolic of the full seasonal cycles of life and the idea of closure, and it engages the elements of earth, air, wind, fire, and akasha (the soniferous ether from which the other four elements are created). It is an excellent activity to do with family, colleagues, or a close circle of friends, though it can also be accomplished in solitude.

ASHES TO ASHES, DUST TO DUST RITUAL

Juniper or cedar twigs and dry grass like sweetgrass or lemongrass (kindling)

Mesquite or other fragrant wood

3 to 4 cups white ash (available at many traditional Asian incense suppliers or collected from grill or fireplace)

4 tablespoons incense; choose from Byakudan and Byakudan Kokoh leaves and Zuikun Jirushi, Tokko Jirushi, or Sutoko Jirushi chips (see qualities of each on page 175)

Matches

Jug of water (to extinguish fire)

Clear away brush and debris. Place the kindling down first and then the heap of wood on the cleared area. Light wood and grass from beneath. Sit down (in a circle if working with a group, and tell stories about the event that has brought you together). Gaze at the flames; imagine the fire as a source of transformation and healing. When the fire dies down, completely spread white ash, making a circle around the wood. Sit and reflect on the circle; consider the seasons and the cycle of life. Concentrate on closure while breathing slowly and deeply.

Face south and sprinkle a tablespoon of sandalwood on the ground. Face each of the remaining cardinal directions (east, north, and west), sprinkling more of the incense every five minutes. Remember the person, animal, or thing that is the source of longing, mourning, and grief. Contemplate, relax, and pray for the release of bottled-up energy. Welcome tears as they come. Let the tears bless and extinguish the heat of the smoldering wood (you can also use water if needed).

Remembrance Altar

Afterward, collect some of the cool, dry ash and place it in a small earthenware bowl. Place the bowl on a mantel or table, along with a sandalwood candle and fresh flowers; this is the beginning of a remembrance altar. Add more significant objects until the altar feels complete. Visit the Remembrance Altar to reflect and remember.

**The mangrove forests are a terrestrial paradise.
I will do whatever is necessary to save them.**[2]
—*Wadja Egnankou*

In part I of this book, I wrote quite extensively about ashe. Remember that ashe is the liquid energy within healing plants. The masa are conduits for ashe to travel and become accessible. Masa are masters of the waters. They travel the air and waterways on a magical boat that travels to the moon. Masa free up energy to allow magic to take place. They are the points between the lwa connecting them. They are formed from a combination of astral light and water. Masa appreciate the type of libations we will explore at the end of this chapter. They also like offerings of glass bottles, which in Kongo cosmology suggest the *funfun* realm of ancestor and spirit—crystal clear yet remote. They love bath salts as they contain healing elixirs from the sea—one of their favorite places.[3]

Olokun: Sea Father of Benin

The Ijo of Nigeria have two types of nature spirits, called oromo: one is of water, the other of the land. The water spirits are seen as beautiful and kind. Conversely, grass and forest spirits are seen as nasty, ugly, and malformed.[4]

The water spirits appear in the seasonal masquerade festivals as aquatic creatures or quasi human beings. The coastal people and riverine cultures create elaborate masks and full-body costumes. In the Niger Delta region, marine animals are depicted as humans with fish features. People believe the dances imitate the activities of the water spirit. Sometimes, to further the illusion, the masked dancers enter and exit by way of the water.

Lanky, fair-skinned spirits with shining ornaments hung all over their bodies represent water spirits; they are naked otherwise. They are men, women, and children, some good and some bad.[5] The association with Europeans—the Portuguese, for example—is partic-

2   Quote provided with permission from Wadja Egnankou through the Goldman Prize.
3   Sallie Ann Glassman, *Vodou Visions* (New York: Villard Books, 2000), 162–63.
4   Martha G. Anderson and Christine Mullen Kreamer, *Wild Spirits, Strong Medicine* (New York: Center for African Art, 1989), 41.
5   Anderson and Mullen Kreamer, *Wild Spirits, Strong Medicine*, 49.

ularly important along coastal areas where trade takes place. Africans associate Europeans and other foreigners with the water creatures because of their appearance and the fact that they arrived by sea.

In Benin, the light-skinned European spirit is depicted as Olokun. The Portuguese visited Benin, bringing luxurious items like coral, cloth, and brass. These items became associated with Olokun in Benin. Olokun is king of *oba* (waters) and he works with Yemaya—in Santería you would not mention one without the other, thus I hyphenate the two. The oceans of the world into which rivers flow are a source of earthly wealth capable of helping economies, the environment, and of course our health.

Water spirits prefer exotic (imported or nonlocal) offerings. This lends a sense of eclecticism to African tradition. Olokun presides over the underwater realm. Olokun's symbols come from the riverbank, the place where earth and water meet. It is a liminal zone of mudfish, pythons, chalk, and clay—all of which are associated with him. Cowries and eagle feathers are used in Olokun rituals, and vessels made of riverbank clays are used in the sculptures that represent him.[6]

The underwater villages, and the spirits that inhabit them, are phenomenally wealthy. They are also mischievous and sometimes vengeful—drowning people and stealing children. Overall, they are considered more playful than dangerous. Water spirits have a strong preference for white. White befits Olokun as one of the cool, less aggressive orishas of Benin. The Olokun cult in Benin represents peace, purity, long life, prosperity, and happiness. Interestingly, the bronzes that record the riverain water spirits date from the ninth to the fifteenth century—this is prior to known European contact.[7]

Mami Wata

Mami Wata is a female siren-like spirit with followers in a large part of Africa, especially Southeastern Nigeria, as well as various locales in the diaspora. Mami Wata is seen as a light-skinned, long-haired, voluptuous half-woman, half-mermaid. Some people think her imagery was inspired by a German print of an Indian snake charmer. Mami Wata is one of

---

6   Anderson and Mullen Kreamer, *Wild Spirits, Strong Medicine*, 49–50.
7   Anderson and Mullen Kreamer, *Wild Spirits, Strong Medicine*, 50.

the most powerful female deities, and she is held in awe. I spoke with a Nigerian informant, whose people are the Igbo. She reported that she was raised to have a fear and great respect for Mami Wata. This informant lives in the United States now and is studying for her PhD, yet she still holds fast to the traditional beliefs about Mami Wata instilled by her parents. Mami Wata combines modern and traditional imagery and eclectic practices from around the world, including elements drawn from Christian, Hindu, Buddhist, and astrological beliefs.[8]

Basil (Sacred or Holy) "Tulsi" (*Ocimum sanctum*): A Sacred Herb of Obatala for Hearth and Home

Aromatherapy and alternative spirituality have a way of coming together to open up new dimensions in pleasure, health, and happiness. Like most people, I had a fixed perception of basil. In the West, we have a tendency to think of basil primarily as a culinary herb used in Thai and Italian cooking, or in a salad or perhaps a sandwich. In India, one species of basil is considered a sacred herb. The Latin word *basilicum* supports this Indian conception; *basilicum* translates roughly as "royal" or "princely." In India, the herb is commonly called tulsi. It is also referred to as *bhutagni* ("destroyer of demons"). Tulsi is thought of as a divine incarnation of a goddess; worshippers of Vishnu perceive the plant as the goddess Lakshmi; devotees of Rama see tulsi as Sita; and Krishna bhaktas view the herb as Vrinda, Radha, or Rukmini.

There are numerous legends, called *pura-katha* ("ancient tale") or *divya-katha* ("divine story") in India that revolve around sacred basil. In the *divya-katha* ("Churning of the Cosmic Ocean"), Vishnu obtains tulsi from the rough ocean waves as an aid to the health of all beings.

In Sanskrit, the sacred herb is regarded as an incarnation of Tulasi. Tulasi was the wife of a celestial being, blessed by Lord Krishna so everyone could worship her. Offerings are not complete unless they include Tulasi's blessings. Many types of incense are named for these goddesses, graced with the names Tulsi, Tulasi, Lakshmi, and Laxmi.

Obatala is an elder orisha of mountain and wood. He embodies *funfun* as a representation of all that is pure, balanced, cool, even-tempered, mysterious, deep, and immaculate. Orisha Obatala, one of the oldest and most respected orishas of the Yoruba pantheon, is master of the *funfun* realm. Obatala is beyond human emotions or concerns. He is one to visit to understand the authentic self. In these ways, he is a Yoruba spirit. Understandably, one of his esoteric herbs is basil, released by way of the water. To approach Obatala's energy, his basil must be used in baths, healing, and washes.[9] Obatala energy, released by the masa, is all that is pure, moral, strategic, intelligent, peaceful, ethical, and immaculate.

Healing Qualities of Tulsi

We will explore Obatala's esoteric herb, basil, in its sacred incarnation in India. Use of Indian herbs such as tulsi is greatly enhanced by a basic understanding of Ayurveda. According to Ayurvedic practice, the mind exerts profound influence on the body. A well-balanced, tranquil mind can free the body from illness. This is an absolute tenet of Ifá and many of the healing practices in the diaspora, particularly Jamaica. Acute awareness is central to achieving the necessary balance required for healing. The elements—as well as nature, talismans, amulets, and symbols—each play an important role in Ayurvedic healing.

One of the most promising qualities of Tulsi within the ancient Indian system of medicine is *moksa-prade*. *Moksa-prade* substances keep the body healthy and the mind free from worry, enabling concentration on spirituality and inner peace.

Basil is grown widely in the African diaspora. Several types of basil, including the standard *Ocimum basilicum,* called *eme* in Ghana, are grown in Ghana. In Ghana, eme is used to treat various ills. An infusion of the leaf is used warm to promote perspiration and break fever. It is also used to treat gas and as a carminative.[10]

Basil is looked upon as a panacea in Jamaica where East Indian influence is marked. Authors of *Jamaican Folk Medicine,* Payne-Jackson and Alleyne, highlight the qualities and uses of basil by Jamaicans of African descent:

- Basil is used as a vermifuge because of thymol, an anthelmintic, and eugenol[11]
- It is used as a treatment for tuberculosis because of the alpha-bisabolol it contains, which is antitubercular[12]
- Basil contains numerous constituents that ease the symptoms of colds, flu, fever,

---

9   Ra Un Nefer Amen, *Metu Neter* (Brooklyn, NY: Khamit, 1990), 267.
10 Abbiw, *Useful Plants of Ghana,* 162.
11 Payne-Jackson and Alleyne, *Jamaican Folk Medicine,* 168.
12 Payne-Jackson and Alleyne, *Jamaican Folk Medicine,* 167.

and bronchitis: including analgesics, expectorants, antibronchitic agents, and decongestants, as well as medicines to boost immunity and fight infection: antivirals and viricide.[13]

- Basil is used to treat mental illness and depression—the menthol it contains is a stimulant for the central nervous system.[14]
- An abscess, ulcer, and boil medicine is also contained in basil.[15]
- Basil is a panacea because of the anethole, which is an immunity booster.[16]
- Basil is useful to the Haitian people spiritually where it is hung in dried bunches for protection and as a tribute to Erzulie, lwa of love. The tea is consumed for a host of cross-cultural medicinal purposes as well.
- Basil is used as a headache treatment because of the anodyne it contains.[17]

Growing and Using Tulsi

Tulsi is a member of the Labiatae family of mints. Headquartered in Africa and Asia, it also thrives in the pleasant climate of the Caribbean. In South Africa it is called *basielkruid*. Transvaal basil, which is *O. canum*, is used for seasoning. Zulu basil grows in the Natal and Transvaal through tropical Africa, where it is used aromatically. Sweet basil is used in South Africa as a sedative, a treatment for headaches, and an aphrodisiac, as well as to relieve tension.[18]

In temperate zones, it can be grown from seed, beginning indoors during April in a moist, peaty soil. This herb is a vigorous grower, usually reaching eighteen inches tall. It should be placed outdoors in mid-June in pots or window boxes or directly in the garden. Grow tulsi outside your home or business as a natural amulet to encourage blessings and as a protective plant. Pinching back the top of the plant ensures healthy growth and prevents an unattractively tall, leggy appearance. Use pinched clippings in culinary or magical recipes.

---

13 Payne-Jackson and Alleyne, *Jamaican Folk Medicine*, 157.
14 Payne-Jackson and Alleyne, *Jamaican Folk Medicine*.
15 Payne-Jackson and Alleyne, *Jamaican Folk Medicine*, 149.
16 Payne-Jackson and Alleyne, *Jamaican Folk Medicine*, 166.
17 Payne-Jackson and Alleyne, *Jamaican Folk Medicine*, 176.
18 Palmer, *South African Herbal*, 120.

TULSI BUNDLES FOR PROSPERITY

A simple, fragrant, and magical use of tulsi is to create a natural amulet using a tied bundle of the herb.

Take a few clippings (approximately 10 to 12 inches long) from the plant, tie firmly in a bunch with a green (symbolizing healing, love, and life) ribbon. Hang the tulsi bundle upside down, away from direct sunlight or heat, in the home—especially the kitchen. Tulsi bundles attract prosperity, health, and good spirits. They are ideal for hanging just before the New Year or the changing of the seasons or in a new home or workspace.

RELAXING APHRODISIAC

To create a brew that is a stimulating aphrodisiac:

Steep a few tulsi leaves in 2 cups red wine overnight. Strain. Share a glass of this love potion with your partner or companion at room temperature.

TULSI FLOOR WASH

In many ATRs, particularly Candomblé (Brazil) and Hoodoo (United States), floor washes are used to spiritually cleanse the home and charge the air with a wealth of fragrances. We typically use Italian basil because it has been widely available. I suggest trying tulsi, now that it is more widely available, since it matches up with the conception of Obatala. This will help bring additional power and spiritual strength to the brew.

To create a tulsi floor wash, fill a stockpot loosely with fresh tulsi. Fill the pot almost to the top with water (rainwater will give this a special fertility energy). Bring the pot very close to a boil. Cover, reduce heat to low, and steep for 25 minutes. Remove from the heat and steep 10 more minutes. Strain to remove tulsi. Pour into a wash bucket. Add a few drops of chlorophyll (green food coloring used very sparingly is OK as a substitute; not too much colorant or you'll stain your floors). Add ¼ cup castile soap or Murphy's Oil Soap. Drop in 10 drops sacred basil essential oil. Mop floors.

This floor wash should bring good luck and prosperity as well as inspiring creativity. It is great for spring-cleaning or to spread blessings, hope, or the spirit of renewal.

White Willow (*Salix alba*)

Obatala addresses the white fluids of the body. White willow is another of Obatala's healing herbs. White willow grows in North Africa, Central Asia, Europe, and the Northeastern United States. It has rough gray bark and grows to seventy-five feet, though it is also maintained as a shrub.

White willow is a balancing herb associated with magic and witchcraft. It is also a plant with tremendous healing potential. For over two thousand years, white willow has been used to alleviate pain. It contains the constituent salicin, an aspirin-like medicine that helps reduce inflammation. Traditionally, willow has been used to treat rheumatism, internal bleeding, gum and tonsil inflammation, and eruptions, sores, burns, and wounds on the skin. The bark is collected in the spring. Between 1 and 3 teaspoons of bark is infused in cold water for 2 to 5 hours. Only 1 cup per day is recommended.[19]

---

19 John Lust, *The Herb Book* (New York: Bantam Books, 1974), 486.

Obatala White Mountain Elder and Clay

In Santería, Obatala is the father of orishas. He represents the traditional way of life, balance, and ideal character, also called *iwa*. Ashe is a type of mystical coolness. When Obatala's iwa and ashe come together, white clay immediately comes to mind, along with the unique healing medicines it possesses.

Rhassoul mud (also called ghassoul)—Africans and Africans in the Americas have a lengthy history of using clay for cleansing and nutrients. These days, there are numerous beauty products that contain rhassoul. Rhassoul is ancient clay believed to have formed millions of years ago. It is buried deep within the Atlas Mountains of Morocco. Rhassoul is called a swelling clay: it has a tremendous capacity to absorb water, herbal infusions, and oils. Rhassoul viewed in a mystical way is ancient earth plus Obatala (orisha of the mountains), brought to life by way of the masa, who imbue the clays with ashe. Rhassoul mud is an excellent cleanser and detoxifier for the hair and skin because of these qualities. Covering yourself in mud sounds more like a way of getting dirty, but it really does cleanse by drawing out impurities. Most mud formulas bring together the earth, air, and water elements. Rhassoul affords an excellent opportunity to encourage intimate contact with a wide variety of spirits including Obatala, Oshun, Yemaya-Olokun, Nut, and Isis. This of course would depend on the ritual performed in the creation of the mud, along with the selection of ingredients connected to individual deities or orishas.

Other clays—Mud baths are relaxing and help clear pimples that arise from hormonal fluctuations. Ran Knishinsky, author of *The Clay Cure,* touts the numerous benefits of eating clay—an activity that African and African American people have been engaged in for centuries. Pure white clay as an emblem of Obatala regulates the bowels, reduces headaches, and fights acne while also ridding the body of all sorts of toxins. Eating the refined pure clay, montmorillonite (also referred to as bentonite), is recommended as a part of inner cleaning regimens.[20]

---

20 Ran Knishinsky, *The Clay Cure: Natural Healing from the Earth* (Rochester, NY: Healing Art Press, 1998).

The Way of the Lotus

Lotus (*Nelumbo nucifera*)

Lotus plants and the oil extracted from them were held in high esteem in ancient Egypt. Women wore lotus flowers as hair ornaments, on necklaces, or on top of their heads. *Nymphaea caerulea* is the species most frequently depicted in Egyptian art. Pure lotus oil of the type favored by the Egyptians is believed to be extinct; nevertheless, the species currently available, *Nymphaea lotus,* is quite exquisite.

The scent and physical structure of the flower is likened to hyacinth, and it was used to symbolically refer to the sexuality of women. The white lotus, *Nymphaea lotus L.,* only blooms at night, a metaphor for sensuality and sexuality used by the Egyptians who thrived on puns. For the Egyptians, the lotus was synonymous with love and became the focus for the mythic tales of creation—after all, it grows in water.

Lotus represents the fertility and rich soil of the Nile. The blossoms were placed on statues of Osiris, god of vegetation and regeneration. The lotus was linked with the immortality attributed to Osiris and his son Horus. God of light and the soul, Horus was pictured with the lotus blossom in ancient art.

The plant oil is slightly narcotic, causing sedation, deep relaxation, and the release of anxiety and inhibitions when used at full strength. This type of lotus oil comes from blue, white, and pink flowers—each has a distinctive aroma. Pink is rare, highly sought-after, and quite expensive—its scent may also be an acquired taste as it is very unusual. I suggest the white or blue flower lotus oils as an introduction: they oscillate between earthy, watery, and ethereal. White or blue lotus oil is slightly musky and very sensual, with a distinct, though attractive, aroma.

The lotus was the primary accessory of women from the Old Kingdom until the decline of ancient Egyptian civilization. Of course, the Yoruba attribute the aromatic women's flower to our lady of sweet waters, Oshun. To access Oshun energy, remember that she appreciates invocation by way of water (lotus baths) as well as lotus oils and incense. Oshun's chakra is the pubic region. Using this flower will open this center while putting the user in touch with kundalini energy. It is also a perfect way to switch from the left or analytic/masculine brain to the right, which is considered more creative and feminine. Using lotus will inspire artistic projects and give the radiant energy of beauty to the living or working environment. Understanding the symbolic power of the lotus plants makes the journey into the asana (yoga poses) easier because it is truly a sublime plant.

The lotus is a celebrated plant among Australia's Aborigines and Africans, as well as in Asian cultures, particularly India. In Ghana, lotus is eaten and used medicinally. The ground parts of *N. lotus,* simply called water lily, are eaten. The stems and roots of *N. lotus* are infused in water to treat sexually transmitted infections (STIs). The leaves are prepared in Ghana as a lotion, whereas *N. micrantha, N. lotus,* and *N. maculata* are used decoratively.[21] Perhaps the reason this singular plant has captivated the imagination of many is that while lotus plants grow in water, the leaf itself never actually gets wet. In an ancient shloka from the Bhagavad Gita, the paradox of the lotus serves as a metaphor for human wisdom, also called *gyaani*—the lotus is described as remaining blissful, unfettered by our world of sorrow and change:

Brahmanyaadhaaya karmaani
Sangam tyaktvaa karoti yaha
Lipyate na sa paapena
Padma patram ivaambhasaa.

Roughly translated: "He who does things as an offering to Brahma, abandons attachment and is not tainted by sin, just as a lotus leaf remains unaffected by the water or mud it grows in."

Like the lotus flower, our bodies have energies described in the Yoga Shastra as chakras. Our chakras relate to lotus petals structurally. The sahasrara chakra (top of the head) opens when a yogi attains self-realization; this is represented by the lotus with a thousand petals opening to the light of the sun.

The lotus is a symbol for the relationship between creation and spirituality. A lotus grew from the navel of Lord Vishnu. Lord Brahma originated from it and went on to create the universe from his lotus home.

---

21 Abbiw, *Useful Plants of Ghana,* 147, 152.

Papyrus, Called *Mhyt* or *Twfy* in Ancient Egyptian, *Burdi* in Modern Arabic[22]

Papyrus once grew abundantly in Egypt along the River Nile. The aquatic plant called papyrus is very attractive. The stem grows ten to fourteen feet tall and is triangular in cross-section, with several short-fibered leaves growing around its base. It is smooth, without any knots, and tapers gently toward a flowering cluster that is quite large, fragile, and tassel-shaped. The plant grows abundantly in stagnant shallows of lakes and rivers in many parts of Africa.[23]

Thin coats or pellicles of the papyrus, from which the paperlike substance is made, are separated with a long pin or pointed mussel shell and spread on a table that has a thin layer of water. The first layer is followed by a cross-layered sheet. Papyrus is a very productive plant; as many as twenty-two strips can be pulled from a single stalk. It was a very popular writing surface from the fifth to the third century BCE.[24] Each layer was laid in an opposite direction to the previous one, eventually forming the dense fiber that was durable and strong. The fiber was woven into sails and cloth mats or twisted and used to make rope and straps for sandals. Papyrus was used as a jar top and to make children's balls. The mature stems were the ideal foundation for elegant bouquets, so beloved by the ancient Egyptians in their temple and tomb decorations. Herodotus tells how the lower part of the plant, about half a meter, was eaten as a delicacy, particularly when baked in a clay vessel over an open fire.[25] Papyrus was the main writing material used in Egypt for approximately four thousand years. It was used for many purposes including receipts, petitions, and private and official letters.[26] The Egyptians chewed papyrus raw and boiled or roasted it; they would swallow the juice and spit out the quid, just as their contemporary counterparts utilize sugarcane today in Egypt. In pharaonic medicine, papyrus was used with other herbs to created cast-like bandages to secure limbs. The plant was also used to make eye compresses. The Copts used the ashes of the plant to make tooth powder. They also treated tumors with the ash of the plant. In Islamic medicine, the ash of papyrus is applied to open wounds to dry them out and used to treat mouth ulcers; it is also macerated with vinegar to make a poultice for nosebleed.[27]

---

22 Manniche, *Ancient Egyptian Herbal,* 99.
23 Vance Studley, *The Art and Craft of Handmade Paper* (New York: Dover, 1977), 16–17.
24 Studley, *Art and Craft of Handmade Paper.*
25 Manniche, *Ancient Egyptian Herbal,* 99.
26 Sophie Dawson, *The Art and Craft of Papermaking* (Asheville, NC: Lark Books, 1992).
27 Manniche, *Ancient Egyptian Herbal,* 99–100.

In contemporary Egypt the ashes of the papyrus plant continue to have many healing applications quite similar to those found in ancient times. Ashes of the plants are used to check malignant ulcers, keeping them from spreading in the mouth or throat. The plant is macerated with vinegar and burned, then used to treat wounds.[28]

Many artists, including me, continue to utilize this strong earth-water substance for painting, writing, and drawing. Healers can use their own creativity writing out love spells on papyrus with dove's blood or dragon's blood ink to conjure. Incantation or invocation of the ancient Egyptian god Horus or goddesses Isis or Nut would be effective using the same materials, as would a call to Oshun if you need her energy.

Luckily, papyrus is still widely available in many countries as a prepared surface, ready to use for gift-giving, writing out petitions, creating magical squared amulets, spellwork, letter writing, and other creative ways of touching the spirit of others.

The following lwas and orishas are the incarnation of various energies of the sea.

Yemaya-Olokun

Sea mother and father orishas Yemaya-Olokun have a variety of medicines, healing energy, and nourishment swirling about them in the sea. Since we have previously visited Olokun, we now go to Yemaya to learn of her possibilities. Yemaya is the first of the many sea mothers of the African diaspora. Her symbol is the round fan because in the Ifá kingdom she restored peace between the orishas numerous times. The round fan suggests the vessel that carries sustenance, as it is similar in shape to the rounded home used by many African people, the cast-iron pot used to create nurturing meals, the rounded belly of pregnancy, and its symbol the calabash. Yemaya is also noted for protection and mystic retribution against evil, as are many riverain orishas and goddesses.[29] Yemaya in her various other incarnations is intimately connected to the art of transformation—she is the witches and sorcerers' orisha. In a broader way, she is creatrix and Great Mother. Thus, like the more frightening Kali, she is orisha of life and death. All these aspects explain why the water orishas, gods,

---

28 Boulos, *Medicinal Plants of North Africa*, 82.
29 Thompson, *Flash of the Spirit*, 73.

and goddesses are loved and feared. It is important to understand her complexity and not just see her as one-dimensional.

Yemaya is associated with the sexual and reproductive organs. Her ewe includes kelp, spirulina, plantain, and peppermint (discussed in depth in chapter 12).

Agwe

Olokun's Haitian counterpart is Agwe, king of the sea. Agwe is married to Lasiren and is guardian of seafaring vessels. He is the ideal husband image: strong and sustaining like the sea. Like the undulating waves, Agwe's energy is sexual, sensual, dangerous, riveting, and deeply spiritual. Agwe likes seashells, seagrass, white chickens, sea glass, and stones from the ocean.[30]

Labalen—Whale

Labalen is a whale lwa who is the protective womb and a nurturer that holds sea energy. Her body can encompass, protect, or devour us. She moves from the water's depths and can also travel the crossroads. Labalen appreciates algae like the blue-green spirulina we will discuss soon, as well as fish, octopus, ambergris, whale images, and salt water.[31]

Fish

Fish have always held a place in our spiritual symbolism and on our soul food menus. Many African people flourished on coastal regions, and when we were enslaved we were first brought to the coastal towns with useful ports for transport. When I was growing up, my family, clustered on the Northeastern Coast of the United States, ate plenty of freshwater

30 Glassman, *Vodou Visions,* 122–23.
31 Glassman, *Vodou Visions,* 121–22.

fish like bass, sunfish, and pike; we were also in close proximity to the Atlantic, so we could have ample blue crab, whiting, and porgy. Each season we were given cod-liver oil as an immunity builder and systemic tonic. Today we know that fish, particularly the cold-water ocean fish, have numerous vitamins, minerals, and healthful oils like essential fatty acids, which assure cardiovascular health and total well-being. It is just important to know the source of the fish to make sure they have not been contaminated by human activities.

Salts

While it is true that salt is overused in processed food and when we eat outside the home, salt remains an elixir of life that plays an important role in our health and healing. Salt has gained a bad rap as a contributor to high blood pressure and obesity, yet several important research projects have shown that there is nothing wrong with salt used in moderation; the fault is more in the lifestyle of abstaining from whole foods while eating mostly processed food. I use salt for regenerative baths and several different types of sea salt, sparingly, in meal preparation. I recommend natural flavor enhancers such as herbs, lemon, and other citrus fruit to add sass to a meal, with a sprinkling of choice sea salts used frugally.

Salt is one of few known substances used as a preservative in ancient times. Egyptian mummies were preserved in a saltwater solution called natron or "birth fluid." Salt was accepted as a substitute in Egyptian burial rites for a mother's regenerative blood since it comes from the sea (womb).[32] There are a wide array of types and sources of salt.

Sea salt, or sodium chloride—the crystallized compound that comes from the ocean, such as the fine white salt that comes from the Pacific Ocean. Sea salt is harvested from seawater.

Table salt—to which iodine is added, is bleached and refined and contains anticaking agents. Salt is harvested from inland deposits left by ancient oceans in a mining process to yield table salt.

---

32 Walker, *Woman's Encyclopedia*, 886.

Kosher salt—can be fine- or coarse-grained. It does not contain additives, but that is not why it is called *kosher*. It is kosher salt because it is permissible to use it to cure kosher meats. Kosher salt absorbs more moisture because of the large surface area of the grains. I find that it needs to be used very sparingly to avoid oversalting food.

Sel gris (gray sea salt)—comes coarse or fine. It contains clay from the salt marshes from which it is harvested. It is naturally high in minerals like magnesium. It is slightly moist and processed mechanically.

Fleur de sel (flower of salt)—a hand-raked gray salt rich in minerals. It is a gourmet salt, used for adding a finishing touch to a dish near the end of cooking to preserve its natural sweetness.

Dead Sea salts—renowned for their therapeutic benefits since ancient times because of their high mineral content:

- Magnesium combats stress and fluid retention and serves as an antioxidant.
- Calcium prevents water retention, increases the circulation, and strengthens fingernails.
- Potassium energizes the body and balances skin moisture.
- Bromides ease muscle stiffness and relax the nervous system.
- Sodium is important for lymphatic fluid balance.

Benefits of Dead Sea salts have been proven in several clinical trials,[33] showing them to be beneficial to patients with osteoarthritis, tendonitis, and psoriasis in as few as 3 to 4 baths a week at a very low dilution (5 percent for skin ailments and up to 10 percent dilution for osteoarthritis and tendonitis). You can calculate the desired concentration of your solution by weight and volume, or consult packaging instructions on purchased salts.

---

33 J. Arndt, "Salt from the Promised Land Helps Psoriasis Patients," *Ärztliche Praxis* 34, no. 48 (1982); I. Machtey, "Dead Sea Balneotherapy in Osteoarthritis," *Proceedings of International Seminar on Treatment of Rheumatic Diseases* (1982); and Amy K. McNulty, "Salt Information FAQ Sheet."

Kelp (*Alaria esculenta*), ewe of Yemaya (the orisha that affects the breasts)—is another name for various seaweeds. Kelps include *wakame* and *kombu*[34] (*Laminaria japonica kombu*) and are sometimes called bladder wrack. Kelps contain alginic acid, which detoxifies by removing heavy metals and radioactive isotopes from the digestive tract and bones. Kombu is being investigated in relation to the low breast cancer rate in postmenopausal Japanese women. Evidence suggests it may reduce estrogen; lower estrogen levels provide less fuel for estrogen-dependent cancers like breast cancer. Sea vegetables contain ten to twenty times more minerals and vitamins than land vegetables. Kombu contains vitamins A, B, B$_{12}$, C, and E. Kelp is added to various foods like sushi and miso soup. It is also wonderful in hydrotherapy. I recommend the dried, sifted kelp as an additive to healing bath soaks.

Dulse (*Rhodymenia palmata*)—is a type of kelp that shares a similarity with blackstrap molasses; it is very high in iron. It is also high in calcium, one of the most abundant mineral elements in the body, with a key function to aid our health, strength, and vitality.

Irish moss (*Chondrus crispus*)—also called carrageenan, is a stabilizing and gelling agent in many foods, including puddings, soups, and ice cream. Irish moss is used magically to bring good fortune and it is used cosmetically as a hair gel. Decocting ⅓ cup dried Irish moss per 4 cups water creates hair gel. Simmer 20 minutes, and let steep and thicken an additional 20 minutes. Strain and use immediately.

Spirulina—a blue-green microalga containing beta-carotene, an antioxidant. The green color is from chlorophyll. Dried, sifted spirulina is added to smoothies, soups, and teas by the level teaspoon. It is used in some weight-sustaining and weight-loss formulas. Spirulina is also used in immunity-building formulas to fight cancer, the effects of AIDS, and diabetes.

Preparation and uses for seaweed: To use in a cooked dish such as beans, soups, or grains (rice is popular), the dried seaweed needs to be soaked first. Each packet has its own directions; recommended soaking time varies from 10 to 20 minutes.

---

34 Kombu has been shown in some tests to interfere with thyroid function and contribute to the formation of goiters. It is not recommended for the treatment of HIV/AIDS.

Libations

Libations are liquids that contain ashe, poured on the earth or in bodies of water while saying a praise chant or invocation to request the blessings of various orishas or deities. Libations suitable to the orishas discussed in this chapter are:

Fresh water—for Oshun energy or to consult with the masa.

Sweet waters—like cologne, Florida water, rosewater, orange water, and lavender water, as well as potions of Oshun.

Salt water—belongs to Yemaya-Olokun, Agwe, the simbi, Lasiren, and Labalen. Salt water, considered the tear of Isis, is also suitable to her.

Use this holistic healing method to invoke water spirit when assisting others in recovery, replenishment, and repair of a mental, physical, or spiritual nature.

CHAPTER 10

The Sacred Wood

TREE MEDICINES IN FOCUS

- Pines
- Oaks
- Iroko
- Kapok / mapou / silk cotton tree
- *Helichrysum gymnocephalum* (DC.) H. Humb
- *Psiadia altissima* (DC.) Benth and Hook
- *Bryophyllum proliferum* (Bowie) ex Hook, Crassulaceae
- *Brachylaena ramiflora* (DC.) Humbat, Asteraceae
- *Sigesbeckia orientalis* L., Asteraceae
- Shea
- Cacao
- Neem
- Pau d'arco
- Banana
- Plantain
- Avocado
- Guava
- Pineapple
- Soursop
- Sweetsop
- Custard apple
- Peach
- Mango
- Magnolia
- Palms
- Coconut

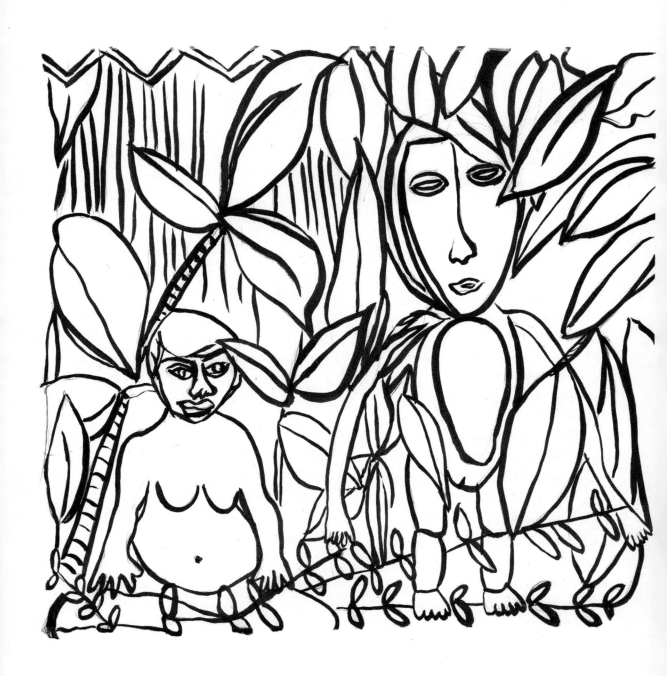

A Piney Story

I'm sure you have heard the idioms before "hicks from the sticks," "country bumpkin," or just plain "hick" (to rhyme with *stick*, of course)—meaning people who hail from the forest. Most people from the Pine Barrens are called Pineys, so here is my Piney story.

I never really felt shame about being associated with the forest. Just as in fairy tales, where the wood holds mystery and magic that take place nowhere else, so too is my story of the wood.

I owe my early affiliation with the woods for my patience, willingness to search, and love of mystery. These are three woods-acquired habits that led to my passion for art, writing, and dance. Some of the folks that would visit us were afraid for the sun to set on them in the wood; they were much older than me. Now that I've matured, I understand the reason. These were Black folk, our relatives, whose relatives in turn had heard of the lynching in trees, and some were directly affected. This connection between human and tree is the grim story of the way people—innocent or sometimes not—would find judge, jury, and ultimately punishment hanging from a tree. It is shameful that a people could turn tree-loving people against the wood, but this is just what happened to a certain extent in the case of my people.

Billie Holiday sang to perfection a bittersweet song written by Jewish English teacher and political activist from the Bronx, Abel Meeropol, called "Strange Fruit." This song, which *Time* magazine named "Song of the Century," is an ode to the lynched person, casting a spotlight on injustice. Rich in metaphor, "Strange Fruit" likens the swinging, dull, lifeless bodies of our people to a strange fruit. Deep inside, I could never fault anyone, particularly a Black man of an older generation, for being afraid of the wood. This fear is the source of some of our "*country*" blues, and I don't mean that in a musical way; rather, it is the malaise we feel in colonized lands that was not present in the same way in the Motherland. We feared animals, reptiles, wild spirits, and foreign warrior clans, but not aliens who would kill us simply because of the color of our skin.

I am undeterred. While others have made their way in the urban jungle, my grounding and centering remains in the forest, as lush and mysterious as it is forgiving yet foreboding.

Trees of Life

When those folks would come and go from our home in the summer after a weekend barbecue, they would take off from the three swamp oaks; wacky and weird as those trees are, they were still an emblem of home. To this day the trio of oaks bear marks: the marks of my siblings and me as we played games growing up, our numerous dogs' and cats' scratches on them, cars as well as a few pickup trucks that came too close to the trees in their hurry to return to the bright lights of the big city.

For us, trees, with their medicinal bark, their shade so cool, the breeze from their leaves always welcome, served as visual markers. Trees are my way of knowing where I am, where I am going, and where I have been in a personal and historical way. Growing up in Salem County, one of the annual field trips during grade school was to see our old oak tree, with its ever-widening girth and tales of how it began its life over four hundred years ago. Salem County is rich in history; it is one of the original colony's oldest counties, established in 1694. The tree is believed to be the place where John Fenwick signed a treaty with the local native group, the Lenni Lenape, to purchase the land. Since 1681, the Religious Society of Friends (an offshoot of the Quakers) has owned and maintained the land where the tree grew. It has been a Friends burial ground for hundreds of years. At the seat of the county, the Salem Oak there was an anchor for the town; people died, and stores closed, but the tree was an emblem of continuity in a sea of change for hundreds of years, having finally passed on in 2019.

For years I internalized all of these connections to the wood; they were there, but I didn't quite understand the feelings until moving to a loft in the inner city in Chicago's Mexican American Pilsen community, where there was barely a tree over five years old. I literally thought I would die. How would I know when it was winter, when spring was just about to return, or even when the sun was about to set, without trees? Trees are my marker—a guidepost in life. Our home on the lake has been demolished so that the wetlands can be preserved. The area is earmarked to become a state preserved area. Nothing is left, except memories and the trees that I grew up with. The last time I visited the area, a magnificent wild holly with a wonderfully triangular growth was in full color, covered in rich red berries.

The state tree of Illinois is a reminder of home—it is an oak. It is no mistake that the urban place where I now reside has an entire department of forestry to manage the trees of the urban forest, and it has been noted by the National Arboretum Society as one of the country's top tree towns. Where else could I live? Outside my house is a weird and wonderfully twisted oak tree that lets me know the time of day, the season, and the mood of our land. This chapter explores the trees (and a few treelike large plants) of the greatest importance to people of the Motherland. We begin with the humble pine—another tree of my heart and home.

Uplifting Pine: A Closer Look

In the early days of life in the Americas, African slaves, sharecroppers, and freemen insisted that a tree was planted on a burial site. The tree was usually a conifer that served as a reminder of the persistence of life. The trunk, branches, and leaves exist in the realm of humans, while the life force of the tree—the roots—lies beneath the earth. Evergreens are a metaphor for the interaction between departed spirits and their living community.

According to Professor Robert Farris Thompson in *Flash of the Spirit*,[1] pine (*Pinus* spp.) and spruce (*P. picea*) trees in particular play a key role in traditional Southern US burials—this owing to their availability in the region. To early Black Americans, the green scent of evergreen trees contained *medicine* to heal the body and the spirit. Ethnobotanist Dr. Faith Mitchell lists a variety of conditions pine treated in *Hoodoo Medicine*: stuffy nose, fever, stomachache, whooping cough, bacteria, parasites, and fatigue. The indigenous people of the Southeast Coast used pine tar for swelling, burns, itching, sore throats, colds, and consumption; these applications influenced African American root doctors as well.

The German Expanded Commission E states that while various pines have been used medicinally, including shoots of black spruce, dwarf pine, and longleaf pine, a medicinal-grade pine needle oil is derived from the steam-distilled essential oil of *Pinus sylvestris L.*, taken from fresh needles, branch tips, or a combination. The commission approves pine needle oil used therapeutically as a treatment for catarrhal diseases of the respiratory tract and externally as a rub for rheumatic and neuralgic ailments, and recognizes its use as a fragrance in cough and cold remedies. Those with bronchial asthma or whooping cough are advised against using it. Irritation of skin or mucous membranes might occur with the use of pine, so testing and observation periods are important before using therapeutically. Recommended as an aromatherapy agent, several drops of the oil are added to hot water and

---

1   Thompson, *Flash of the Spirit*.

the steam inhaled.[2] Use according to an ND or herbalist's prescription, or in self-treatment infusion; the ratio should be at 2 grams pine needle to 150 milliliters water. Tinctures should be 1.5 (g/mL) to 10 mL alcohol solution. Pine is available as a prepared product and I have listed some of those later; it is also included in various soaps (pine tar), shampoos, conditioners, baths, and salt soaks, as well as prepared as an ointment rub.

My grandfather, who was born on a plantation in Virginia in the late 1800s, used tiny portions of oil of turpentine, a by-product of pine, as an antiseptic. In fact, he swore by the stuff, claiming it could make just about anything feel better, from a cut to the common cold.

The Pine Barrens are so named because they contain many stands of pine forests as well as pine/oak forests. The entire lower half of New Jersey is designated as a pine plain, and the trees grow readily there. Alloway, the tiny town where I grew up, is one of the isolated, outer areas of the Pine Barrens. Pine was all around and thankfully it remains so. On our drives to the (sea) shore, you could see the sparse forests of pine. Sometimes they had succumbed to spontaneous fire; burnt wood springing from marshes and swamplands lend an eerie quality with the aura of spirit realm. Directly outdoors behind our home was a sparse forest, populated by pine. It was used as a wall covering (knotty pine), for firewood, and to clear our environment. In addition to the indigenous holly and laurels I have mentioned, wild blueberry bushes also grow quite well. The trees of the barrens include:

- Shortleaf pine (*Pinus echinata*)
- Virginia pine (*P. virginiana*)
- Red cedar (*Juniperus virginia*)
- Black oak (*Quercus velutina*)
- White oak (*Q. alba*)
- Chestnut oak (*Q. prinus*)
- Post oak (*Q. stellata*)
- Blackjack oak (*Q. marilandica*)
- Scarlet oak (*Q. coccinea*)
- Southern red oak (*Q. falcata*)[3]

---

2   American Botanical Council, "Pine Needle Oil," in *Expanded Commission E report.*
3   Jack McCormick, "The Vegetation of the New Jersey Pine Barrens," in *Pine Barrens: Ecosystem and Landscape,* ed. Richard T. T. Forman (New Brunswick, NJ: Rutgers Univ. Press, 1998).

Prayer for the Cedar
Our greatest hope was that this land would not be developed and filled with condominiums or luxury homes. The goddess has granted this wish.

Working the Pine

When my mother was nesting, she used pine floor wash to prepare for her new baby. Pine floor wash makes the home feel energized and has some antibacterial agents, lending further to the feeling of freshness. This is a tradition I continued with the birth of my children and to the present day when there is a stale feeling to the air. Many African Americans grew up with the smell of freshly scrubbed floors, tiles, and bathrooms. Some now reach out for commercial products, but it is not really necessary; as you will see in a bit, you can easily prepare your own pine-scented products.

When I am cooped up indoors, in the middle of winter, my spirits grieve the lively spirit of autumn. Pine floor wash has a remarkable influence on the emotions. The floor washes below are recommended as a winter tonic and for grief, mild depression, and fatigue. These two updated formulas featuring essential oils are antibiotic, antiseptic, and antifungal.

LIFT-ME-UP PINE FLOOR WASH

An infusion of pine needles treats cold symptoms when taken as tea. Pine infusion makes a fine hair rinse or a mouthwash for sore throats and laryngitis. Chewing white pine freshens breath; the needles contain vitamin C.

Clip and fill a stockpot ¾ full of pliable shoots from spruce, pine, or juniper trees (can be a combination). Bring to a boil. Reduce to medium-low, cover, and decoct 25 minutes. Cool, then strain. Drop in essential oils: ½ teaspoon white pine (*Pinus sylvestris*), ¼ teaspoon lemon (*Citrus limonum*), and ¼ teaspoon juniper (*Juniperus communis*) oils. Add 3 tablespoons liquid castile soap.

Sprinkle Pine Floor Wash on a broom, and sweep. Or dip a mop into a bucket of Pine Floor Wash and cleanse the environment physically and spiritually.

Prepared Products

The Grandpa Soap Co.'s pine tar shampoo treats scalp disorders that arise from drying winter winds. Pine soap helps dry, itchy, flaky skin.[4]

Kneipp makes an uplifting pine bath useful for replenishing energy drained by winter holidays.

Tree Whisperers

Even in the United States, where enslaved Africans suffered what was arguably the greatest spiritual restriction and ardent conversion to some form of Christianity, people found sanctuary for their spirituality amid the brush and arbors of the deep forest. It was to the forest that early African Americans stole away to form congregations to sing and pray.[5] As the practice of tree-talking demonstrates, we also maintained the custom of communication and learning based on tree knowledge.

Masters of Jiridon

Learning the proper way to mix plants and the elements takes many lessons. The lessons are not taught through an apprenticeship with a human, as much as they are learned directly from the trees and plants themselves. Jiridon is the science of the trees. To learn Jiridon, the seeker, whether hunter, warrior, or shaman, must spend ample time alone in the wilderness, observing the workings of nature, including the expression of animals and the whispers of the trees.

In early African American historical accounts, there are reports of people who spoke the language of the trees; they were called tree whisperers. Tree whisperers in the United States spend time living with and studying a single tree. The apprenticeship takes place with nature, not a human, as is the custom in most paths. Tree whisperers are highly observant. They listen attentively to the reactions the tree has to the lashing of wind and its reactions to sunny, warm days. Eventually the tree whisperer can hear the tree speaking quite

---

4   Warning: pine is a known allergen. Wear gloves when handling pine essential oils and test skin for allergic reaction twenty-four hours before use. Not advised for sensitive skin; most people should use pine products sparingly.
5   Fett, *Working Cures*.

clearly to them. The tree teaches those who will listen to be Masters of Jiridon. Masters of Jiridon are also master herbalists and adept ecologists.

In 1930 Ruth Bass, a white Mississippian, collected a fascinating firsthand account of a tree talker in the Bayou Pierre swamplands. I share the story of the ancient practice, told by African American tree talker Old Divinity, in *Sticks, Stones, Roots & Bones: Hoodoo, Mojo & Conjuring with Herbs.* According to the folklorist Bass, "the basis of tree-talking is to develop fellowship with a particular tree—any type of tree will do. It is simply magic, a magic that is still found in the Bayou Pierre swampland today (as of 1930s)."[6]

Working the Oak

There is a magical type of oak called live oak (*Quercus virginiana*) that has become a part of the spiritual ethos of the Gullah people. On the Gullah islands, there are forests where oak dominates, often moss-draped, making it seem evergreen. There is a huge serpentine live oak on John's Island, South Carolina, called Angel Oak. Live oaks spread rather than grow upward, so the tree is 65 feet tall and 160 feet wide, creating enough shade for 17,100 square feet. The tree branches go underground and resurface, lending it the distinctive air of a grove rather than being a single tree. Angel Oak predates the planter family for which it was named and the enslaved people whose spirits claimed it. The tree is haunted by the souls of murdered African Americans who were lynched on it. The tree societies I have spoken with, brought to the area to work the land, came to be known as the Gullah people because of the unique customs and dialect they retained from Africa. After lynching, people who had the caul (a gift for seeing into the spirit realm) saw spirits in and near the tree. The Gullah call these spirits angels and go to the tree to make offerings and pray, just as our people have done and continue to do in the Motherland. Angel Oak can be visited free of charge. It is the oldest tree east of the Mississippi. Having begun its life during the time of King Arthur, Angel Oak is believed to be more than 1,400 years old.[7] If the idea of "Strange Fruit" makes your spirit ache, perhaps you would like to go pay homage to the spirit of those bereaved people by making a discreet offering at Angel Oak in South Carolina.

---

6   Bird, *Sticks, Stones, Roots & Bones.*
7   T. Pakenham, *Remarkable Trees of the World* (New York: W.W. Norton & Company, 2003), 142.

Igboro-Egun: Trees in Africa and the New World

Pine and cedar were readily available to us as newly transported enslaved people in North America. The use of trees for spirit medicine and religious observance is a very important part of African culture. The Yoruba people make groves, which are regarded as sacred, to honor some of the deities and to serve as consecrated workshops. The ancestral groves are called *Igboro-Egun* ("grove of the ancestors") and are sacred to the spirit of the ancestors. Another type of grove is specifically for orishas, for example the *Igbo Osayin* is a sacred grove of the orisha of herbalism, Osayin. The omiyolo tree and the iporogun and atori shrubs are among the most sacred trees to the Yoruba.

Before cutting down a tree, one must address the tree spirits because evil spirits can also dwell in trees, according to Yaya Diallo, a master drummer of the Bamana. In his book *The Healing Drum*, Diallo tells the story of a family that became mentally ill because they did not adequately follow the protocol for tending to the tree spirits. A tamarind tree next to this particular family's home held spirits that were not evil or good. When the father of the family died, the children decided to cut down the tree. Two of the children became disturbed and irrational as soon as the tree was cut. After the spirits lost their tree house, they did not want to live alone, so they decided to live within the children and family on whose property the tree grew. Diallo reports that their speech was incomprehensible and they cried without provocation.[8]

The Bamana people, which Diallo refers to as Minianka, live in a southeastern circle of Koutiala and Yorosso between the Bani River and the Banifing River. The Minianka subgroup of the Senufo tribe lives in Southeastern Mali or Côte d'Ivoire and Northwest Burkina Faso. *Minianka* means "those who refuse the master"[9] and refers to the fact that the fierce warriors of the area would not relinquish their land or freedom during the French conquest. The people remain primarily animists; they have refused to adopt Islam, a major religion of the area, or Christianity, the minority religion.[10] According to Diallo, "Cultivating a great respect for nature is the ultimate goal of all the customs concerning the sacred wood."[11]

---

8   Diallo and Hall, *Healing Drum,* 61.
9   Diallo and Hall, *Healing Drum,* 8.
10 Diallo and Hall, *Healing Drum,* 9.
11 Diallo and Hall, *Healing Drum,* 20–21.

Diallo makes outsiders privy to a fascinating custom of the people of Fienso and Minianka villages, the idea of the firstborn tree grove. A small forest or grove, in the middle of which you can find a special tree called the firstborn, is a characteristic of villages of the Fienso and Minianka people. These groups of people believe trees and plants have ancestors just as humans do. The firstborn is considered the first plant of the creator god, called Kle, and it is the ancestor of all the other plants in the area. Entire groves exist to offer sanctuary to the firstborn. Only the most qualified initiates know exactly which plant is the firstborn and it is shrouded in secrecy. Most often no one can enter the sacred wood carrying metal (like an axe to cut down a tree or plant) or matches. Some folks believe evil spirits shelter in the wood, so it is unwise to enter without a spiritually grounded guide. Severe punishments are dispensed to anyone who dares to disturb the growth or habit of the firstborn tree of the sacred grove.[12] If the sacred wood burns, it is considered a very bad omen for the entire community. If such a catastrophe were to occur, a great effort would need to be made to save the firstborn tree so that its role as ancestor to the forest would be preserved, allowing the area to thrive.[13]

Iroko: Brazilian Tree of the Sacred Wood

When Africans were transported to various areas of the New World, we brought our belief systems with us; stripped bare of physical contact or the social positions held in the Motherland, we nevertheless maintained a strong oral history that held our ATRs. We observed the healing ways of the indigenous people to the areas where we were transplanted, but the development of African Caribbean and African American ethnomedicines were not taught to us by others; we adapted our ways to a new land as other immigrants have. By and large, we learned through experimentation, testing, and direct observation, as has been the way of herbalists and shamans around the world from time immemorial.

The notion of the sacred tree offers a good example. Iroko (*Chlorophora excelsa*) is one of the most respected spiritual trees of Brazil, inspired by oloko, the sacred silk cotton tree of West Africa. In Candomblé, oloko represents the god of time and eternity since he resides within the tree. The male deity of time is also associated with peace and settling disputes between humans. Temples were built wherever it grew. The New World iroko germinates

12 Diallo and Hall, *Healing Drum*, 20.
13 Diallo and Hall, *Healing Drum*, 21.

spontaneously, growing quick and strong where other trees take their time, lending even more mysticism to the tree.

This approach to trees harkens back to the Yoruba liturgical plant taxonomy, a notion that, though sharing some resemblance to Native American, Amerindian, and fellow indigenous practices, remains distinct. The Yoruba evaluate medicine primarily based on the sensory attributes of the tree, what it does, how it appears, and how it grows and moves, as well as its countenance, smell, and feel.

Professor Robert Voeks gives an intricate analysis of the Yoruba relationship to the forest and its development in the New World of Brazil in *Sacred Leaves of Candomblé*. According to Voeks, the type of belief system the Yoruba brought with them to Brazil was animistic to the core. Unlike universal religions of conversion and salvation like Christianity and Islam, which use proselytizing, spiritual hegemony, and geographic expansion as central codes of belief, the Yoruba have a system that is firmly rooted to place. The Yoruba deities, called orishas in West Africa and orixa in Candomblé of Brazil, are nature gods and goddesses (as well as a few hermaphrodites) that personify the elements: wind, thunder, water, trees, and soil. Reverence and meaning are attached to sacred places and parts of nature, including villages, hillsides, forests, mountains, rivers, the sea, stones, and specific trees.

Voeks calls the Yoruba belief system "myopic" and describes it as a closed and fixed religion, where close inspection to details of the land dominates. Enslaved Africans in Brazil successfully introduced their sacred trees, obi (*Cola acuminata*) and akoko (*Newbouldia laevis*).[14] Other trees with a significant place in their ritual and ceremonies were also established.

While there is similarity between the climates, terrain plant families, and genera of some areas of Brazil and West Africa, not all of the spiritually significant liturgical plants could be transplanted. Substitutes were made and added to the oeuvre of Candomblé medicines. A Brazilian substitute for the African iroko is usually *Ficus* spp. or *Gameleira branca*. Both trees are in the mulberry family; both bleed latex when cut. They are formidable, broad, commanding trees with multiple niches and buttresses, just right for placing offerings to the spirits, ancestors, and various deities. Latex from iroko has many medicinal applications, including the reduction of swellings[15] and tumors.[16]

---

14 Robert Voeks, *Sacred Leaves of Candomblé: African Magic, Medicine, and Religion in Brazil* (Austin: Univ. of Texas Press, 2010), 160–61.
15 Abbiw, *Useful Plants of Ghana*, 191.
16 Abbiw, *Useful Plants of Ghana*, 194.

Silk Cotton Tree (*Ceiba pentandra L. Gaertn*)

The silk cotton tree is a native of South America, but now it has spread to primary rainforests of West Africa and parts of Asia. It goes by many names, including ceiba (pronounced "say-ba") tree. This tree holds a lofty position in West Africa and New World healing medicines. It is a massive, rapidly growing deciduous tree that can reach more than eighty feet and in some regions up to two hundred feet tall and a diameter of five to eight feet above its buttresses. The buttresses are up to ten feet tall and extend ten feet from the trunk. Large spines grow from the trunk, discouraging damage to the trunk and lending a spiritual aura to the tree.

Silk cotton tree is called an emergent tree, since it is the tallest tree of the Amazon rainforest and it plays a very important place in the rainforest ecosystem. The tree is broad, with a flat crown of horizontal branches. The leaves are palmate compound with five to nine lance-shaped leaflets that range from three to eight inches long. The tree loses all its leaves in the tropical dry season (winter in the northern hemisphere). During the wet season, it produces five-part white-to-pink-colored flowers in dense clusters, blooming before leaves appear. The interior wood is pale pink to ash brown with a straight grain.

The tree hosts many aerial plants, insects, birds, frogs, and other animals and plants that use its height to obtain sunlight. Silk cotton tree produces three-to-six-inch-long elliptical fruits. The fruits contain numerous seeds encased in a dense mat of cotton-like fiber. The fibers are dispersed into the air when the fruit ripens like downy snowflakes. The fibers are largely made of cellulose; they are light and airy and resistant to water penetration, with a low thermal conductivity. While silk cotton tree fibers cannot be woven, they are used as a stuffing fiber; to insulate, pad, and create life preserves; and for stuffing mattresses and pillows. The oil is very useful for cosmetics, massage, and hair and skin care.

Libaka, Ngombe Tree of Covenants

Libaka is the name for silk cotton trees used by the Ngombe people of the Democratic Republic of Congo. Libaka is the sacred tree that serves as a symbol for the union between the seen and unseen worlds. It is the site where the living community converges with the ancestors.

When a new village is being established, it cannot become an official living space until the chief plants Libaka. At the end of the first hunt, each hunter cuts a special stick that he plants in the ground close to Libaka. The sticks are all tied together with a special cane, fixed with seven knots. Libaka is treated with respect. Two important covenants are peace and friendship. It is essential that these agreements be made at Libaka, for then the ancestors witness, participate in, and share in all covenants.[17] Elsewhere in West Africa, silk cotton trees are dressed with a ring of palm leaves around the trunk as an offering to various orishas.

Silk Cotton Tree in the Diaspora

Silk cottonwood tree is called kapok in Puerto Rico, where it is the national tree. The tree has been planted in many of the plaza centers for shade, and it is valued as a honey tree. Puerto Rican practitioners of Santería, a faith inspired by Yoruba beliefs, use the tree in their rituals in six ways:

1. Leaves are used in love magic.
2. Roots are the place for offerings and sacrifices.
3. The trunk is used for hexing and curses.
4. The bark is used medicinally in brews and potions.
5. The soil is used in magic.
6. Shade attracts the spirits, lending supernatural power to those buried beneath.

In Jamaica, practitioners of Obeah also believe spirits of the dead, called duppies, live mostly in silk cotton or almond trees. The tree is not to be planted too close to the house because duppies who live in them have an otherworldly temperature and their heat brings discord to people. Duppies are temperamental and mischievous and can hurt people if disturbed.

Cuba is a part of the West Indies, situated in the Antilles Archipelago. Many Africans were enslaved and brought to Cuba to work the fields. Cuba has a rich flora with nearly three thousand endemic plants. Ceiba grows well in Cuba and has an important role in the magical traditions there. African Cuban followers of the Yoruba-inspired ATR called Lucumí form agreements, make petitions, and perform invocations, rituals, and ceremonies beneath the silk cotton tree.

---

17 Harold Scheub, *A Dictionary of African Mythology: The Mythmaker as Storyteller* (New York: Oxford Univ. Press, 2000), 124–25.

In Suriname there are people called Maroons,[18] who quickly escaped their captors before they could be enslaved. These people retained a great deal of the social traditions, communal customs, and healing ways of West Africa. The traditional medicine of the Suriname people includes many uses for the tree, which they call kapok. Kapok seeds, leaves, bark, and resin are used to treat asthma, dysentery, fevers, and kidney disease and to regulate menstruation.

The Cautionary Tale of Mapou, Haiti

I have shared some of my personal forest story and that of African people in a broader sense. I have described how my kinship to trees developed and where I am with it now in hopes that it might inspire those without such a relationship to cultivate one. The role of trees in spirit medicine has been introduced, but they also have myriad other implications. Some people feel that trees and kinship toward them is a luxury they cannot afford. People want to utilize trees for what they have to offer: food, medicine, fodder, fire, lumber, or currency. Often this concern usurps interest in the contribution that the existence of trees makes to our overall well-being. Continuing to explore the silk cottonwood (*Ceiba pentandra*), the majestic native of West Africa, the Caribbean, and North and South America, might just change some minds.

The people of Haiti called silk cottonwood mapou. Mapou has a lengthy history as a sacred tree. It was once illegal to fell the trees. Instead, offerings were laid out at the base, within the buttresses, nooks, and crannies of mapou, just as they are with the Angel Oak and other trees throughout Africa and the diaspora. As a sacred tree, mapou is believed to be the container of the ancestors. The roots are said to contain the Vodou lwas and spirits. When a child is born, the father buries the umbilical cord of the baby at the mapou. The tree holds the baby's soul, and as we know, children are the future generations of societies to come. This brings us back to Libaka, the notion of the sacred union of spirit and living beings by the silk cottonwood tree.

The Taino people, who are indigenous to Haiti, named the tree *mapu,* meaning "large

---

18 Maroons have a sizable presence in Jamaica as well.

red tree." Mapou grows to an enormous size in places where most trees remain saplings. The trunk is hollow with numerous branches and cavities. It requires a reliable water source. It does not supply a good source of lumber and was traditionally valued as a source for shade, spiritual engagement, folklore, and mythology, as well as spirit medicine.

Eventually, it was discovered that it is a good source for charcoal. Charcoal was sold for pennies per pound to bring income, however tiny, to very impoverished people. The place named for the great tree, Mapou, Haiti, does not have a single mapou left. A period of massive deforestation severely disrupted the ecosystem and holistic environment in Haiti. The primary beliefs of the people and homage to their ancestral spirits were severed along with the trees. Whether one believes in tree spirits or not, the fact remains that an estimated 2,500 people were killed by a great flood in June of 2004. Approximately 1,600 victims came from Mapou and its environs. Trees serve the spirit; they offer medicine and an opportunity to commune with the ancestors. As the cautionary tale of Mapou, Haiti, shows, trees also have a very important ecological function. Their roots soak up water and forests form barriers, stemming the tide of erosion. In short, trees play an important role in balancing our ecosystem and sustaining life.

Mapou Mouri, Kabrit Manje Fey

Translation: "When the mapou dies, goats would eat its leaves."

This Haitian proverb in Creole attests to the role of mapou in community abundance compared to poverty. Mapou had a very important place in the cycle of life, continuity, and balance in Haiti; unfortunately a notion of a different type of survival based on economics disrupted this.

Lessons of the Sacred Forest from Africa

The forest is our home; when we leave the forest, or when the forest dies, we shall die. We are the people of the forest.[19]
—Old Moke, a BaMbuti Pygmy of the Ituri Forest, Congo, Central Africa, recording in the early 1960s

Often the indigenous people around the world are spoken of in the past tense. It is as though they are all gone and their ways of life are only a part of our collective past. With the significant numbers of indigenous people in Africa and the Americas, there is nothing further from the truth. Nevertheless, locked into this mindset, based more on an agreed-upon mythology than fact, people look to Westernized societies for lessons of how to live in harmony with nature. Two Canadian men, Dr. Bill Mollison and David Holmgren, coined the term *permaculture* in the early 1970s. It is a descriptor for a sustainable way of life.

Permaculture—or permanent agriculture, as it is known today—is the conscious design and maintenance of agriculturally productive ecosystems that are diverse, stable, and resilient. It is also a way of bringing together landscapes and people, creating a symbiotic relationship. Environmental harmony is created when people, animals, and the environment have their holistic needs met through permanent agriculture. This circular relationship in turn becomes sustainable.

When I wanted to learn from a culture that has practiced permaculture for thousands of years, I did not look to North America; instead, I headed off to Australia for extended study with various Aboriginal cultures. The Aborigines are numerous, diverse groups who live in vastly different ecosystems. They have managed their land and ecosystems respectfully in accord with steeped tradition for over fifty thousand years. While some live in tropical coastal environs, many people have managed over the generations in harsh desert environments.

Increasingly, other people from various walks of life are paying attention to environmental programs modeled after the traditional ways of life of the indigenous cultures. As you shall see in the following examples, there are lessons for how to live a healthful life being developed and disseminated from the Motherland to this very day.

---

19 Turnbull, *Forest People*, 260.

Sacred Grove of the Malshegu Community of Ghana

Over centuries, indigenous Africans have lived close to their environment. Their holistic, traditional, scientific knowledge, drawing on experimentation, observation, and innovation, continues to evolve. Taboos based on spirituality and traditional value systems have protected the biodiversity of various communities in Africa, including the Malshegu community of the Northern Region of Ghana.

Malshegu is located in the northern administration region of Ghana with five thousand people. It is situated in the savanna. The settled area came into existence as a way to escape the oppression and rule of Arab invaders from the Sudano-Sahelian region. The Malshegu people are members of the Dagbani ethnic group. Their migration began after the fall of the great empires of ancient Ghana in the twelfth century.

The people have maintained sacred groves of forest, surrounded by Guinea savanna. Women do most of the tending of the crops. They use animal manure to assure soil fertility; crop rotation and intercropping with legumes allow six-month fallow periods. Women use hoes and animal traction to prepare the soil. Chemical fertilizers and pesticides are seldom used.

The Malshegu people have set aside 0.8 hectares of existing open canopy of the forest for their god, Kpalevorgu. Kpalevorgu is in the form of a boulder, under a large baobab tree. The Malshegu believe the tree has helped families over the years and protected them from invaders. The grove has its own priest to tend to it, called Kumbriyili, who is also the village leader. As the god's sanctuary, this area offers a respite from the daily goings-on of mundane life, as well as peace and quiet. It also provides an overview of the village.

The Malshegu sacred grove is one of the few remaining examples of non-riverine, closed-canopy forests in Ghana's savanna. The Malshegu sacred grove and Kpalevorgu fetish god form part of a rich and complex traditional form of conservancy. The grove is a vital habitat preserving much of the area's fauna and flora and forms a physical focus for the Malshegu's spirituality. The sacred grove is an important location for seeds and seed dispersers vital to traditional cultivation practices. It is naturally the home of medicinal herbs for healing, as well as medicines with social and religious functions. The grove ensures that the water table remains high in the immediate area. The baobab tree that anchors the grove indicates a high localized water table. The forest protects the Malshegu from wind, rain, storms, brush fires, and potential flooding. According to environmental engineering student Edmund Asare, the sacred grove is an example of ways traditional culture combines religion and cultural practices and can lead to successful environmental management, preservation, and sound resource management.[20]

Indigenous-Led Alpine Rainforest Conservancy in Madagascar

While well-intended, conservation efforts, often led by people who are from outside areas, fail for numerous reasons. Recently, there is more support and attention paid to conservation and sustainability efforts that are led by indigenous people. Seacology is a not-for-profit organization that supports indigenous-people-led research projects dealing with island ecosystems around the world.

Seacology supports the work of Professor Elisabeth Rabakonandrianina (or Bako, as she is affectionately called), who works diligently to protect Mount Angavokely. Mount Angavokely is a 1,717-acre oasis of intact, high-altitude rainforest just fifteen miles outside the capital city of Antananarivo, Madagascar. As it stands, Madagascar is the fourth largest island in the world. Eighty percent of its plant and animal life are endemic (they grow no place else on earth). Madagascar is isolated on the Indian Ocean, 250 miles east of the Mozambique coast.

Bako's passion is to record and preserve the high-altitude rainforest. It is home to more than 120 species of rare and endangered orchids. The forest forms a watershed for three local communities of indigenous people totaling twenty thousand inhabitants. Seacology and Bako are working with a Malagasy organization called ARCVERT, faculty from the University of Antananarivo and Uppsala University, and the Service des Stations Forestieres to create a new national park at Mount Angavokely for recreational purposes and research opportunities.[21] Often there are stakeholders from a variety of facilities, making this the optimal way to work.

Several medicinal herbs have been found on Mount Angavokely, including these members of the Asteraceae family:

Helichrysum gymnocephalum (DC. H. Humb)—used as an aphrodisiac, antiseptic, and stimulating treatment for bronchitis.

---

20 Edmund Asare, "Traditional Knowledge in Forest Conservation: Case Study of the Malshegu Community in Ghana," paper (Tampere, Finland: Tampere Polytechnic, 2002).
21 Karen Peterson, "Seacology Helps Conserve Medicinal Plants of Madagascar," *Journal of the American Botanical Council* 65 (2005): 20.

Endemic *Psiadia altissima* (DC. Benth and Hook)—used as a dentifrice, to make toothpaste, and as a treatment for eczema.

Endemic *Bryophyllum proliferum* (Bowie ex Hook. Crassulaceae)—used for coughs.

Brachylaena ramiflora (DC. Humbat, Asteraceae)—used to lower malaria fever.

Non-endemics include the fascinating *Siegesbeckia orientalis L.* (*Asteraceae*), which is used to stop bleeding and heal wounds. According to Bako, the indigenous name for the plant, *Satrikoazamaratra*, means "I am happy to have wounds because it heals real fast."

A problem that leads to the poaching and deforesting of precious trees is the drive to find fuel wood that makes good charcoal. This issue affects just about every indigenous culture and has not left Madagascar unscathed. To prevent massive destruction, Bako developed and introduced an alternative charcoal using forest litter and rice hulls (which are grown locally) instead of hardwood. Bako won the Seacology Prize for her outstanding work in the Manafiafy Forest, a 1,730-acre area comprised primarily of one of the last standing littoral forests of Madagascar palm.

Sacred Kaya Forest of Kenya

Along the southern coast of Kenya, the sacred kaya forests of the Mijikenda are a long-standing legacy of the people's history, culture, and religion. For centuries, these once-extensive lowland forests have shielded these areas, called *kaya*, meaning "homesteads," of the Mijikenda. The kaya is a shield against invaders, while also serving as a space for sacred activity.

As with the Malshegu people of Ghana, and the work of countless groups in all points of the Motherland, social taboos have prohibited the felling and removal of trees and other forest vegetation for all but a few purposes and only by trusted individuals. The kaya's protected status allowed it to become a repository of biodiversity, harboring many rare species of plants and animals. Still, challenges and conflicts between traditional and more Western ideals persist in causing a struggle to preserve the area.

Kaya forest is the domain of nine Mijikenda groups—the Giriama, Digo, Duruma, Rabai, Kauma, Ribe, Jibana, Kambe, and Chonyi—from forced migration from southern Somalia.

The groups used the thick belts of forest to protect themselves. The entire community lived within a central clearing. A protective talisman called a fingo, which represents the community identity and history, is buried in a secret spot within the kaya clearing. Burial sites located within the surrounding forest and shrines honor graves of great leaders. Social protocol established and enforced by kaya elders regulate activities that could otherwise damage the kaya. Cutting trees, grazing livestock, and collecting or removing forest materials was strictly forbidden. A code of behavior, emphasizing decorum, respect, and self-restraint, protects the surrounding ecosystem.

More than half of Kenya's rare plants grow in the coastal region. Over fifty years of ever-growing demand for land and resources have dramatically reduced the size of the kayas and completely eradicated some of the smaller groves. Many factors play a role in the destruction, including population growth and expansion, the hotel and tourist industry, mining, agriculture, livestock, and the erosion of spiritual traditions. There is a decline in knowledge of the cultural values, thus they are pushed aside, often to the detriment of the holistic health of the community. The spread of Islam and Christianity has had a negative impact as well.[22] Today, sacred groves and sites are gaining recognition once again for the vital role they play in biodiversity, sustainability, and conservation.

Tree Medicine

Shea Tree

You have undoubtedly heard a lot about shea, finding shea butter in your shampoos, conditioners, soaps, lotions, and creams. I find that, as an herbalist, it is always useful to also know where a particular ingredient, especially something as new to our marketplace as shea butter, comes from.

The shea tree is a member of the Sapotaceae family, *Vitellaria paradoxa C.F. Gaertn*, formerly called *Butyrospermum paradoxum* (also used as a synonym). Shea trees are found exclusively in the African Sahel, a semiarid region south of the Sahara Desert. Shea tree is native to Benin, Burkina Faso, Cameroon, Chad, Côte d'Ivoire, Ghana, Guinea, Mali, Ni-

22 Anthony N. Githitho, "The Sacred Mijikenda Kaya Forests of Coastal Kenya and Biodiversity Conservation," paper, 27–35.

ger, Nigeria, Senegal, Sudan, Togo, and Uganda, where it is distributed in parklands, dry savannas, and forests. Shea trees grow for between 150 and 200 years. The nut of *Vitellaria paradoxa* is almost 50 percent fat.

Shea butter is one of numerous nontimber forest products (NTFPs) that makes significant contributions to rural African societies. Shea butter, known locally as *karite* in the Dioula language, is also called women's gold because it brings women significant income. Shea butter has been traded as a commodity since at least as early as the fourteenth century. Today shea butter is the third-highest export product in Burkina Faso. It is one of few economic commodities under women's control in Sahelian Africa. The trees have been tenderly cared for by women farmers and their children for hundreds of years, yet with the steady rise in popularity of shea butter in international markets, some concerns have arisen. Agroforestry and environmental organizations fear that overharvesting of the shea nut could contribute to land degradation, eventually leading to desertification. This is one of the reasons I also advocate for the use of alternative butters like mango butter, which will be discussed later.

While in the West we utilize shea almost exclusively as a cosmetic additive, in Africa it has diverse uses. For the Mossi people of Burkina Faso, shea butter is the sole source of fat. Groups in Burkina Faso and elsewhere use shea to make soap, healing balms, cosmetics, candles, lamp oil, and waterproofing putty for housing. Shea wood is used for creating tools, flooring, joinery, chairs, utensils, and mortar and pestles. The wood also creates a fierce heat and can be prepared as a substitute for kerosene, yet the trees' destruction for fuel is discouraged because of its more prominent medicinal uses and economic contribution to African villages. The root and bark are used medicinally.

Many types of imported chocolates contain shea. Shea butter is exported to Japan and Europe to enhance the pliability of pastry dough and to enrich chocolate recipes. In Africa and around the world, shea butter is utilized for its ability to soothe children's skin, soften rough skin, and protect against sunburn, chapping, irritation, ulcers, and rheumatism.

The Making of Shea Butter

Creating shea butter from nuts is a monumental, labor-intensive task involving huge amounts of water and wood, as it is made on an open wood fire. West African women almost exclusively run the production of shea butter processing, with the assistance of their children. Manufacturing takes place during the rainy season, a time when harvesting duties are already intense for women. Preparation takes several days. Nuts are collected, boiled, sun-dried, hand-shelled, roasted, and then crushed with a mortar and pestle. Water is added and a paste is formed. Several women knead and beat the paste in a pot until a skim floats to the surface. The fat is cleansed repeatedly, yielding white foam. The foam is boiled for several hours. The top layer is skimmed once more, and this yields the white shea butter we use.

Golden Shea

Shea butter is called women's gold by some because of the economic benefits it brings through women's work. Recently, I had the opportunity to try a lovely shea with a golden color imported by African Shea Butter Company. I enjoy the golden shea butter immensely because it retains the smells of the open wood fires on which it is created. This is likely to be a sentiment shared by those who work herbs because it reminds us of the power of the elements.

Delving into a jar of golden shea can spiritually transport the user back to the African village in which the shea was processed. Those of you who seek a more unprocessed product with a lively spirit still intact would be wise to avoid ultra-refined shea butter, which is stripped of its contact with its source.

Cocoa Butter (*Theobroma cacao*)

One of my earliest introductions to the botanical world was through cocoa butter. I remember visiting with my cousin in the 1970s. She lived in a primarily African American city in northern New Jersey. As most teenage girls do, we were experimenting with styling our hair using hot combs and hot curlers. Of course, quick as a wink, I had a burn on my neck. Just as swiftly, my cousin produced a push-up tin of cocoa butter. She pushed up the cocoa butter and gently dabbed it onto the burned area. It was quite soothing. I became curious about cocoa butter and was shown by other members of my family how it could also be applied directly to the skin to keep the skin pliable to lessen the severity of stretch marks—also useful information to a fast-growing adolescent girl.

The *Theobroma cacao* tree is grown in the tropical rainforests of Central America and

Africa (particularly Ghana), where it makes a significant impact on the local economy. I recently saw a cacao tree. The tree is a remarkable sight. It has dark-brown bark, resembling the color of chocolate. Curiously, white flowers grow directly from the branches and trunk of the tree. The delicate, light-colored blossoms create a sharp visual contrast against the deeply colored, rough-looking bark. In fact, the cacao tree is one of the more unusual trees that I have seen. The scent the tree emits is quite subtle, not the rich chocolate aroma you might expect. The part of *Theobroma cacao* utilized in natural beauty products is also edible and is derived from the processed beans.

Cocoa butter is created from hydraulic pressings of the cocoa nib or cocoa mass from cocoa beans that are further refined through filtering or centrifuge. The scent of cocoa butter is removed using steam or a vacuum. Some herbalists, massage therapists, and aromatherapists prefer the scentless substance called deodorized cocoa butter.

Using Cocoa Butter

Cocoa butter is a useful ingredient for vegans (those who prefer no animal products, including beeswax) since cocoa butter is a serviceable hardener, thickener, and counterbalance to stickier ingredients like shea butter. An additional gift of cocoa butter is that no solvents are involved in its manufacture; it is a human-food-grade, edible ingredient. The edible aspect is appealing to those who desire wholesome, nurturing ingredients in homemade potions, creams, and healing balms. Cocoa butter is widely available, ships well, is reasonably priced, and has a shelf life of two to five years.

Cocoa beans are 15 percent fat. The oil is very attractive as an ingredient in herbal cosmetics. Cocoa butter has been traditionally used as a skin softener, emollient, belly rub, and soothing substance for burns. It is useful as a superfatting[23] agent in soap. Cocoa butter has an SAP value of 0.137. To superfat cold-processed soap, add ½ teaspoon melted butter per pound of soap.

The high stearic composition of cocoa butter allows it to increase the hardness in handmade soaps and healing balms. In a pinch, I have substituted it for beeswax with good results. It can also be used as a base oil in soapmaking and is best combined with other oils, such as coconut oil, for a productive lather. The addition of coconut, palm, or almond oil

---

23 Superfatting is a process used in cold-processed soapmaking, accomplished by adding liquid fat once soap reaches trace, or just before trace. These oils tend to have a therapeutic effect and add nutritional benefits to the soap, since they have had limited contact with the lye water.

helps create a looser healing balm or salve that melts faster. A hard soap, containing large concentrations of cocoa butter, lasts for a long time in the bath. Cocoa-butter-enriched soap will also hold intricate patterns of elaborate molds. (One of my favorite chocolate cocoa butter soapmaking recipes is in part III.)

One of my favorite ways to use cocoa butter is to hold a small chunk of the butter in my hand as I run hot water in the bathtub. The cocoa butter melts and then acts as a skin softener as I bathe. After the bath, particularly in the fall and winter, I find cocoa butter useful on areas of rough skin. I apply it nightly to my heels after a bath and then promptly put on cotton socks, for an evening of foot softening as I dream. This also works well on calloused hands after gardening, housework, artmaking, and crafts.

Black Cocoa Butter

One of my newest enthusiasms is black cocoa butter. Most of you are probably familiar with the eggshell-colored cocoa butter that has been widely available for quite a while. Most of the ordinary cocoa butter that comes from Africa is processed before the seeds are allowed to germinate. With black cocoa butter, the cacao pods are germinated first, which produces a deep, espresso-colored butter that smells like roasted cocoa. You might find that, as body butter, it truly lives up to the botanical name of *Theobroma cacao*, "food of the gods." If you want to try something a little different in your skin-softening regimen, consider black cocoa butter because it is softer and more readily malleable than the cream-colored type. Black cocoa butter[24] is very easily absorbed by the skin and a nice addition to soaps, lip balms, and body butters. It is useful as a hot oil treatment to condition the hair.

A Tree of Forty Cures: Neem Tree

Neem has a distinguished history in India. In the Sanskrit language it is known as *nimba*, a derivative of the term *Nimbati Swastyamdadati* ("to give good health").[25] Neem has been naturalized over the past hundred years in coastal East and West Africa. Known as the

---

24 The dark color will temporarily stain light skin. The oil is absorbed readily and, once it is absorbed, no stain remains.
25 Neem Foundation, 1997. See also *International Journal for Innovative Research in Multidisciplinary Field*, Issn 2455-0620, vol. 2, August 2016, p. 124.

"tree of forty cures," neem is called *mwarubaini* in the Kiswahili language.[26] Neem is an eco-friendly tree since its leaves quickly decompose, forming nourishing mulch for plants that surround it.

The leaves, seed kernel, and bark of neem trees are all useful. The tree has antibacterial, antifungal, and antiviral qualities, and there is also the possibility that its use reduces infertility. The neem kernel contains about 45 percent oil, making it an effective emollient. Useful in the treatment of ringworm and other fungal infections, neem is also highly regarded for maintenance of scalp, hair, skin, and nails.

Pau D'Arco (Divine Bark) (*Tabebuia impetiginosa*)

Pau d'arco is native to the Central and South American rainforests. The tree has bright-green oval-shaped leaves with thick golden seams, which cut designs resembling mosaics into each serrated leaf. The tree blooms with clusters of dangling purple trumpet flowers. Early medicine men peeled the trees' bark in long strips. They separated the outer bark from the purple inner bark to make tea, which was considered a panacea for centuries. It is called "the Divine Bark" in Brazil, Mexico, Argentina, and the Bahamas, where it is considered a cure-all. The divinity stems from the fact that it attracts alpha rays that exert a positive electrical charge on human cells since crystalline oxygen is trapped in its inner bark. Pau d'arco contains iron, calcium, selenium, and vitamins A, B complex, and C, as well as the minerals magnesium, manganese, zinc, phosphorous, potassium, and sodium. It contains flavonoids, alkaloids, quinines, and saponins. It is considered to be antibiotic, antibacterial, antimicrobial, antifungal, and antitumor. It is used as an immune-system stimulant and disease fighter. The antitumor agent, lapachol, inhibits cancer growth and lymph congestion. Mucous congestion, psoriasis, eczema, ringworm, scabies, and problems with the throat, mouth, and gums show improvement with pau d'arco tea taken internally or used as a wash. I have used it to replenish the strength of people who are severely ill as well as with cold and flu.

---

26 Mwarubaini, The Plant That Can Cure 40 Diseases, Paukwa, https://paukwa.or.ke/mwarubaini-the-plant-that-can-cure-40-diseases.

Banana (*Musa paradisiaca var. sapientum*)

Portuguese or Christian missionaries probably introduced sweet banana to Africa. It is cultivated in the forest regions and southern savanna area of West Africa. Banana is a most useful staple in Africa; the multiple-purpose plant is used in the home, medicines, utilitarian crafts, rituals and ceremonies, cosmetics, and trade. The fingerlike fruits are fermented in East Africa and used to make alcoholic beverages. The Gikuyu people of Kenya have traditionally utilized banana as one of their staple foods.[27] In Nigeria and Côte d'Ivoire, banana brings economic returns as an exported good. The leaves are used as fodder; the stem and peduncle yield useful fiber.[28] Banana leaf is used to make umbrellas, roofing, tablecloths, and plates in Ghana. The leaf is also used in community rituals. Poultices are made from the leaves to treat wounds in West Africa. An antiseptic is derived from the inner peeling. The sap from the tree renders dye. The black seeds are harvested and used to make decorative beads in Ghana. The banana is also a beloved tree of Puerto Rico, among other islands where people of African descent now live. In Puerto Rico, banana is sometimes referred to as "poor man's bread." The plantain is actually peeled, toasted, and eaten just like bread. The roasted or fried banana is cooked while green and served with other foods.[29] Another wonderful gift of banana and plantain is that they are a very sustainable, economic plant. One acre planted with the trees can support fifty people, whereas an acre planted with wheat supports only two individuals.[30]

Eating bananas works wonders for the body. Bananas:

- play a role in the prevention of colon cancer.[31]
- improve the health and functionality of the colon.[32]
- create good bacteria that ferments in the belly.[33]
- reduce high blood pressure.[34]

---

27 https://www.fonazioneslowfood.com/en/ark-of-taste-slow-food/mutahato-banana/ (accessed 11/30/2023).
28 Abbiw, *Useful Plants of Ghana*.
29 Eliza B. K. Dooley, *Puerto Rican Cookbook* (Richmond, VA: The Dietz Press, 1948), 99–100.
30 Dooley, *Puerto Rican Cookbook*.
31 Carper, *Food—Your Miracle Medicine*, 102–3.
32 Carper, *Food—Your Miracle Medicine*.
33 Carper, *Food—Your Miracle Medicine*.
34 Carper, *Food—Your Miracle Medicine*.

- reduce plaque formation in the arteries (anticlotting).[35]
- build bone density.[36]
- are a dense source of carbohydrate.
- act as a natural diuretic.
- make the body excrete water and sodium.
- are useful for irregularity.
- are used as a sweetener in hot cereal (oatmeal).
- are a useful addition to smoothies, adding body, fiber, good taste, and nutrition.
- are a tasty addition to fruit salads, with good texture, sweetness, and rich taste.
- make a moistening hair conditioner and hydrating face mask.
- are a lovely sight, soothing to the senses and inspirational where they grow.

The daily value (DV) of banana is as follows:

- 33% DV vitamin B
- 15% DV vitamin C
- 13% DV potassium
- 11% DV fiber
- 9% DV vitamin A
- 8% DV magnesium
- 6% DV folate

Plantain (*Musa x paradisiaca*)

Plantain is a native of tropical Asia believed to have been introduced to Africa through Egypt. In Ghana, plantain is cultivated in forests and used as a staple. Plantains are not cultivated in East Africa, but they grow well in the area on their own. There are twenty-one varieties in three main groups. The cultivars of plantain that are cooked prior to eat-

---

35 Carper, *Food—Your Miracle Medicine.*
36 Carper, *Food—Your Miracle Medicine.*

ing are French, French horn, false horn, and horn.[37] Plantains are eaten in just about any imaginable way: boiled, eaten when unripe as ampesi, pounded into fufu, or sometimes mixed with cassava. They are eaten roasted and served with peanut butter, which is called groundnut, and eaten unripe but mostly ripened. Fried ripe plantain is a favorite dish with bean stew made with *Vigna subterranea*. Unripe plantains are fried as chips or dried and powdered as kokonte. Ripe ones are pounded with corn dough and other ingredients and fried as tatare or kakro or used alone with porridge or as a sugar substitute. Stems yield fiber for fishing tackle and for a sponge and towel used by elderly women. Burned peelings of fruit yield potash used in local soapmaking.[38]

In Puerto Rico, the plantain is peeled, toasted, and eaten like bread. It is roasted, fried, and combined with other foods. It is cooked while green or allowed to mature. A flour is made from the plantain in Puerto Rico by drying and grinding plantain; this flour is used in porridge and gruel. It helps most stomach disorders and is easily digested by babies. A quick and easy Puerto Rico plantain recipe is to fry[39] it in butter until brown, then sprinkle with a smattering of sugar and a pinch of cinnamon and ground nutmeg. For a healthier alternative, bake the plantain whole until soft; serve with the main course.

Plantain is similar to banana but starchier, so they are often eaten cooked. Plantain is actually richer in vitamins and minerals than bananas. The daily value of vitamin C is 28 percent; it contains 19 percent of the DV of B_6, 10 percent of the DV of folate, 20 percent of the DV of potassium, and 20 percent of the DV of fiber.[40]

Avocado (*Persea americana*)

Avocado belongs to the laurel family and is related to cinnamon, camphor, and sassafras. The edible part is more of a nut than a fruit. It contains 1.5 to 2.5 percent of the DV of protein and 13 to 22 percent of that of oil.[41] "Avocado pear," as it is called in Jamaica, grows well on the island and has many medicinal uses because of its various constituents:

---

37 "*Mus x paradisiaca: Plantain*," Kew Royal Botanical Gardens, accessed November 30, 2023, https:www.kew.org/plants/plantain.
38 Abbiw, *Useful Plants of Ghana*, 30.
39 Be sure to fry in a monounsaturated oil like canola, olive, or even coconut oil.
40 Carper, *Food—Your Miracle Medicine*, 102–3.
41 Dooley, *Puerto Rican Cookbook*, 109.

- Chlorogenic acid lends an analgesic effect, hence it is used as a headache treatment in Jamaican folk medicine.[42]
- Chlorogenic acid also provides a diuretic quality.[43]
- The paraffin it contains serves as a laxative.[44]
- Caffeic acid is an antiviral, bactericide, are viricide.[45]
- Pinene is a bactericide.[46]
- Nonacosane is antiviral.[47]

Guava (*Psidium guajava*)

Guava is one of the most nutritious fruits. It is higher in vitamin C than citrus fruits, particularly if you eat the rind. It contains an appreciable amount of vitamin A, along with some iron and pectin, which is used to make jam and promote digestion. The leaves and bark have a long history of medicinal uses. An infusion of the leaves or decoction of the bark is used by traditional people to treat diarrhea, dysentery, and vertigo, and to regulate menstrual periods. Guava contains natural chemicals that lead the Jamaicans to utilize this tasty fruit as a healing medicine: quercitrin is an antihemorrhagic constituent, gallic acid adds anti-inflammatory and astringent actions, the quercetin is also anti-inflammatory, ursolic acid lends an antihistamine quality, and citral is antiallergic and antihistaminic, which is useful for insect bites and hives.[48] Guava contains beta-bisabolene and has antibronchitic, antiviral, viricide, antirhinoviral, and antiviral qualities, making it useful if something like COVID-19 or RSV arises. The ripe fruit is easy to juice in a cold-pressed juicer. It is used to treat ulcers and boils.[49]

Pineapple (*Ananassa ananas*), Also Called *Pina*

The pineapple is a native of South America and it is partially naturalized in tropical Africa and extensively in West Africa. The wild varieties grow in the forest, although the crop

42 Payne-Jackson and Alleyne, *Jamaican Folk Medicine*, 162.
43 Payne-Jackson and Alleyne, *Jamaican Folk Medicine*, 163.
44 Payne-Jackson and Alleyne, *Jamaican Folk Medicine*, 154.
45 Payne-Jackson and Alleyne, *Jamaican Folk Medicine*, 153.
46 Payne-Jackson and Alleyne, *Jamaican Folk Medicine*.
47 Payne-Jackson and Alleyne, *Jamaican Folk Medicine*.
48 Payne-Jackson and Alleyne, *Jamaican Folk Medicine*, 163–64.
49 Payne-Jackson and Alleyne, *Jamaican Folk Medicine*, 149.

is basically of the savanna and particularly strong in the southern savanna of Ghana.[50] It is a part of the economy of Ghana as an export. Puerto Rico has long been famous for the pineapple. The sliced fruit is placed in salt water before eating in Puerto Rico and the West Indies. Anabasine is the active principle. The juice is healing to catarrhal affections and recommended for sore throat. It is indigenous to tropical America. The stem and stump are rich in starch. Pineapple has a very positive effect on regulating menstrual flow, especially when that flow is too heavy, due to its high manganese content. Consuming foods high in manganese, like pineapple, prevents abnormally heavy menstrual periods.[51] The manganese-rich pineapple also keeps bones strong. Lack of manganese is implicated in bone metabolism in tests.[52] The ripe fruit can be consumed as a juice or eaten raw. The juiced form is especially easily absorbed by the body. It has a beautiful shape and color that has come to symbolize the spirit of welcoming and hospitality.[53]

Soursop (Annona muricata)

Soursop is a member of the family Annonaceae, comprising approximately 150 species, a few of which are discussed below. The tree is only about twenty feet; the leaves are leathery, very dark, shiny, and green. The leaves have a pungent odor when crushed. It yields yellow flowers. Soursop, also called guanabana, has a fruit that is oblong, somewhat curved, around thirteen inches long, and weighing up to eight pounds. The fruit has numerous black seeds. The creamy, aromatic pulp is juiced and used to make ice cream. It is rich in vitamins B and C. It has a musky, acidic flavor. This native of tropical America is grown on small plantations or in private gardens. The leaves are medicinal and contain several phytochemicals, as do the seeds and stem. These parts are thought to have cytotoxic action on several types of cancers. There is research going on concerning the cancer medicine it contains and an effort to isolate the chemicals it contains with the strongest anticancer and antiviral activity. It appears to seek and destroy actively reproducing cancer cells, while leaving the other cells undisturbed; the seed oil kills lice.[54] In Jamaica's folk medicine, the fruit is used as an antihypertensive to treat high blood pressure because of the coreximine

---

50 Abbiw, *Useful Plants of Ghana.*
51 Carper, *Food—Your Miracle Medicine,* 405.
52 Carper, *Food—Your Miracle Medicine,* 338.
53 Dooley, *Puerto Rican Cookbook,* 125–26.
54 Abbiw, *Useful Plants of Ghana,* 45.

it contains.[55] The caffeic acid in soursop is used for its sedative qualities, whereas the reticuline serves as a stimulant for the central nervous system, thus it is used to treat "nerves" in Jamaica. Soursop juice is used in baths; the procyanidin it contains is antibiotic, antiviral, and antibacterial. The malic acid it contains is a bacteriostat.[56] In Suriname's traditional medicine, a tea is created from its leaves and used to treat nervous tension and hypertension. It is also used as a treatment for flu and fevers. The fresh leaves are used to alleviate insomnia in Suriname.

Sweetsop (A. squamosa)

The ripe fruit of this member of family *Annonaceae* is sweeter than soursop but the taste is not as rich. Sweetsop contains borneol and is used as an analgesic in Jamaica.

Custard Apple (A. reticulata); Cherimoya in Spanish

The reticuline in custard apple serves as an analgesic. It is a tasty treat used to make ice cream.[57] Eaten on its own, it tastes like banana and ice cream. Custard apple is considered an effective treatment for colds; it is also used to build regularity in Jamaica.[58]

Peach (Prunus persica)

Peaches grow in many temperate and warm regions around the world. In the United States, the dominant peach producer is California. We had plenty of peach orchards in the surrounding towns and counties of South Jersey. The trees are generally small if left to their own devices—twenty to twenty-five feet tall—but the orchard trees are kept much shorter. The leaves are thin, serrate, and oblong-elliptic to lanceolate. The flowers are a delicate pink. The leaves are medicinal with diuretic, expectorant, laxative, and sedative qualities. Peach tea leaf is used for chronic bronchitis and chest congestion. It has a strong laxative action and is not recommended during pregnancy. The powdered leaf is used to heal wounds. Use 1 teaspoon leaf to 1 cup water; 2 to 3 cups per day or a tincture with 2 to 15 drops in water, 30 minutes before meals.[59] American folklore espouses the use of peach leaf for hair conditioning and as a hair growth aid

55 Payne-Jackson and Alleyne, *Jamaican Folk Medicine*, 164.
56 Payne-Jackson and Alleyne, *Jamaican Folk Medicine*, 151.
57 Payne-Jackson and Alleyne, *Jamaican Folk Medicine*, 161.
58 Payne-Jackson and Alleyne, *Jamaican Folk Medicine*, 154–55.
59 Lust, *Herb Book*, 303–4.

used as a water-based infusion. I have used peach tea infusion with good results on dull hair that lacks body. Peaches contain a lot of boron, which boosts steroids in the blood. The boron in peaches increases 17beta-estradiol, the most active form of estrogen, making the fruit useful to consume during menopause or after a hysterectomy. Peaches are also believed to decrease occurrences of osteoporosis and increase testosterone because of the boron.[60] A collaborative study by US government scientists at the Agricultural Research Service with South African and Israeli/Palestinian colleagues has found that the natural oil in peaches that lends them their scent also kills fungi and other pests in the soil. It is being investigated as a pesticide that is safer for animals, people, insects, and the environment.[61] Peach kernel oil has some vitamin A and minerals. It is used as a carrier oil in aromatherapy and as an emollient in hair or skin treatments. The juice, oil, pit, and fruit itself are used in magical love brews because of the aphrodisiac quality of peaches.

Mango (*Mangifera indica*)

The mango is a native of the East Indies and Myanmar and is now naturalized in tropical West Africa. In Ghana, it grows better along the coastal savanna. The fruits are rich in vitamins and the starchy kernels are edible when roasted. The fruits are eaten green as a vegetable. The tree yields gum, some tannin, and a yellow dye. The seeds, leaves, bark, and root have varied medicinal uses.[62]

Magnolia (*Magnolia glauca*)

Also called swamp laurel, swamp sassafras, and white bay, magnolia is an evergreen tree found in the Atlantic and Gulf Coast states. Its beauty is especially visible in the Southeastern United States. The tree has soft, leathery leaves, which are alternate, elliptical, glossy, deep green on one side, and pale underneath. The flowers revive the spirits and bring a warm, comforting atmosphere with them inside the home or as a blooming specimen in the yard. The creamy flowers are beloved by artists and seem to soothe the mind and calm the spirit. One of the most beautiful renditions of the magnolia is an oil painting by the Hudson River School painter, Martin Johnson Heade, done in 1888. The dried leaf is used in

---

60 Carper, *Food—Your Miracle Medicine,* 410.
61 American Botanical Council, "HerbalGram," no. 48 (Austin, TX, 2000) 10.
62 Abbiw, *Useful Plants of Ghana,* 44.

Hoodoo as a natural amulet to instill monogamy and faith in marital relationships. The leaf is put in between the mattress and acts as a charm.

The bark is a medicinal part with astringent, diaphoretic, febrifuge, stimulant, and tonic qualities. The bark is also good for dyspepsia, dysentery, various skin disorders, and as a douche for leukorrhea. It has been used in folk medicine to treat tobacco addiction. To use, the bark is gathered in the spring and summer. Whenever gathering bark, gather sparingly with respect to the future growth of the tree. Decoct the bark using 1 teaspoon bark to 1 cup water. Take only 1 cup a day. For external treatments, simmer 1 tablespoon bark to 1 pint water for 10 minutes. Let cool, then apply to the skin with a cotton ball.[63]

Palms
Date Palm (*Phoenix dactylifera L.*)
In modern Egyptian Arabic, the tree is called *nahl* and the fruit is *balol.*

The date palm has grown in Egypt since prehistoric times, and it is still a predominate feature of the Nile Valley landscape. The fruits are eaten fresh or dried. Dates are distilled for various aperitifs and liquors. The insides of the top of the palm trunk are edible and taste like celery. Soldiers ate it in Greece and now in Iraq. In classical pharaonic eras of ancient Egypt, wine was made from palm dates and, along with honey, the juice of the fruit was one of the major sweetening agents in the days before sugar beet and sugarcane. Today health-conscious people trying to reduce sugar consumption continue to utilize dates as a food and drink additive. Wine was drunk and used during mummification rituals and was used to wash the mummy's body. The fruits were, and still are, pressed into blocks and hung on strings and used as currency to pay workmen in Egypt. The wood is used for roofing, fibers for basketry, and leaves for brushes and ropes. Dates are used herbally in several processes: infusion, potions, suppositories, unguents, and poultices. One poultice is used to fill the nostril with dates as a remedy for sneezing. A poultice is also used to reduce the swelling of legs.[64]

---

63 Lust, *Herb Book,* 263.
64 Manniche, *Ancient Egyptian Herbal,* 133–34.

Nut-Producing Palms (the Family Arecaceae)

There are about 225 genera, with 2,650 species, of palm; only a few are used and the most famous is the edible coconut.

Coconut (*Cocos nucifera*)

Coconut is a major African crop benefiting the economies of Ghana, Côte d'Ivoire, Kenya, Nigeria, Mozambique, Togo, Somalia, and Tanzania, among other African countries. Copra, the dried coconut endosperm, is a cooking oil that is also used cosmetically. Copra is called *mbata* by the Swahili people and *igi agbon* by the Yoruba. Whatever the name, it provides villages with milk used for cooking and beverages, a base for molasses, and precious oil. Coconut-oil-based soap works well, forming a thick lather even in salt water, making it popular with seafaring people for hundreds of years. During early African American history, Black people had many uses for coconut. The shell was pulverized and drank with wine as a systemic tonic. It was used to accelerate movement of the blood and was deemed a favorable herb for the elderly. Like the calabash explored in chapter 4, the shell was made into numerous household tools such as cups, measuring containers, spoons, and small plates. The coconut groves were a place where enslaved people went to commune with nature and relax in the Caribbean.[65]

Coconut oil can be a polarizing substance in the herbal community—some love it while others despise it. It is said to be drying to the skin, particularly if used as a large part of a soap oil base. Many African body butters are thick emollients that might overwhelm normal or combination skin; coconut oil is a welcome alternative. Coconut soaps are very useful for cleansing oily skin as they make a frothy cleansing lather. For those who enjoy a light moisturizer, coconut cream or other coconut products may well do the trick. Coconut oil can be combined with cocoa butter or shea butter to create a balanced soap that is neither too astringent nor excessively emollient. Coconut cream is gaining popularity as a natural botanical for skin and hair care.

Using Coconut Oil

Another type of coconut skin care treatment is coconut cream, and not the type in the food aisle. Coconut cream is available from Togo, where women villagers hand-press coco-

---

65 Grimé, *Ethno-botany of the Black Americans*, 106.

nuts to extract creamy oil. This virgin coconut oil is pressed from fresh coconut milk and meat rather than copra. Coconut cream works well as a massage therapy oil because of its silky texture. In Africa, coconut cream has been used traditionally as a hair conditioner, strengthener, and growth aid. The oil is rubbed into the scalp and may also be applied to the ends. Melted oil, cooled slightly and then applied to the scalp and ends as a hot oil treatment, followed by a shampoo, is preferable for those with oily scalp. See "Hot Shea Butter Hair Treatment" in chapter 13 for the application procedure. I find that, when applying coconut cream to my face and hands, it is a butter that disappears within a minute or so, without leaving a trace of greasiness on the skin in the way shea butter can.

African Palm (*Elaeis guineensis*)

Palm oil is the quintessential West African oil used commercially and in households to make soap, cook, and create healing balms. African palm originated in Africa and is now cultivated throughout the tropics. It is by far the most important source of edible palm oil. The oil is made from the nuts of three varieties of palm: dura palms, pisifera palms, and tenera palms. Dura palms have kernels with a thick shell. Pisifera palms have kernels with no shell. Tenera palms have kernels with a thin shell. Varieties are distinguished by the color of their seeds. Orange-colored seeds produce the finest oil but from small kernels. Brazilians call this oil *dende*. The others contain less oil but larger nuts, which are roasted and eaten. Numerous Brazilian and West African dishes contain *dende*.

Argun Palm (*Medemia argun* Württemb. ex Mart)

The argun is a fan palm, like the dom palm previously discussed, but its stem is not branched. It has an ellipsoid edible fruit of a deep purple color with yellow flesh. The tree grows sparsely in the Sudan. In ancient Egypt, it was a garden tree. Fruits of argun have been found in burials of the fifth dynasty.[66]

Argan oil is from *Argania spinosa*. It is rich in antioxidants, flavonoids, and tocopherols. Argan oil contains 56 mg/kg of polyphenols and almost double the amount of tocopherols of olive oil. The tree is native to southwestern Morocco near Agadir. The plum-sized fruits are eaten by goats who climb the trees—women used to harvest the kernels from the goat droppings. Nowadays, modern technology has eliminated older processes. The kernels

---

66 Manniche, *Ancient Egyptian Herbal,* 119.

are stripped of fruit by a machine and cold-pressed to express the oil. The oil has a specific aroma and is considered gourmet in Morocco.

Coquilla Nut (*Attalea funifera*)

The coquilla nut is one of the forty kinds of palms found mainly in Brazil. They have an especially hard shell covering the four-inch dark frame. They are a substitute for ivory in buttons, knobs, and jewelry, and other species furnish hard brooms and brushes.

Cork Palm (*Microcycas calocoma*)

Cork palm is in the Cycad family, and like several cycads, it is considered a living fossil. It grows in the Pinar del Río region of the Viñales Valley, an area that dates back three hundred million years. The rare Cuban prehistoric plant began life during the Cretaceous Period and is considered a valuable link to the history of plant life on earth. UNESCO has declared cork palm a World Heritage plant. It is the type of plant that speaks to our akashic self by providing spiritual commune with the natural world.

Palmyra Palm (*Borassus flabellifer*)

An eighty-foot tree from tropical Africa and Asia, palmyra palm is one of the most useful palms for durable wood. The leaves are used for thatching roofs and for writing paper. Palmyra palm is used for making mats, bags, baskets, umbrellas, and many more utilitarian objects. The tender seeds have a soft, sweet, gelatinous, pulpy nature with a little liquid, which is relished during hot summer months. The pulp gradually hardens into a bony kernel that develops into a fibrous coat and a cream-colored substance with the consistency of cheese and a pleasant taste. The seedlings are two to three inches and send out tender shoots, which are eaten and which supply the foundation for making starchy flour.

Peach Palm (*Bactris gasipaes, Guilielma gasipaes*), Also Called Pupunha and Pejibaye

Peach palm grows from Central America to Ecuador, where it is an important food crop. The fruit weights up to twenty-five pounds and contains a high percentage of oil. Peach palms are extensively used, especially in Costa Rica, where their hearts (heart of palm) are processed, eaten, and exported.

Rattan (*Calamus* spp.)

Climbing palms belong to several genera from West Africa. The stems and leaves are barbed with vicious curving spines that hook onto plants. The inner part of the shoots can be eaten. The fibers make a tough and reliable material for furniture. Pulverized calamus root is used as a preservative for potpourri and herbal blends, in homemade botanical powders, and in Hoodoo magic as a love-drawing herb.

Wax Palm/Carnauba (*Copernicia prunifera*)

A very famous vegetable wax is removed by shaking the tree. This wax is suitable for vegans who do not use beeswax and is a suitable replacement for the beeswax in some cosmetic formulations. The wax is used in records (vinyl), candles, and floor and fine furniture wax. Young seeds from the kernels can be eaten.

Palms are explored elsewhere in this book, including an exploration of palm nuts used in divination and the North American medicinal, and the palm saw palmetto is also featured in "Dudu Awo" (chapter 11).

Dudu Awo
(Black Secrets)

HEALING MEDICINES IN FOCUS

- Dudu osun
- Black seed
- Benne
- Deer's tongue
- Devil's shoestring
- L'herbe a malo
- Job's tears
- Tonka beans
- Kola nut
- Palm
- Cotton
- Quassia
- Asafetida
- Boneset
- Buchu
- Saw palmetto
- Myrtles
- Patchouli
- Pawpaw
- Poke
- Rue
- Cayenne
- Maize
- Guinea corn
- Corn plant
- Peanut
- Citrus: lemon, orange, and neroli

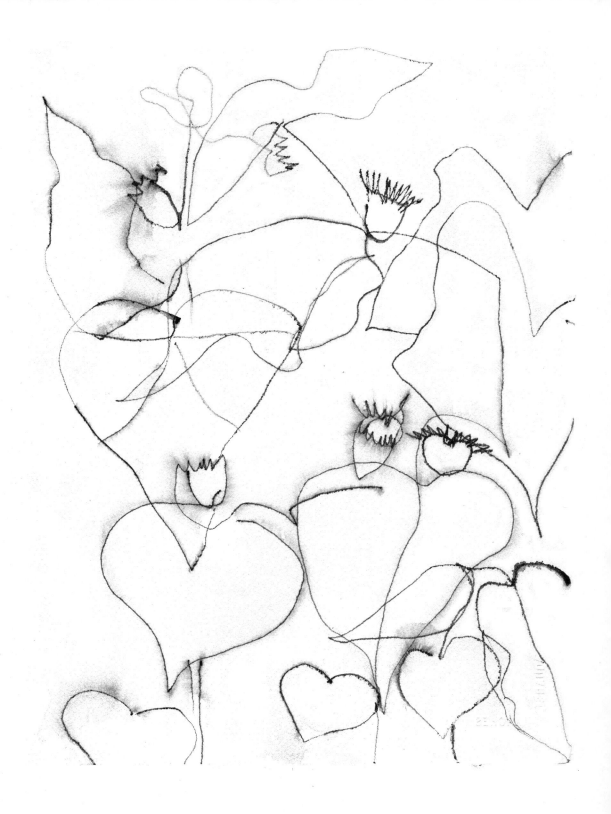

African Healing Traditions

In the black seeds (cumin) is the medicine for every disease except death.
—Arabic proverb

Earlier, I voiced the hope that someday African healing traditions would take their rightful place alongside the other great healing ways of the world. Often the question arises in our community, Why aren't we there already? After all, humans come from Africa. The Motherland is the seat of the oldest civilizations on the planet. Why are our traditions not considered more widely as a valid method of healing?

Of course, since many of us have a history of enslavement or colonization, the thought of racism arises. We cannot help but wonder whether it could be that we are so loathed and looked down upon that our traditional medicine remains systemically ignored, treated as inferior, and attributed to other cultures or appropriated.

Gaining recognition as a people with a valid and valuable healing tradition is staggering. Professor Voeks states the sentiment felt by many ATR healers in *Sacred Leaves of Candomblé*. This quote refers specifically to the situation in Brazil, but has implications throughout the diaspora: "The widely held conviction among Europeans and their descendants that African American herbal medicine was somehow inferior to its Amerindian counterpart was not a question simply of ethnobotanical expertise. Spanish and Portuguese colonists and their descendants were equally ignorant of New World flora and yet their folk medicinal skills were seldom alluded to with the same level of contempt as that leveled at African healers. African based medicine was and is cognitively codified as a form of 'deviant science.'"[1] He goes on to state his deep-seated belief that the attitude toward our healing ways is a visceral reaction built around fear of the African mastery of magic and sorcery. Moreover, according to Voeks, the indigenous American cosmology seems to have been perceived as a blank slate upon which Europeans could fill in their own religious message.

Conversely, the worldview held by Africans was so thoroughly steeped in a different way of thinking: what was seen as idolatry and superstition was an allegiance with supernatural

---

1   Voeks, *Sacred Leaves of Candomblé*, 45–46.

powers that an army of priests could not erase. Indeed, magic was one of few weapons of resistance Africans had, and it created anxiety in the Portuguese community of Brazil. Brazil is not alone. African magic—and the fear of it—was a potent force anywhere large numbers of enslaved people were held, as illustrated by the following examples:

- The high priest Boukman carried out chants and Vodou rituals during the Haitian rebellion to immunize his followers against the white man's magic.[2]
- Priest and doctor, Gullah Jack was a principal organizer in the Vesey Rebellion of 1822 in South Carolina.[3]
- Henry Bibb, a North American enslaved person, described how he used Hoodoo conjuring powders and roots to control his "master."[4]
- African sorcerers in eighteenth-century Suriname entered trances and encouraged slaves to murder their captors.[5]
- White Roman Catholics in colonial Venezuela called on African witches to exorcise the devil from parishioners.[6]

In short, according to anthropologist Alfred Metraux, "The witchcraft of remote and mysterious Africa troubles the sleep of the people of the big house."[7] This sentiment summarizes the feeling toward ATR by empowered white Americans during the antebellum South. Sad to say, traces of the way of thinking remain today regarding ATR.

In another poignant statement, African American ethnopsychiatrist, professor, and author, Wonda Fontenot addresses the issue of our place in the world's healing traditions in *Secret Doctors*. Fontenot says her research and healing practice were fueled by a healing wish. Displeased with the fact that African American medical practices were viewed in bad taste, whereas healing traditions of Latin Americans and Chinese Americans warranted

---

2   C. L. R. James, *The Black Jacobins: Toussaint L'Ouverture and the San Domingo Revolution* (New York: Vintage Books, 1963), 86–87.
3   M. W. Creel, *A Peculiar People: Slave Religion and Community-Culture Among the Gullahs* (New York: New York Univ. Press, 1988), 148–65.
4   B. Jackson, "The Other Kind of Doctor: Conjure and Magic in Black American Folk Medicine," in *American Folk Medicine,* ed. W. D. Hand (Berkeley: Univ. of California Press, 1976), 259–72.
5   J. Stedman, *Expedition to Surinam* (London: Richard Clay, 1963 [1796]), 212.
6   A. Pollak-Eltz, *Vestigios Africanos en la Cultura del Pueblo Venezolano* (Caracas: Universidad Catolica "Andres Bello," 1972), 9–98.
7   Alfred Métraux, *Voodoo in Haiti* (New York: Pantheon, 1989).

attempts to respect culturally diverse thought and appeared to excite the [white] intellect,[8] she set out to make a difference in her work.

Today, we are frequently portrayed in black and white—helpless victims or wanton criminals. The view of Africans and people of the Caribbean, particularly Haitians, is portrayed in major media sources as a people out of control, with few resources and, frankly, without much sense. This endears the heart of the type of people seeking support for their vision of "other" as helpless, ignorant, and the noble savage.

In the Michael Moore's film *Bowling for Columbine*, a combination of cartoon and actual news coverage footage is used to tell the story of how hostility developed toward us and how it is currently acted out. The cartoon *South Park* shows the history of Africans in the United States; weaved into the story was the element of fear—fear of Blackness. Then there is the "news" footage of the explanation of the African bee invasion, an invasion that, though predicted, never occurred en masse. It is easy to see the comparison between the *South Park* cartoon's view of American history and the non-story/story about the African bee. African bees are described by scientists in the clips as being bigger, inherently more aggressive, and swarming in groups, unlike the gentler European and American types. The African bee was most likely a metaphor for African Americans (Bs as in Blacks), to speak in codified language about the perception of our temperament and behavior. Underlining this mini-story in *Bowling for Columbine* is a fear of us and a fear of what is perceived as different in general.

Another difficulty that I have personally experienced is that reputable organizations dedicated to herbs and herbalists have a system of screening prospective professional members that is prohibitive to practitioners of ATR. Many African-descended people, including myself, are taught orally, by family. We supplement this with independent research (comparing notes with other healers, conducting field studies in natural environs, and utilizing books). Our lessons are not formalized; they are incorporated into how we live, which is the essence of holism. We do not keep written records—that would be completely out of place. Our tradition is handed down, and it is largely oral. This is true for almost all African healing traditions, apart from those of ancient Egypt, which is probably why we know—or at least, think we know—so much about Egyptian healing.

The fact that spirituality, the supernatural, and the metaphysical are woven into our

---

8   Wonda L. Fontenot, *Secret Doctors: Ethnomedicine of African Americans* (New York: Bloomsbury, 1994).

practices along with the arts used therapeutically puts practitioners of ATRs at a further distance from many other forms of healing. As there is a swift movement toward "evidence-based herbalism," the magical element is eroded further, replaced by "science," making herbal treatment not much different from taking a pill. This approach is diametrically opposed to ATR. You will notice throughout this book I recommend parts of the plant, fruits, vegetables, waters, and salts, but not encapsulated supplements.

Our ways do not qualify in the eyes of herbal organizations as "professional" or "certified." Most of the programs that offer certification have inherent practical problems.

- As "schools" that are not recognized by state or federal government, financial aid is unavailable, excluding people with low incomes or those with families to support.
- The teaching methodology systematically overlooks our traditions, our medicines, and our ways with medicine, which include the spirit and supernatural.
- The herbal and aromatherapy school certificates have little, if any, validity in the real-world, mainstream professional or medical establishment. Being a certified herbalist means nothing legally, and little economically, particularly in our community. In many ways, paying for such an education is a luxury we cannot afford.
- In short, for most of us, attending school to become practitioners of ATR is not a valid option.

Moreover, as a proud people, humiliated repeatedly by empowered whites, we would be the last people to accept an investigation of our techniques or accept "sponsorship" by a member of the organization who is not a member of our community. This kind of policy and protocol of so-called herbal schools and many of the herbalist organizations automatically excludes us. ATRs continue to be misunderstood. For all of us sharing this planet, cultural exclusion, however it is disguised, is a lose/lose proposition because there is a great deal that can be gained by all through communication and sharing.

In a modern society that wants to see certification and scientific proof for just about everything, the fact that systems like ATR lie outside the mainstream protocol for validation means we are further away than ever in terms of being integrated into CAM. This is at least partially responsible for the lack of understanding—or honor, for that matter—regarding our healing ways. Still, I cannot help but look on in chagrin to see the lack of people of

African descent represented in the "alternative" health movement. I wonder, "alternative" to what? I read healer conference brochures and alternative spirituality newspapers with sadness at the lack of Black representation.

The notion of invisibility is entertaining when watching a Harry Potter movie, but in the context of Black culture, it amounts to little more than psychological genocide. Our methods are ignored, undocumented, discredited, and overruled, making our mark as healers an invisible one. I cannot state enough that this is a loss for everyone involved, not just African-descended people. By means of intercultural research, collaboration, cooperation, and sharing, perhaps healers could come together to tackle some of the horrendous illnesses that threaten our vitality as a global society.

I will say, though, that there are many organizations that do very positive work. Seacology is an organization dedicated to island environments. They support projects on islands all over the world that are initiated and maintained by indigenous people. The organization I am proud to be associated with, the American Botanical Council, consistently highlights and initiates activities that revolve around healing and the plants of Africa.

The Black Secret

The gentler part of my mind wants to see situations in a less exclusive light. A cultural phenomenon that may have also kept our practices outside the boundary of consideration is our own preference for secrecy. I have mentioned this in terms of our client/practitioner relationship and how the traditions are taught. Even the plants and other healing medicines we have identified and created uses for go under the radar, and this is in part by choice, as it is dudu awo—the black secret.

In Fontenot's exploration of the Southwest Louisiana secret doctor or treater,[9] she tells the story of how early African Americans from her area used herbal remedies to deal with ailments. As I have stated repeatedly throughout this book, however, ailments in the case of ATR are of a biological (natural) or supernatural (unnatural) origin. While enslaved people endured biomedicine and were treated like chattel, they also maintained their own medicine,

---

9   Treaters are generalists, while secret doctors usually have an area of specialty, like bone setting, antidotes for snakebite, or mind reading, which she attributes to a unique area of ethnopsychiatry (Fontenot, *Secret Doctors*, 35).

shrouded in the cloak of secrecy, hence the name secret doctor. These doctors without degrees or certificates hid their knowledge about medicine and administered their remedies that include herbs, amulets, prayer, and incantation, all dispensed behind closed doors.[10]

This chapter explores secrecy and how it has been used in the Motherland and beyond to help and harm. The notion of dudu awo is addressed in terms of what needs to be done about "secrets," to heal rifts within ourselves and our relationships with others. The combination of Blackness, or *dudu,* with secrets, called *awo* in Yoruba, is a rich theme not just in Africa but in the Black Caribbean and Americas as well. *Awo* is used in ways that are good, bad, and just plain ugly. We will go through the ways of using secrets succinctly, stopping off as usual to explore the gifts from the plant world with healing secrets of their own. The chapter ends on a bright note, looking forward to productivity in the future.

Hunters' Vests and the Notion of Secrecy

ATR keeps its client-patient relationship private, and its medicine is guarded almost as though under the cloak of secrecy. The revered priests of the Odù and ways of Ifá are actually called "Keepers of Secrets." They are the Babalawo. Herbalists, of many different names previously discussed, also keep secret recipes, formulas, incantations, and rituals.

Exploring the cloak of secrecy is rich in metaphor, yet there are also physical objects that address this notion. West African hunter jackets are cloak coverings with numerous tiny pouches filled with natural charms such as herbs and animal parts used for protection and to build strength and confidence.

You may wonder how or why a hunter's shirt would be loaded with magic? It is the hunters who traditionally brought back sustenance to the community. The job is extremely important, requires a great deal of skill, and is very dangerous. In traditional West African societies, the main arbitrators between humans and spirits are the hunters and warriors. For the most part, their clothing easily identifies them to the animals, deities, spirits, and humans as a warrior on all fronts.

The tea-stained magical shirts worn by Mande, Asante, and a few other groups set them apart from normal citizenry. Hunter and warrior shirts are garments laden with amulets,

---

10 Fontenot, *Secret Doctors,* 30.

knotted cords, animal teeth, claws, horns, cowrie shells, and bits of glass—each of these objects has symbolic significance. The shirts are naturally dyed, leaving an earthen tone, created from the stains of tree bark teas. The tree bark decoction is blessed with protective incantations as it is prepared. The sacred clothing, covered by amulets and animal substances, helps the warrior blend in spiritually and physically with the wilderness. For the warrior, these are more than just cloaks; they are shields from predators and weapons, while also serving as spiritual camouflage lending invisibility.

Hunters and warriors understand that every animal is full of *nyama*. Nyama is the unpredictable energy and action that flows through everything in the universe. Nyama is always present—it can be useful or dangerous. Hunters attempt to understand and control the flow of nyama, and in that way they are engaging the spiritual and metaphysical. The idea of using snake venom and snake medicines explored in chapter 5 are arts requiring one to master nyama. Old-timers had this gift; they knew how to use venom to both harm and help people.

There are lessons for us as we observe the hunter/warriors of Africa, for though far removed in some aspects from that world, we still hunt, gather, and fight wars, albeit of a different type. It is critical that we don't become drunk with our own power. Traditional warriors feel a tremendous responsibility for their actions. They spend many years learning herbalism in the wilderness in the "science of the trees" called *Jiridon*, which is discussed in the previous chapter. Warriors use Jiridon to study and honor the power of their opponents or prey.

The hunter/warrior shirt reflects the experiences of the hunter, by visually documenting his research of various medicines and tactics. The shirts contain knowledge of extracting venom from spiders and snakes among other dangerous ordeals. There is even a specific type of amulet that captures the tears of its prey, called a *nyi-ji*.

Examining the nyi-ji, or tears amulet, helps us understand the staying power of amulets in African diasporic magic and healing. Nyi-ji grows out of the hunter's desire to hunt responsibly. A secret ritual is performed to redirect the nyama (life force) of the animal after it has been killed. Roots of seven specific plants, dug from seven separate footpaths; the flower of a baobab tree; a large nicotiana blossom (from a tobacco plant); the staff or cane of a blind person; fiber from a hibiscus plant used to wash a medicine pot; and a lady's personal washcloth are the main ingredients for the nyi-ji. All of these objects are burned down to white ash. The ashes are placed in the cavity of a horn. The stopper for the horn is pierced with a piece of iron and then the blood of a white rooster is poured over it. Pointing it at an animal activates the nyi-ji amulet. The concentrated power of the nyi-ji, combined with the strong intent of the warrior, makes the animal's eyes water. The tears obscure the animal's vision, allowing it to be trapped.

Once the animal is killed, the hunter rushes up to it and waters an iron staff with the animal's tears. This is but one of the powerful amulets that a warrior/hunter wears on his shirt. The numerous bulging pockets filled with amulets attest to the prowess and bravery of the wearer. The amulets announce that a spiritual force has been captured and is now working for the wearer of the cloak. Some of the pockets contain special blessings (magical squares), a verse or prayer from the Holy Koran. These magical squares are folded a prescribed number of times, according to the desired deity correspondence being invoked, and placed in some of the amulets. Asante wear these shirts for battle, rather than for hunting.[11]

Dudu Osun: The Hidden Medicine

One of the founding principles of Yoruba medicine is a separation of the hidden from what is revealed. The hidden is the spirit, soul, and inner workings of the body. The revealed is everything we can observe on the exterior, with some of the focus on male and female bodily fluids. As I have mentioned, *dudu* is the Yoruba name for "black." Black is one of the three significant color symbols; the others are red (blood and the earth) and white (sperm and spirituality). The Yoruba notion of black includes green and blue, the colors of nature, and as you can imagine it is also used to describe the people of African descent. Dudu is the color of the soil and it represents the concept of burial within the soil, as in planting seeds. Black represents skin as the container of the soul, and the water lies beneath it—dudu is the interior of the self and how we should tend to it.

Tending to the skin is very important in African healing because it is a strong indicator of health. Medicinal soaps are an important way of preparing herbs. In Yoruba, medicinal soap is called *ose*. One of West Africa's great healing medicines is *dudu osun*, commonly called black soap in the United States. To this day, its ingredients and preparation remain a

---

11 Bird, *Sticks, Stones, Roots & Bones*, 101–4.

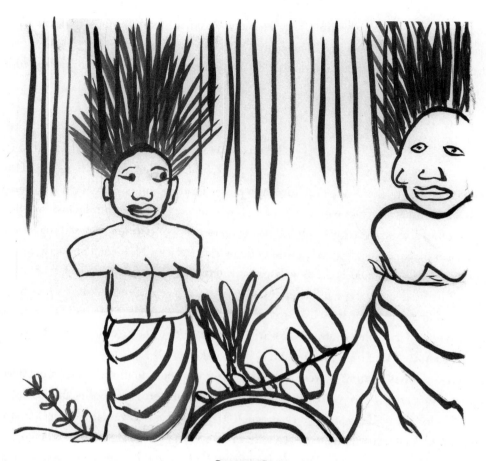

Osun and Eziza

well-kept secret. We do know its rich black color is created through the use of the unique herbal preparation technique called *etu* (burnt medicine), wherein ingredients are slowly charred. It contains palm, a highly prized holistic health tree, used in cooking, beauty, health care, storytelling, and divination. In dudu osun, palm oil is saponified.[12] It contains ashe (liquid medicine with healing force) from lime and lemon and other indigenous herbs as well. While the exact recipe for the medicine within dudu osun stays hidden, its healing benefits have been revealed.

Dudu osun is used to treat numerous skin and scalp irritations, including eczema, seb-

---

12 This means it is made into soap using a catalyst like wood ash or lye.

orrhea, psoriasis, itching, burning, wounds, acne, dandruff, boils, lesions, and leprosy. It is used as a soap, shampoo, and conditioner. While we can buy proprietary blends of the soap base to make something akin to it, for now the truth about dudu osun is wrapped in the cloak of secrecy.

Amulets

Amulets are objects that exercise control and power for the good of the person who wears them. The intimate contact with the wearer allows the person to exert influence over how the amulet is directed. Amulets can be entirely man-made or natural. One of the most famous natural amulets used cross-culturally is garlic. A very well-known man-made amulet containing natural amulets is the mojo bag. It is interesting to note that a mojo is also called a flannel because of the type of material used for the exterior of the amulet (soft cotton). Fabric and fibers are frequently used to create man-made amulets. The textile tradition is very strong in Africa and continues in various forms in the Black Atlantic, most notably with African American quilt making and Gullah basketry.

The amulet has healing power in the treatment of illness (natural or unnatural) because the sickness of the wearer is transferred to the object. Nowhere is this easier to see than with the walking stick (carved cane). Treaters in Southwest Louisiana actually create the sticks for their patients, often with a protective, totemic animal carved on them, like a snake. In this way, amulets are for curing and prevention as well as protection. Components of the amulet typically have names connected with divinities, spirits, or the trickster. Archangel root is a good example of an herb associated with the higher order of spirits—angels.

Natural Amulets
Black Seed Called Tepenen and Black Seed Oil
Black seed is a health amulet that is considered a panacea by many African people. It is believed to be an indigenous Egyptian herb, used for a host of ailments and applied as a lotion or unguent. Ethiopians mix black cumin seeds (*Nigella sativa L.*) with butter, and then wrap the body in cloth or inhale the herbal mix for headaches. Strewn among linens,

it serves as a moth repellent. To this day, cumin is an important African herb.[13] It is used for skin, nail, and hair care, as well as in botanical cosmetic formulations. In short, black seed oil is a multipurpose health oil.

Benne (*Sesamum indicum*)

Commonly called sesame seed, this is one of the herbs brought to the Americas by enslaved people. It is associated with one of the most feared and respected orishas, Sonponno and his cult, who all wear red. Sonponno is a wind orisha that whips up evil storms that disperse smallpox. You can imagine the power of Sonponno if you visualize smallpox as the welts left behind after a tornado blew sesame seeds at someone's face. Benne is eaten atop wafers, mixed into candies, and as cookies. The oil is used in cooking and massage. Benne has been used historically as a natural amulet to protect against theft when planted at the end of the rows of a garden. This has been recorded in the American South, particularly in gardens tended by the Gullah people of South Carolina and Georgia's Low Country. Benne also has a West Indian connection to Obeah, repelling thieves and other intruders.[14]

Deer's Tongue (*Frasera speciosa, Liatris odoratissima*)

Certain herbs are also named for animals because they embody some of their spiritual qualities. Deer's tongue has a scent similar to vanilla, or what we might imagine an innocent deer's breath to smell like. Deer's tongue can be worn in a mojo bag, purse, briefcase, or backpack, or in shoes or pockets. It is thought of as a lust-inducing herb and aphrodisiac. For this reason, it is also sprinkled under and on top of the bed.

Devil's Shoestring (*Viburnum* spp.)

Devil's shoestring is a holistic herb and natural amulet. It grows in the woods, and we have explored the connotations of the forest in African medicines in the previous chapter. The shoestrings are derived from *Viburnum alnifolium*, called hobblebush; *V. opulus*, called European cranberry or cramp bark; and *V. trilobum*, called highbush cranberry; among others of the species. Medicinally it is used as a cramp treatment, especially as an antispasmodic

---

13 Stephanie R. Bird, "African Aromatherapy: Past, Present and Future Applications," *International Journal of Aromatherapy*, 2003, https://www.academia.edu/8362714/African_aromatherapy_past_present_and_future_applications.
14 Ira Berlin and Philip Morgan, *The Slaves' Economy* (New York, Taylor & Francis, 2016).

for painful menstruation. In this capacity, it is readily used as a tea or tincture. As an amulet, devil's shoestring is either soaked and pierced with a very strong needle, pierced by a jeweler's Dremel tool, or tied with string and worn around the neck or ankle. Wear this necklace against the person (underneath clothing) as a protective shield and luck-drawing amulet. Wearing devil's shoestring as an anklet is believed to trip up the devil and bind evil intent, especially when used in Hoodoo foot track magic. Devil's shoestring is also added to mojo bags.

L'Herbe a Malo (*Sagittaria platyphylla*)

Treaters, practicing behind the closed doors of their bedrooms, cut this root indigenous to the area's swamplands at the joint into nine (a magical number in Africa) pieces. They string the root, which is also called arrowroot, on white cord. This amulet is placed around a baby's neck to help with teething and to reduce fever and pain.

Job's Tears or Prayer Seeds

Job's tears are a common name for *Coix lacryma-jobi*, a species of grass of the *Maydeae* genus. The part of interest appears to be the seed but is actually the plant's fruit. The plant is a native of India, but is widely spread throughout the tropical zone. It grows in marshes and has a place in the "secret doctor" medicine of Louisiana and Hoodoo.

Job's tears is also called bead plant because it is used to make necklaces, Mary's tears because it is used to create rosaries, and teardrops because of its shape. It is more commonly referred to in African cultures as Job's tears, so I will use that name here. The idea of creating seed jewelry has been recorded since early times. In Africa, bodies buried during the fifth dynasty of Egypt have been found adorned with seed necklaces. The seed necklace is used against evil for mummified bodies and worn by those who were alive to ward off illness in ancient Egypt.[15]

Job's tears are indigenous to tropical regions. The plant looks like a small version of maize, which it is related to. The plant produces teardrop-shaped light/dark-gray shiny beads that miraculously even have a hole in the center just right for making necklaces. The beads are beautiful in their natural state. Job's tears can also be stained with natural dyes.

Job's tears have been grown by various cultures for hundreds of years and were histor-

---

15 Kathryn Moore, "Seed Jewelry: Seeds Used as Beads: Facts and Folklore," *Plant Lore* 6 (1982): 19–27.

ically an important food source. Today, the seeds are used as herbal supplements and as an ingredient in some foods and beverages, including Japanese sake. Hoodoos recommend carrying the tears as a type of wish bean. The person making the wish is asked to carry three concealed beads for luck, throw seven beads in a fresh water source, or place a string of beads around a baby's neck to help with teething pain.

Job's tears are easy to grow, though not many people grow them anymore. They are annuals, easily raised from seed, though the tough outer shell requires soaking the seeds for a full day before planting. Job's tears is a plant with flexible growth needs. They thrive in either full sun or partial shade. Job's tears should do well in any climate in which corn thrives and can tolerate wet areas with poor drainage, though that is not preferred.

Tonka Beans (*Coumarouna odorata*)

The tonka bean tree is big, growing more than 120 feet high, and is exported from Venezuela. The wrinkled parts called beans are actually the fruits. The fruit is a rich black color, between two and three inches in length, and contains a single seed. Tonka beans have a very romantic, aromatic, musky fragrance that is at once sweet and sultry. Tonka bean is used as a scent preservative in potpourri, sachets, and other handmade botanical blends. It is also used in perfumery.

Magically, tonka beans are used as talismans in Hoodoo to attract a lover, and I must say they have a very good record of success. Medicinally, the tonka bean is used as an anticoagulant because it contains coumarin. The wood is used for heavy, durable construction such as shipbuilding. In Suriname's traditional medicine, a decoction of the seeds is mixed with sugar and used to deter the common cold. Tonka beans were, and may still be, used as an adulterant to vanilla, which is dangerous because too much coumarin becomes unhealthy. The beans are used to flavor tobaccos and snuffs. The essential oil is widely used in the perfume industry.

A total mind, body, and spirit fruit, tonka bean is used to elevate the mood and it is considered to be balancing. Tonka bean is very important in love-draw magic and serves as an attraction agent and aphrodisiac.

Nut Rituals

Devotees use sacred palm nuts (with a Babalawo doing the reading, or alone) for prayer. Palm nut is sacred to the almighty Orunmila. Kola nuts are sacred to Obatala, the old, wise one, and Shango, the thunder orisha. Palm is used as an offering to the trickster orisha Elegba, while warrior orisha Ogun desires palm wine and palm oil. Nut divination typically supplies "yes" or "no" answers, though more complex readings are sometimes also given.

Kola Nut (*Cola acuminata*)

Cola tree is *C. nitida,* which yields the kola nut, and a sweet beverage called *bese* is made from bitter cola. Cola is indigenous to the forests in Ghana, cultivated in Sierra Leone and the Niger estuary in Nigeria. The nuts of *C. nitida* are the richest source of caffeine, and one of the nut's major uses is as a stimulant. Kola nut has been exported from Ghana to the northern savanna regions since prehistoric times. Kola nut was once an ingredient in Coca-Cola, although now the flavor and stimulant come from different sources. The nut is chewed fresh or more commonly dried for its stimulating effect, reducing drowsiness. It is also chewed to aid weight loss; it controls hunger and thirst because of its alkaloids, caffeine and theobromine.[16] Cola twigs are used as a dentifrice, even though they have a very disagreeable, bitter taste; they are used to clean the teeth and gums.[17]

Kola nut is exported around the world for use in drug manufacturing for methylxanthine-based drugs. These drugs are used to treat preterm infant apnea, chronic obstructive pulmonary disease, and particularly asthma. The alkaloids it contains relax the bronchial passages and stimulate the central nervous system and cardiac muscle.[18] The *German Commission E Expanded Edition* approves the nut for mental and physical fatigue as well as to elevate some depressed moods. It must be avoided with gastric or duodenal ulcers and by those with a serious diagnosed psychiatric disorder under medical treatment. It can

16 Abbiw, *Useful Plants of Ghana,* 72.
17 R. Trindall, *Ethnobotanical Leaflets: The Culture of Cola: Social and Economic Aspects of a West African Domesticate* (Carbondale: Southern Illinois Univ. Herbarium, 1997).
18 Louis Sanford Goodman et al., *The Pharmacological Basis of Therapeutics,* 8th ed. (New York: Pergamon Press, 1990).

cause insomnia, overstimulation, nervousness, and gastric irritation and can disrupt sleep patterns, so it should be used under the supervision of an ND or traditional herbalist.[19]

Typical usage: chewing the twigs, infusing 2 g in 150 mL water; 2 g per day powdered, crushed, cut, or whole; tincture: 1:5 (g/mL) in 10 mL alcohol.

The Metaphysical Dimensions of Palm

There is so much to write about palm from an African perspective that it could truly fill a book. We have covered some of the medicinal, utilitarian, and food uses of palms already. This is primarily a discussion of the palm nuts of Ifá called *ekuro Ifá* or *ikin Ifá*. These nuts are different from ordinary palm nuts. Ordinary palm nut is called *ekuro* and comes from the oil palm (*Elaeis guineensis*). The multipurpose palm nut is *ikin Ifá*. The sacred palm nut is from *E. idolatrica* and is used almost exclusively in ritual, hence its Latin name *E. idolatrica*. *Ikin Ifá* tree is branched, its nut has four eyes or more, and the oil overflows from its black cast-iron pot, causing a grease fire rather rapidly. Because of its tendency to overflow from its sacred containment, the black pot that is likened to a womb, it has a great deal of mysticism attached to it. Sacred palm is feared and respected. The branches, called *ori* or heads, can have as many as sixteen eyes. *Ikin* has only about four in contrast. *Ikin Ifá* are shiny, black, beautiful, sumptuous, and sensual—a promising container of dudu awo.

Rituals are varied; one is to collect the young palm fronds that stand erect (a positive symbol), encircling the *ori* of the plant to make wine or oil used in ritual. These same types of fronds are used to set apart sacred groves, which are discussed in the previous chapter. Their presence indicates that divinity or spirit may be present. The blackness within symbolizes the sacred awo.[20]

As a central object to Ifá, *ikin Ifá* are presented to each Babalawo when training is completed. By gaining understanding of *ikin Ifá,* understanding is also gained of the divine nature of the palm tree itself. Sixteen black palm nuts at the heart of an Ifá ritual are kept in their special container when not used for divination.

Palm is associated with Sonponno in the spiritual beliefs of the Yoruba. Sonponno is a feared orisha associated with smallpox, whipping winds, diseases of the skin, and epidemics. Palm wine called *emu* keeps Sonponno away.

---

19 American Botanical Council, "Cola Nut," in *Expanded Commission E report.*
20 Buckley, *Yoruba Medicine,* 124.

Here are a few other ways palm is used on the spirit realm.

- A broom made from the midribs of the palm frond is used to symbolize the smallpox epidemic.
- Sometimes these brooms are bewitched to make a bad person, usually a thief, tire themselves by sweeping until they pass out.
- A palm frond broom is smeared with red camwood and kept in the smallpox victim's room.
- Palm oil is a spiritual antidote to smallpox.
- Palm kernel oil, called *adin*, is an offering to Sonponno to tease and annoy him so he will go away, curing the disease.
- During the smallpox epidemic, people drank the palm wine to chase the orisha away. It is a preventative.
- Palm wine is splashed around the yard, courtyard, or verandah as a libation to keep Sonponno away.
- Obatala, on the other hand, is a white orisha who likes to consume white things, so he drinks raffia palm called *oli oguro*.
- Palm wine is associated with revelation, which destroys internal order.[21]
- The Babalawo uses both palm nut and cola nut as tools of divination.

Cotton: Crossroads of Enslavement, Freedom, Feminism, and Discovery

Cotton is the most important economic botanical plant in the world. It was a major impetus for the need of an ample, unpaid labor force that inspired slavery in the American South. Even the story of how the plant migrated is full of intrigue and controversy. My favorite is the story of how it probably became a stowaway in some long-ago vessel that was making its way to the New World.

Cotton was a major force in the antebellum South economy and culture. During the 1930s, more than half the world's cotton was produced in the United States. Even today, with machines thankfully replacing enslaved people, over a million bales are produced in America's cotton boll states. The leading producer is now Texas, followed by California, Mississippi,

---

21 Buckley, *Yoruba Medicine,* 108–11.

Louisiana, Arkansas, and Arizona. We are sixth in production these days behind China, India, Pakistan, Brazil, and Turkey. Species of cotton grow and are processed in West Africa as well.

Cotton and Africans came together in a brutal way, under the poorest possible conditions. Still, enslaved Africans carried out the orders of their owners, planting, picking, and helping to process more cotton than what was thought humanly possible. African women, who were charged with a great deal of the health care responsibility on the plantation for Blacks and whites, particularly women's health as midwives, soon discovered cotton root's abortifacient qualities. This discovery enabled midwives to induce labor for already-deceased (stillborn) fetuses. Cotton root decoction also allowed the women who endured rape by planters and their associates, as well as the prospect of having their offspring sold away into slavery, the ability to terminate unwanted pregnancies. Please note, before you get any ideas, this is a very dangerous activity (abortifacient herbalism). I am not suggesting for anyone to self-treat using cotton root bark because the results could be lethal.

Cotton (*Gossypium herbaceum*) is a biennial or triennial herb with a round branching stem of about five feet tall. It has a hairy palm-shaped leaf and yellow flowers. The fruit is a three-to-five-inch celled capsule where seeds are held. Cotton is an Asian native cultivated throughout the world. The inner bark of the young root was used historically. Cotton was recognized between 1863 and 1916 by the USP (United States Pharmacopeia) for its effects on the uterine organs. During the nineteenth century the active constituent was called *gossypin*. African American uses were reported as early as 1840, wherein the enslaved people were found to use the root bark as an abortifacient. In Euro-American medicine, the bark of the root was used in cases of difficult labor, uterine inflammation, sterility, vaginitis, and suppressed menstruation.[22] Today we use cotton as a styptic; to hold medication to wounds; to cover fresh wounds so they can still breathe; to hold poultices, infusions, decoctions, vapors, and rubs; to cleanse the face and apply makeup or sacred ornamentation; to secure henna tattoos, letting the stain seep into the upper layer of the skin; to blow our nose; cover and clean our ears; and of course for clothing. Organic cotton is a wholesome option available today that is less likely to irritate delicate skin, and it is kinder to the environment than cotton processed commercially. Organic cotton is expensive. To cut costs, seek organic cotton garments or bedding in resale shops or as bulk fabric to design and sew your own apparel.

---

22 Mitchell, *Hoodoo Medicine*, 54.

Herbs and Secrets

The Secret of Quassia (*Picrasma excelsa L.*)

Quassia is pronounced *"kwosh-u."* Quassia is a pure bitter once sold in wooden cups made of the herb. Water extracts and dilutes the quassia readily. It was used to discourage thumb-sucking. As an intense bitter, it is used as a substitute for hops in making beer. It is used in bitter tonics and for winemaking.

The secret of quassia is how it came to our knowledge. Quassia is also called slave wood. An enslaved person named Quassia held the secret to this medicine from his native Suriname for quite a while; in the end he sold the secret to Rolander, a Swede, around 1756. Some accounts say the secret medicine held in the tree was revealed from the spirit realm and shared with Quassia. White doctors looked on as Quassia "doctored" people of all races, reducing what would have been a deadly fever. He gave it freely but did not want to reveal what was contained within the potion. Eventually he sold it; some accounts say it was for a large sum of money while others say it was in exchange for his freedom. Quassia was very important as a cure for dysentery in 1713, when it was sent to France. Between 1718 and 1725 an epidemic flu prevailed in France, which resisted all the usual medicines. Quassia was tried and was very successful. The so-called slave wood became a sought-after medicine in Europe during the eighteenth century. It is used by West Indians and was a time-honored European cure for fever, malaria, snakebite, dysentery, dyspepsia, venereal diseases, rheumatism, alcoholism, intestinal worms, and cancer.

Quassia is a West Indian and South American tree. A Jamaican quassia is *Picrasma excelsa* and it grows in the West Indies. The West Indian type is taller than the Surinamese, Brazilian, and West Indian types. It grows in French Guiana and the islands of Dominica, Martinque, Saint Lucia, Saint Vincent, and Barbados. The name given by the founder of the genus was *Carib simarouba*. The tree is sixty feet or more, with many long, crooked branches covered with smooth, grayish bark. The leaves are nine to twelve inches long, and the flowers grow in small clusters with thick, off-white petals. The bark is usually found in pieces several feet long; the roots are long, horizontal, and creeping. The roots are odorless and difficult to pulverize. It is frequently imported from Jamaica in bales.

Quassia contains a bitterness identical to quassin, as well as a resinous matter, a volatile oil, malic acid, gallic acid, and small amounts of other constituents. It restores lost tone in the intestines, promotes secretions, diminishes insomnia, and is used to kill lice in the hair of children. It is sometimes set out in saucers as an infusion and used to kill flies, mealy bugs, and gnats. Most important, it is an herb that eases the later stages of dysentery when the stomach is not affected. This is helpful to people who prefer herbal remedies and useful to those who have little access to reliable biomedicines.

Asafetida, Also Called Devil's Dung

Because it is so acrid, asafetida is thought of as an aid to dark forces in the Americas, hence its moniker devil's dung. It is also a mainstay in African American folk medicine as a panacea for a variety of ills, including that very-hard-to-describe *spiritual heart pain* discussed in chapter 8. The way folks use asafetida varies but typically includes taking a piece the size of the end of the pinkie, rolling it in a ball, dropping it in hot water to infuse, then straining and drinking it.

How to use: asafetida—or dasa-foetida, as it is sometimes called—is infused in whiskey, with garlic buds added for good measure, to serve as a general health tonic. Used in this manner, only one teaspoon is taken every other day.[23]

Boneset (*Eupatorium perfoliatum*): Gullah Treatment

Boneset is called *break-bone fever* by the Gullah. It is a bitter tonic, used to treat cold symptoms, fevers, body aches, influenza, and rheumatism.

How to use: add 1 teaspoon dried herb to 2 cups very hot water, cover, and steep 10 minutes. Strain. Add lemon. Boneset tea is used therapeutically at 4 to 5 cups per day.

Buchu

Buchu is a small South African shrub that grows between two and three feet tall. It is an aromatic, carminative, diaphoretic, and diuretic stimulant that has been used for hundreds of years by the Khoisan people. Growing primarily on the Cape of Good Hope, buchu brings the hope of relief to men suffering from prostate disorders and urinary infections. A strong tea is made of the dried leaves and taken for painful urination, gravel, and catarrh of the bladder. It is also taken for leukorrhea. An infusion of buchu leaves is taken in South Africa as a stomachic and stimulant tonic.

---

23 Snow, *Walkin' Over Medicine*, 21–22.

How to use: 1 teaspoon cut and sifted leaves per cup of very hot water. Steep half an hour. Take only 3 to 4 tablespoons 3 to 4 times per day. As a tincture, it is taken by the dropper (10 to 20 drops) in water 3 times per day.[24]

Saw Palmetto (*Serenoa repens*), Palm Cabbage

Saw palmetto grows in areas where the Gullah people have lived for several hundred years, the Carolina Lowlands. Gullah people have a tradition of using saw palmetto in their sweetgrass basketry, and this tradition continues today. There is a history as well of creating a palm wine called *maluvu* from the sap, juice, or center of the top of saw palmetto, which the people call palm cabbage. Secret doctors and treaters of Louisiana use saw palmetto, which grows there, in their healer's repertoire. This Southern United States plant grows in Alabama and south throughout Florida. It grows abundantly in Florida as an understory plant of the forest and beach growth. Saw palmetto also grows along the Caribbean coastline and has some uses as a beverage there as well. It is commercially harvested from the wild, which is quite a dangerous production because it is a prickly plant, protective of its precious berries.

The Seminole, which have a concentration of African ancestry,[25] recognized saw palmetto fruits as a food, though tart, and used it as a medicine as well. Seminoles prepare infusions of the berries to treat stomach upset and diarrhea and as a diuretic and sexual stimulant. An additional multicultural people who identify as Native American, the Lumbee, have a long history of using saw palmetto medicinally.

Parts used: fronds are used for decorating, weaving, and basketry; berries are used medicinally and as wild food.

How to use: the ratio is 1 teaspoon dried berries to 1 cup water, decocted 20 minutes. Strain, sweeten if desired, and drink.

Saw palmetto is used to treat the prostate. Benign prostatic hypertrophy (BPH) diminishes the quality of life for men, and over 50 percent of men over the age of fifty experience this. It is an herb that provides relief for many people. The most studied phytomedicine

24 Lust, *Herb Book*, 136.
25 Intercultural mixing occurred when enslaved people escaped their owners and were taken in by the Seminole community. The Seminole are one of the more prominent groups of "Black Indians," an admixture of Native American and African American people.

for prostrate are extracts of saw palmetto fruit. The fruit is also associated with improving libido in both sexes and reducing impotence in men.[26]

Hidden beneath many a saw palmetto is the eastern diamondback rattlesnake. Whether it is a totem or protector of the plant remains to be found. What we do know is that each year people are bitten when they do not realize that saw palmetto is the secret hideout of the diamondback rattlesnake.

Myrtle, Also Called Khet-Des

Myrtle was used for skin disorders and sinus infections in early Egypt.[27] Myrtle is used to inspire peace and invite blessings and generosity. Grown since early times for the fragrant flowers and leaves as well as the aromatic bark, myrtle contains antibacterial phenols. Spiritually, myrtle symbolizes Venus and other love goddesses. It is used medicinally to treat tumors, breasts, and genitals. Iranians make a hot poultice for boils, and Algerians use it to relieve asthma. North Africans use the dried flower to treat smallpox.[28] The Gullah people use an indigenous form of myrtle (*Myrica cerifera*), an aromatic evergreen that grows in wet, sandy pinelands and bogs in the Carolina Lowlands and Sea Coast Islands, for diarrhea, dysentery, and uterine hemorrhage and as a gargle.[29]

How to use: African Americans use myrtle by inhaling warm vapors from the tea or making a poultice to relieve head pains caused by a severe cold or flu.[30]

Sweet Myrtle (*Myrtus communis*)

Sweet myrtle is one of the most revered love herbs. This type of myrtle is used as an amulet to assure fidelity and cultivate joyous unions.

How to use: used as a wedding amulet, it can be worn as a hair ornament or on the bride's veil or integrated with the bouquet. This plant is recommended for nuptial gardens and to bless new properties with love.

---

26 Steven Foster, "Men's Health and What You Need to Know About Saw Palmetto," Steven Foster Group (2000).
27 Manniche, *Ancient Egyptian Herbal*, 122.
28 Duke, *Herbs of the Bible*, 1999.
29 Mitchell, *Hoodoo Medicine*, 75.
30 Anna Riva, *Magic with Incense and Powders* (International Imports, 1985), 27.

Patchouli (*Pogostemon cablin*)

Sultry, earthy, dark, and noted for its ability to attract love, patchouli is a base for many perfumes.

How to use: this earth-kissed herb has many useful functions, including:

- Reducing libido
- Aiding relaxation and sleep
- Patchouli leaves are good additions to potpourris, dream pillows, and wool or cashmere storage containers. The leaf acts as a scent preservative.
- Patchouli essential oil will quickly transform an ordinary bath into a nurturing, sensual experience. There is a warm, moist darkness to patchouli, suggestive of the dudu awo of the Dark Mothers and Earth Mother.

Pawpaw: Secret Weapon for Digestion

Pawpaw (*Carica papaya*) is an herb that is beloved in Africa, the Caribbean, and the Americas. It resembles the palms, with seven-lobed leaves, and produces an oblong, yellow-orange fruit somewhat like a melon, thus it is also called melon tree. As I have stated, however, pawpaw is not a tree, though it resembles one. It is considered a gigantic herb and is nonwoody with a hollow trunk three to eight meters tall and twenty centimeters in diameter. The trunk is simple and unbranched and bears large triangle- and diamond-shaped leaf scars. The leaves, trunk, and fruits exude a white, milky sap when injured. It is used in digestive health because of the papain it contains, a digestive protein; it also contains pepsin to aid digestion, vegetable enzymes to digest milk proteins, and another enzyme to handle starches. It is used to treat acid reflux, indigestion, and constipation. The cardiovascular system shows some improvement due to the carpaine pawpaw contains. It cleanses the lymph system and fights infections. Pawpaw is used in weight-loss programs as it aids sluggish digestion and elimination and it is also nutritious.

How to use: the leaves, fruit, deep-black seeds, and juice are all consumed for nourishment and used medicinally. It mixes well with banana, coconut milk, pineapple, orange juice, and strawberries in a blender with some ice to make a tasty smoothie. Pawpaw has a wonderful, pungent aroma and sweet taste—medicine that is beautiful to look at, interesting to the nose, good for the body, and invigorating to the spirit.

Pokeroot (*Phytolacca decandra*, *P. americana*), Also Called Poke

Poke is a common plant native to the Eastern United States. It is a foul-smelling perennial weed that can reach nine feet tall. The large white root extends from a purple stem, and its leaves grow up to one foot long. The newly sprouted poke leaves are eaten as greens. This forest medicine is found primarily in damp fields and open woods.

Contains: triterpenoid saponins, resins, alkaloid, phytolacca acid, formic acid, oleanolic acid, and amino acids.

Actions: purgative, emetic, anti-inflammatory, decongestant, and alternate. Pokeroot has a duplicitous position, beloved by some and loathed by others. The secret about pokeroot is that some people, particularly healers in the African American community, know just how to use it as a curative. Without this secret knowledge, it becomes a very dangerous herb.

Pokeroot is an excellent remedy in the hands of a well-trained practitioner of traditional medicine. It is used as a remedy for the lymphatic system, relieving congestion, swollen lymph glands, and swollen or congested breasts. Breasts are treated using a poultice, which seems to reduce breast lumps and cysts. Poke promotes lymphatic circulation, cleansing, and clearing of toxins and treats tonsillitis, laryngitis, swollen glands, glandular fever, mumps, catarrh, ear infection, arthritis, and rheumatism. It clears skin of acne, boils, psoriasis, eczema, and athlete's foot and is used to detox the body, promote digestion, and relieve constipation. One always has to be extremely careful with herbal emetics and purgatives. Poke contains poisonous constituents, mostly in the roots, and has been known to cause bloody vomit and diarrhea.

Warning: it is to be avoided altogether in pregnancy. I recommend having poke prepared by a traditional healer rather than self-treating.

Rue

Practitioners of Candomblé in Brazil and of Lucumí in Cuba wear rue in their hair with other herbs to deter negative spirits.[31]

How to use: massage directly onto the body to reduce fever.[32]

---

31 Voeks, *Sacred Leaves of Candomblé*, 24.
32 Manniche, *Ancient Egyptian Herbal*, 123.

Cayenne, Hot Sauce, and Hot Foot Powder

Cayenne (*Capsicum frutescens, C. annuum, C. spp.*)

African pepper, a primary component of soul food cooking most notably used in Louisiana Hot Sauce, is also used magically in Hoodoo and as a healing herb. African pepper is used to treat stomachache, sore throat, rheumatism, poor circulation, body aches, sluggish metabolism, and lack of motivation and is also used spiritually by most African people. Cayenne has diaphoretic, rubefacient, and stimulant qualities. Ground cayenne is called chili pepper and has the ability to energize the entire system. The tonic quality and fiery heat of chili stimulate the flow of energy—in short, it is hard to ignore contact with cayenne.

Cayenne: Holistic Uses

Culinary—as an invigorating spice, chili pepper adds intense flavor to stews, vegetables, and even corn bread. Hot sauce featuring cayenne peppers is widely used in African American soul food as an accompaniment. Various pepper sauces are used elsewhere in Africa and the Caribbean.

Medicinal—helps stomachache, sore throat, rheumatism, poor circulation, body aches, sluggish metabolism, and lack of motivation.

Magical and spiritual—cayenne is used by Hoodoos for foot track magic, a practice that clears pathways of negativity. Hot foot powder[33] is full of the element of fire. It is red, it smells acrid enough to burn the nostrils, and if stepped on with bare feet or handled improperly, it can cause major irritation—this is due in large part to its large amount of cayenne. To keep negative influences at bay, hot foot powder is sprinkled outdoors to form a ring of protection. The powder, incense, and oil can be purchased ready-made or created from mixing equal parts of cayenne, salt, and sulfur. Add cinnamon and ground orange peels to improve the smell. (The quantity depends on how much ground needs to be covered.)

---

33 Warning: use a dust mask when creating hot foot powder and wash your hands well afterward.

Maize (Zea mays), Also Called Corn

Maize is an important staple food, particularly in Africa and the Americas, where it has been used to nourish animals and their people for hundreds of years. It is grown widely in the forest and savanna regions of West Africa. Varieties grown include pure white, red, and red and white. Maize is a very important staple in the southern savanna. It is roasted or boiled on the cob and prepared with groundnuts as a dessert. The bulk crop is dried and milled to make corn flour. Corn flour is used to make banku, kenkey, and the porridge dishes agidi (used to nourish those who are ailing) and Tom Brown. Other ways of preparing it include a bread, boodoo, bodongo, and kakro. Maize has a role in annual festivals in Ghana, during which a special dish called kpekpoi is made. Beer, ahei, ngmeda, and tuei are some of the beverages made from corn. Corn oil is used in West Africa for cooking, cosmetics, and soapmaking. In West Africa, a plant glycerin is derived from maize.

Street vendors use maize shucks to create a biodegradable food wrapper for several dishes. One such dish is fante-kenkey, a cooked fermented maize dough wrapped in maize shucks. The shucks are used in Ghana for creating fiber crafts like doormats.

Guinea Corn (Sorghum bicolor)

Also called *atoko* in Ghana, this is the fifth most important grain crop in the world. It is grown in the Sudan and Guinea's woodland and savanna areas. It is a staple food in certain areas. It is prepared as a porridge and brewed into an alcoholic beverage. The mature Guinea corn plant is used as fodder to feed local livestock and chickens.[34]

Maize is a plant around which there is a great deal of cross-cultural sharing, a healing rite that reduces the negative connotations of secrecy. African Americans share both bloodlines and preferred foods with America's indigenous people. Corn bread, corn pone, and succotash of several different types are chief among our shared dishes. The Lumbee use many different parts of the maize plant—which they call Indian corn or big red, since they prefer a red type—for food and medicine. The silk is used as a diuretic tea to treat kidney or bladder stones and as a hair softener. I enjoy using corn silk as a conditioning detangler for kinky or curly hair and find that the diuretics it contains relieve some of the congestions

---

34 Abbiw, *Useful Plants of Ghana*, 23–25.

and discomfort of PMS. The shuck is used for wrapping food and crafts and to make a multipurpose, tasty tea. Lumbee and the people my family blended with, the Cherokee, make whiskey called moonshine from corn, which they used medicinally and as a beverage.[35]

Tied to growth, life, and death, corn is a symbol of fertility and prosperity. Hang dried corn on your front door, place a bowl of cornmeal on your altar, and hang more still by your hearth (stove) in the kitchen. As you gaze upon the dried corn or pass a bit of cornmeal from hand to hand, seek fertility, whether it be in a physical or spiritual sense, and contemplate the goddesses of the corn:

Memu

Memu is the Ugandan creator being whose symbols are corn and beer. Memu, like most goddesses of the harvest, brings love, compassion, and nourishment into our lives.

Odudua

Odudua is the creator goddess of the Ifá pantheon of the Yoruba people of Nigeria. Shrouded in dudu (black, her favorite color), her presence invites fertility, love, and community. Odudua's spirituality is connected to the African American winter holiday Kwanzaa. Kwanzaa is a celebration of the harvest that features corn prominently; it also seeks continued fertility within Black culture.

Corn Plant (*Dracaena fragrans*)

Corn plant is an easy-to-grow, inexpensive, common houseplant used for holistic health. Corn plant is one of the sacred plants of Candomblé, wherein it is called *peregun* in Brazil. The sacred corn plant leaves are placed on the walls of ritual or worship spaces in the form of the crossroads (an X) or placed in a vase. Corn plant brings good fortune to the environment and is used to dispel ghosts.

---

35 Arvis Locklear Boughman and Loretta O. Oxendine, *Herbal Remedies of the Lumbee Indians* (Jefferson, NC: McFarland & Company, 2003), 48–50.

Guba:
Coming Out of Its Shell

Students of African history recognize that an African American man named James Carver "invented" peanut butter. The butter of the guba (peanut), which is more typically referred to as groundnut, has been made into a paste in Africa for hundreds of years. Groundnut is an important African staple food because it is a legume high in protein, making it less expensive than other sources. In parts of Africa, groundnut is pulverized and prepared as a flour that is mixed with skim milk and given to babies as a formula.

Peanuts are rich in phytosterols, about 135 milligrams per 100 grams.[36] They contain ubiquinol-10, also called coenzyme Q10. This constituent helps detoxify bad (LDL) cholesterol. It is one of the most efficient antioxidants and contains phytosterols useful to perimenopausal and menopausal women. It contains up to 38 percent of the DV of protein and is 40 to 50 percent oil. The solid fat is hydrogenated and used to make margarine and cheese. The residue after oil extraction is quite large and is used to make cakes for animal fodder; the green top of the plant is also fed to animals.

Peanuts (*Arachis hypogaea*), like black-eyed peas previously discussed, are an important food in West Africa and the diaspora. Groundnut was introduced from South America as a savanna crop grown in the Sudan and in Guinea. Nigeria, Senegal, and Sudan are the major African producers. There are several varieties. The nut is chewed raw or boiled; it is also roasted as a side dish, usually accompanied by maize. Ground and roasted nuts are used to make groundnut soup and groundnut paste (also called peanut butter).[37] Peanuts are a natural sweetener used to prepare a variety of desserts and breads. Some people have deadly allergies to peanuts, and of course anyone with allergies should avoid the triggers that affect them. It is also a good idea to read packaging well to make sure, if you are allergic, the food you are consuming does not contain nut debris nor was prepared in a facility that handles peanuts. Wild birds and squirrels love peanuts and many wild animal treats feature them.

---

36 Carper, *Food—Your Miracle Medicine*.
37 Abbiw, *Useful Plants of Ghana*, 31–32.

Moving On:
Lemon and Orange

To end this lengthy section of herbal monographs, I leave you with a couple of citrus fruits that offer hope and healing. Their bright appearance and their ability to cleanse, disinfect, lift moods, and fortify the mind, body, and spirit are the perfect way of ending on a bright note, imbued with the fortitude of hope.

Lemon (*Citrus limonum*)

The lemon was brought to Africa and the diaspora from Southeast Asia. It serves in both places as a medicine and food.[38] Lemons are highly touted by the Gullah and Hoodoos. The Gullah use lemon in herbal teas as a natural remedy. Admired in the Black community for the same qualities that attract mainstream aromatherapists, lemons repel insects and detoxify; are astringent, antifungal, antiseptic, and refrigerant; and are high in vitamins A, B, and C and bioflavonoids. Lemons are a useful treatment for fever, high blood pressure, cold and flu symptoms, sinusitis, and lethargy.[39] Associated with positive energy, good spirits, and luck, lemons can be grown indoors. Putting a bowl of lemons out on the table is believed to bring good spirits to the home. In the next part, I will show you how to use lemon in home cleaning and cosmetics.

Orange (*Citrus sinensis*)

We are most familiar with oranges as the juicy fruit consumed during our daily awakening rituals. Orange juice, not coffee, is one of the most invigorating, replenishing breakfast drinks, bringing energy to start the day. I highly recommend orange juice to everyone (who is not allergic or intolerant to it), especially to young people who tend to gravitate needlessly toward coffee for energy. As a symbol of the sun god, Ra, the orange plant is one of nature's most vitalizing gifts, rich in possibilities for healing. Many parts of the orange tree are used for holistic healing and complementary therapies—one of the most intoxicating is the blossoms.

---

38 Grimé, *Ethno-botany of the Black Americans,* 20.
39 N. Purchon and L. Cantele, "Conditions and remedies," in *The Complete Aromatherapy and Essential Oils Handbook for Everyday Wellness* (Robert Rose, 2014), 178, 407.

Oranges in Suriname are of three different types: sour, bitter, and sweet. Originally from Spain and Portugal, they grow readily in warm to tropical regions of the Americas and Africa. Sour orange is used to treat sores and running ulcers.

Early enslaved African people made great use of the sour orange, consuming it raw or smoked (cooked in wood ashes) and using it for dressing (old) wounds in veterinarian medicine, for stopping vermin from entering wounds, and as a vermifuge. It was used as a substitute for soap and for washing clothes.[40] Today, house cleaning formulas and botanical dish and laundry soaps continue to feature orange essential oils because it is pleasant-smelling, uplifting, and has a broad spectrum of cleaning applications. A very positive attribute of the essential oil is that it is good for the spiritual and ecological environment. Whereas some essential oil is very expensive (like the neroli listed below), sweet orange essential oil is affordable for students and others with limited income.

Neroli (*Citrus aurantium, C. bigaradia, C. vulgaris*)

The exquisite and expensive pure neroli oil is derived from the orange blossoms of *Citrus aurantium*, *C. bigaradia*, and *C. vulgaris*. Neroli[41] has a potent scent; used in perfumery, its fragrance is precious, unusual, sweet, floral, penetrating, and alluring. Orange blossom deters dermatitis and stomach upset and is a treatment for menstrual and menopausal discomforts and for infections. Neroli essential oil and orange blossom water are thought to be antidepressant, anti-anxiety, and antihysteric agents, used to ease inhibitions and elevate self-esteem.

On the bright note of orange with all its useful parts, we journey forward from the darkness of dudu awo to the full sun, ready to partake in seasonal recipes and celebrations.

---

40 Grimé, *Ethno-botany of the Black Americans*, 104.
41 Neroli is a heart tonic and must be used under supervision by those with heart disease.

PART III

Wisdom of the Directions

Navigating the Web of Herbal Life

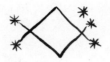

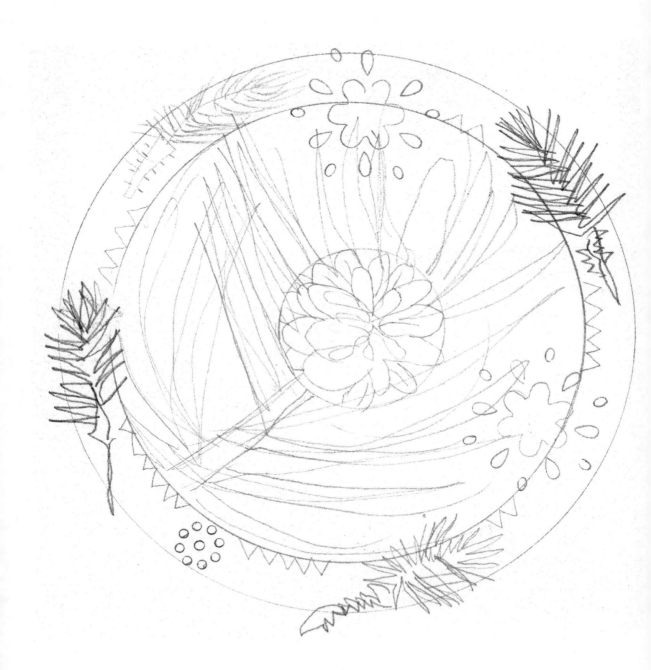

CHAPTER 12

The Web of Life

Safety

Herbs should be used with caution, as many have the potential to be allergens; skin testing is suggested before proceeding whether or not you have known allergies. People taking medications should consult with their naturopath before trying new substances. People with respiratory problems, young children, the elders, and pregnant women should only use incense outdoors and they should be observed for troubling symptoms. Generally if an herb or natural ingredient is very new to you, please be sure to do a skin test or take a small portion, wait twenty-four hours to see whether there is a negative reaction, and then proceed. Herbs do contain chemical constituents, which you could also call drugs, and this is the reason for a cautious approach, especially with the few herbs that I discuss that have contraindications. In closing, none of my suggestions in this segment or elsewhere in the book is designed to replace the professional advice of an MD or ND.

Ananse: Weaver of the Web of Life

So, this last part has an intricate structure; after all, it is inspired by Ananse's handiwork—the elaborate spider web with its elegant design. Within this web that honors Ananse lies a structure built around the seasons of life (life passages), the four seasons of temperate zones, and the four directions. Before we get into all of that, let's familiarize ourselves with Ananse.

Ananse goes by many monikers, including the popular Anansi, Aunt Nancy, Hapanzi, and Nanzi.[1] It is a minor god of the Akan people, who hail from southern Ghana, south-eastern Côte d'Ivoire, and Togo. *Ananse* means "spider" in the Twi language spoken by the Akan, the peoples of the great Akan Empire in the aforementioned countries.

Why is our organizing principle Ananse and its web? Well, for one thing, it is considered a deity, and if not, it's looked upon as an intermediary between the deities, spirits, and people in Akan traditional religion. The religion, known as Akom by the Twi-speaking Akan, spread across the Atlantic Ocean during enslavement, taking a firm root in the Caribbean, in Jamaica especially, where it's related to Kumina, Revivalist, Myal, and Obeah practices.

This book has laid out an intricate vision of our Black healing ways. There is no better way to summarize it, and then put theory into practice, than to turn to the Akan, with which many Africans in the Caribbean and Americas share ancestry. The spider and its web represent wisdom, and we seek this as we come to understand the ways of our ancestors.

As a youth, I learned that my maternal grandmother healed concussions using webs. I wasn't grossed out; I was impressed. Here was a woman who had birthed eleven babies, led a congregation of her spiritualist followers north from Virginia, and at times toted a rifle. This woman, who I understand was barely four feet tall, is legendary in my mind. She is a badass. The fact that she could rely on herself, as determined and wise as she was, and help someone she loved, using webs, may well be what set me on my path to healing.

The web is a design feat that has directionality and a rounded nature, reflecting our lives and the intricacies of the year. Spiders, on the other hand, according to Nancy Mello,[2] an animal communicator, psychic medium, and clairvoyant, have three significant characteristics that are expressed through their symbology: curiosity, wonder, and growth. Kathy Harmon-Luber gives us even more to contemplate in her book *Suffering to Thriving*, where she says that spiders (the embodiment of Ananse) spark many qualities in us that are pertinent to this discussion, including:

- Balance
- Creativity
- Curiosity

---

1   "Ananse," Britannica.com, last updated September 19, 2023, https://www.britannica.com/topic/Ananse.
2   Lauren David, "What to Know About the Spiritual Meaning of Spiders, and What to Do If You're Seeing Them," Mind Body Green, May 19, 2023, https://www.MindBodyGreen.com/articles/spider-spiritual-meaning.

- Growth
- Patience
- Rebirth
- Self-awareness
- Self-sufficiency[3]

You will also find Ananse Ntontan as the logo for the Center of Africana Studies and Culture at Indiana University. According to their website, they made this choice because "the Ananse is associated with a spider's web and it's a symbol of wisdom and creativity." The IU website goes on to say, "Ananse is a wise and cunning figure who is often identified as a symbol of Black resistance to enslavement through its ability to outsmart the plantation structure or individuals who would do harm."[4]

And, regarding Ananse's categorization as a trickster, being that it's a true Africanism and the story demonstrates will and survival, perhaps it's time for that connection to be relinquished. Many African diasporic stories feature a marginalized individual that is disempowered and perceived as a trickster, when in fact it's an emblem of survival. I prefer to consider Ananse a spirit of a dualistic nature; much like the rest of us, it craves the light but sometimes is caught up in darkness. As we tuck into its web, going through seasonal observances, don't discount Ananse as something to trivialize or deem a trickster. Ananse is of the highest ancestry, a child of Nyame (god of the sky) and Asase Yaa (Mother Earth). As such, it's able to petition deities and spirits for humans. It is a deity in its own right. Please consider Ananse, as it has been called "master of direction through indirection, a signifying cultural presence capable of challenging the stability of the linguistic order, as well as the social."[5]

Finally, your signposts will be Adinkra symbols from the kingdom of the Ashanti. They have been chosen because of their succinct way of crystalizing complex concepts as proverbs in Adinkra. These will be your field guilds as you make the way through the seasonal observations and the magic of the four directions.

---

3   Kathy Harmon-Luber, *Suffering to Thriving: Your Toolkit for Navigating Your Healing Journey: How to Live a More Healthy, Peaceful, Joyful Life* (Powell, OH: Author Academy Elite, 2022).
4   "Adoption of the Adinkra Symbol," Indiana University, School of Liberal Arts, https://liberalarts.iupui.edu /centers/casc/about-us/ananse-ntontan.
5   Henry Louis Gates Jr., *The Annotated African American Folktales* (New York: Liveright, 2017, p. 11).

Nkyinkyim ("Twisting"): This Adinkra encapsulates the way resourcefulness, grit, and creativity help us navigate the torturous journey of life

Warming Celebrations
of Winter

The New Year starts in winter in the northern hemisphere, a time in temperate zones when many outward signs of life are dormant. I thrive during this time of the year because I am an interior person. I love nesting and being at home, which our Chicago weather forces upon us at times. Winter has a question: Are you up to snuff, tough enough, to make it through mentally, physically, and spiritually? Each year, I think I know the answer, but each winter also comes with its own set of challenges. This is the time after harvest. In many ways, it is a time that separates the wheat from the chaff.

There are various strategies we can take. We can bond together indoors, enjoying the abundance of the harvest season's fruits and vegetables as friends, lovers, and family. Then, too, there is an abundance of holidays: Kwanzaa and Yule, also called Winter Solstice, which I find to be entrancing. Through the two events, much is laid bare in their different ways. Around the exhausting high holidays, Christmas, Hanukkah, and many other secular and nonsecular observances, Winter Solstice, comes knocking. This noncommercial celebration of Mother Earth—or, in the Akan spirit of this part, Asase Yaa—comes to the fore in our minds. This very dark time of the year, with the shortest day of the year to boot, asks us to see things in a different way. What does the blue-black of the great outdoors have to tell us? Where are the stars leading us, and what is the moon directing us to do? The challenge is, Can we get quiet and still enough to listen to Asase Yaa? Can we honor her or comprehend the universe in which she is situated?

Yule and Winter Equinox

Winter Solstice falls around Yule, and it marks the beginning of winter. It is the darkest day of the year. Winter Solstice is time to celebrate the mysteries of life and how it continues to grow shrouded in darkness. We seek enlightenment and tend to spend more time—more than any other season—near fire: candlelight, smoldering incense, the kitchen stove, or an actual fireside. Here are two different types of ways to incorporate the element of fire.

YULE FIRE AND ICE REFLECTION RITUAL

One of the most enchanting activities in indigenous society is gathering by the fire. This is where meals are cooked, where warmth is provided during the damp, wet seasons, and where seeds are planted in the heads of generations to come. In the West, we have a tendency to depend on the candle more. They are portable and can be burned just about anywhere, as long as they are always tended.

- To celebrate the Solstice, gather your favorite evergreens: choose a few cuttings each of: holly with berries, juniper with berries, cedar, spruce, or pine. These can be gathered from your own property or neighborhood, a forest, or a florist if necessary.
- Fill a flexible container with water. If using a plastic container, add a few small clean cans, such as coconut cream or tomato paste tins (which will later hold your candles). Choose the can size appropriate to your flexible container.
- Weigh down the cans with a few charged stones placed inside each one.
- Place the evergreens in the water.
- Place in the freezer—or outdoors if you live someplace really cold—for a few hours until frozen solid. Let thaw just enough to remove cans.
- Flip container with greens over onto a fireproof plate or old cookie sheet covered with foil.
- Add the candles into the holes left by the cans.

During Yule dinner, light the candles. This beautiful display of fire and ice, which also features the elements of earth and air, is elemental magic at its most basic. Reflect on the fire and ice as you tell stories of what you enjoy the most about winter. I know for some that is asking a lot, but do try—it's good for your spirit. If you are doing this alone, still reflect on joy and winter as you watch the flickering flames and melting ice. This is a gorgeous reminder of the beauty and mystery of winter.

PORTAL OPENER

A portal opener brings quiet, joy, and contentment to your life.

Charcoal
Lighter/matches
A large shell
Fireproof earthenware plate
Skeleton key

4 small frankincense pebbles
1 large chunk myrrh
A piece of copal
Dried orange slices
Red rose petals

Light the charcoal and place it on the shell. Place this atop the plate. Let it get very well-heated; it should turn white in areas. Close your eyes if possible. Clear your thoughts and take deep breaths as the charcoal heats. Decide where you wish to travel. Pick up your skeleton key, close your eyes again, and visualize yourself opening the spiritual door to the locale where you wish to travel. When you feel as though you've gained access (however distant), open your eyes. Gradually feed the charcoal fire each resin, fruit, and flower. Let the aromas take you on your trip to another world.

Evergreens: Symbols of Life, Death, and Renewal

In African American tradition evergreens are a metaphor for the interaction between departed spirits and the living community.

Bring the spirit of continuity, growth, and change into the home by collecting and displaying organic evergreens. Junipers with the berries are lovely. Holly with red berries is symbolic of the Holly King, the traditional Father Winter and Father Christmas. A bouquet, spray, wreath, or garland featuring evergreens energizes the environment as well.

Evergreen Aromatherapy

If you become sick with a cold, bronchitis, flu, or COVID, be sure to add some of these greens to a pot of water. Decoct, then remove from heat. Form a tent with a towel by putting a clean bath towel overhead. Inhale the cleansing vapors designed to open up the nasal passages, bronchial system, and lungs, while also freeing up mucus. Pine infusion also makes a fine hair rinse or a mouthwash for sore throat and laryngitis. Chewing white pine refreshes breath, and the needles contain vitamin C.

AROMATIC PINE FLOOR WASH

When I am cooped up indoors, in the middle of winter, my spirits grieve the lively, spirited colors of autumn. Pine Floor Wash has a remarkable influence on the emotions. The floor washes below are recommended as a winter tonic for grief, mild depression, and fatigue. These two updated formulas featuring essential oils are antibiotic, antiseptic, and antifungal.

Fill bucket ¾ full of rainwater or tap water. Drop in essential oils, using a combination or a single oil: ½ teaspoon white pine (*Pinus sylvestris*) or ocean pine (*P. pinaster*), ¼ teaspoon juniper (*Juniperus virginiana*), and ¼ teaspoon lemon (*Citrus limonum*). Add 3 tablespoons liquid castile soap. Use to mop your floors and to cleanse nonreactive surfaces.

Celebrating Kwanzaa

Christmas: I might as well say it because, whether you celebrate it or not, you are impacted—unless you live off grid in the wilderness and choose not to celebrate. I happen to enjoy the Pagan underpinnings of Christmas. I like giving and sharing with my family and friends. But it gets to me; it drains my energy. And yet, the very next day, another holiday comes about that is built on seven principles; it is called Kwanzaa. I've heard a lot of negative comments about celebrating it. "I'm tired. I don't know how. It seems too complicated." Well, let's take a moment, right now, and sort through the principles and what they could potentially mean in your life.

Kwanzaa is the celebration of the Nguzo Saba ("first fruits" in Kiswahili, commonly spoken by the Swahili people of the Great Lakes Region in East Africa). The dates stay the same each year, as does what it is we are to reflect upon.

This is a relatively recent holiday, founded by Dr. Maulana Karenga in 1966, sparked by the Black Power Movement. Kwanzaa is designed to inspire folks to engage with their heritage. Here's what you need to have on hand and how to perform the ceremony:

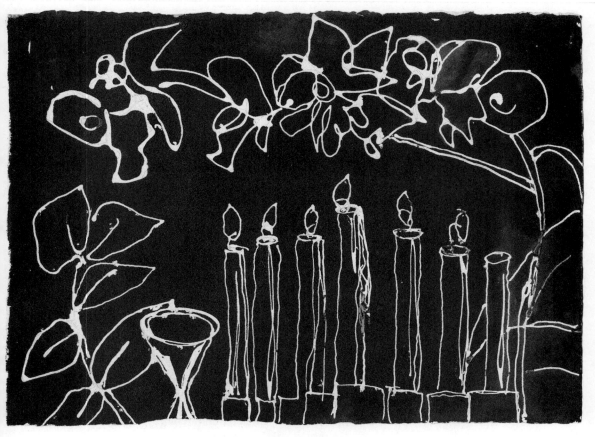

Kwanzaa celebration

- Mishumaa Saba, or "seven candles," of which one is black, plus three each of red and green:
  - The black candle, which is placed in the middle of the kinara, is lit first. It represents unity and the Black people of the diaspora.
  - The red candle to the right of the black candle is lit on the second day. Red represents our blood shed and the struggle.
  - Green goes to the left of the black candle and is lit the third day. Green is Asase Yaa (Earth Mother) and represents the possibilities of the future.
  - Light the candles as follows: on the first day, the black one. On the second day, the red one to the right of the black and the black. The third day you light the

green to the left of the black candle, along with the black and red candle—and so forth until Imani, when all the candles on the entire kinara are bright with the Mishumaa Saba.

- Kinara or candleholder
- Kikombe cha Umoja, or Unity Cup
- Mkeka, or place mat (black or natural woven color)
- Mazao, representing the crops and featuring a cornucopia of goodies
- Muhindi, the all-important ear of corn
- Zawadi, or gifts (preferably homemade; otherwise, definitely bought from a Black maker or business)
- An open heart and patient attitude

Your creativity is welcome during this very open-ended holiday, yet there are a few basic tenets you must follow. Here are the dates, the special words to focus on each day, and a few ideas to get you going. Remember: every day you can say this to someone in the Black community: "What's the word?" And the answer is: "Harambee!" ("Let's all pull together.")

December 26: Umoja ("unity")—as a people, nation, community, and family

- Have dinner with a group of family or friends in someone's home—or, if remote, you will each bring your laptop or smartphone for video conferencing.
- Ask each person to bring a soul food or dish from the African diaspora.
- Hold hands after lighting the candle of the day.
- Each of you starts singing your favorite sacred song (ask others to join in).

December 27: Kujichagulia ("self-determination")

- Make a cup of your favorite herbal tea in an earthen mug (remembering it is made of Asase Yaa). Conversely, a glass of wine is fine.
- As you prepare for Imani, light your candles for the ritual.
- Grab a favorite journal or a couple of pieces of paper and a pen.
- Draft seven ideas for how you can be more independent and self-possessed in the New Year.

December 28: Ujima ("collective work and responsibility")

- Much like the other days, make a comforting, preferable warming beverage.
- Researching in whatever way you prefer, identify a place where you can volunteer to make your community a better place.
- Light your candles for this thoughtful ritual.

December 29: Ujamaa ("cooperative economics")

- Do some research or go out to see what you can do to help the Black community.
- Jot down some ideas or begin your work.
- Light your candles.

December 30: Nia ("purpose")

- Light your candles for the day.
- Pour a red libation for your ancestors, and honor the struggle they had that helps you sit where you are right now.
- In your journal, write out a purposeful declaration about yourself and where you are headed in the coming year.
- Gaze at your candles; see what journey the flickering lights take you on.

December 31: Kuumba ("creativity")

- Outside, pour a libation of the liquor of your choice and reflect.
- Pour a glass of wine, hot toddy, or drink of your choice to sip as you work.
- Light your candles for Kuumba.
- Gather magazines, newspapers, paper, scissors, and a glue stick (or another adhesive) and create a dream or vision board to map out your New Year.
- Use Kuumba to design your New Year of successes!

January 1: Imani ("faith")

- This is a time to exchange your zawadi ("gifts"; preferably handmade or bought responsibly).
- Imani is a wonderful day, the final day of Kwanzaa, to enjoy a soul food or a Caribbean, Brazilian, Puerto Rican, or African feast!

Maize and Kwanzaa: A Celebration of Nguso Saba

When celebrating Kwanzaa, be sure to invite friends and family to potluck dinners. This is a way of maintaining relationships and building community, which is essential to the holiday. As you bless the table, reflect upon the gifts of your ancestors. Remember to eat the foods that enabled them to survive because they continue to bless us with health. The colorful soul foods of our ancestors, rich in antioxidants and available during the winter, include pumpkin; winter squash; collard, mustard, and turnip greens; rutabagas; turnips; parsnips; beets; oranges; and bananas. Make sure to include symbols of the harvest that are important to our African heritage on your Kwanzaa altar including pumpkins, gourds, and dried corn.

Corn plays an important role in Kwanzaa, and rightly so, as it has provided sustenance and nurturing for hundreds of years. In Africa, it has been around for at least five hundred years and it is one of the major crops. South Africa is the largest producer of edible corn in Africa, and this corn is exported to Zimbabwe, Botswana, and Mozambique.[6] In sub-Saharan Africa, it is the most important grain crop. More than three hundred million Africans across the continent utilize maize as a staple crop.[7]

In South Africa, many dishes are featured in the indigenous South African cuisine of the Zulu, Xhosa, Tswana, Swazi, and Sotho. Each tribe has their own version of mielies or pap, corn-based dishes similar to hominy or grits.

- Umphokoqo namasi, also called crumbly pap or amasi, is an easy-to-cook maize meal that is rich and hearty.
- Umxhaxha is corn and squash simmered with salt, sugar, and cinnamon.
- Umngqusho is corn, butter beans, onions, potatoes, and chilis.
- Chakalaka is a unique, delicious brew of onion, garlic, ginger, tomato, carrots, sweet peppers, hot chilis, curry powder, and canned baked beans.
- Ugali is somewhat similar to Nigerian fufu, but it uses maize meal for its starchiness. It is a stick-to-your-ribs side dish to comforting stews in many parts of sub-Saharan Africa.

---

6   "Bumper South African Corn Crop Is a Boon to Import-Reliant Neighboring Countries," Gro Intelligence, April 11, 2023, https://www.gro-intelligence.com/insights/bumper-south-african-corn-crop-is-a-boon-to-import-reliant-neighboring-countries.
7   International Institute of Tropical Agriculture.

Corn Silk Tea

You can just imagine the first people coming across corn silk and thinking it to be so gorgeous that it surely must have a use. Indeed, corn silk is a useful herb and should not be thrown away.

Corn silk is something that has been overlooked and even thrown away. Corn silk is a kind friend to both elders and children. It is a diuretic that helps condition the bladder and reduce bed-wetting. It is particularly helpful to seniors because it helps diminish the buildup of solids that restrict the flow of urine. Corn silk helps to heal numerous ailments and malfunctions of the bladder, including inflammation, which also affects the kidneys and urethra. Corn silk is used as a folk cure for high blood pressure, to lower cholesterol, and to treat arteriosclerosis.

How to use: shuck two ears of corn; reserve shucks and corn for other projects. Bring water to simmer. Add corn silk. Cover, reduce heat to medium, and infuse 10 minutes. Strain and drink. You can follow this same procedure to make a hair conditioner. Instead of drinking it, let it cool and then use it as a final rinse to soften the hair.

HOW TO MAKE SUCCOTASH #1

My mother and aunt would make this dish in a seasoned cast-iron skillet, and you might like to try it as well. As I mentioned previously, cast iron can supply small amounts of iron in the diet, especially when using a recipe like this one that contains tomato or other acidic fruit.

6 ears corn
1 small onion
1 green, yellow, red, or orange
  bell pepper
2 tomatoes

1 teaspoon olive or corn oil
Sea salt and freshly ground
  pepper
Dash of cayenne or hot sauce
  (optional)

Shuck 6 ears corn. Remove silk; set shucks and silk aside for other projects. Hold corn at a slight angle, pressed to cutting board. With a very sharp carving knife and going with the grain, cut corn over the cutting board. Mince a small onion. Remove seeds and interior from green, yellow, red, or orange pepper. Cut in half and mince. Cube 2 tomatoes and sauté them in 1 teaspoon olive or corn oil (using a spraying oil is fine). Add sea salt and freshly ground pepper. Add a dash of cayenne or hot sauce if a spicy taste is desired.

HOW TO MAKE SUCCOTASH #2:
I-YA-TSU-YA-DI-SU-YI-SE-LU

My Aunt Edith, a family elder who was married to a Native American, taught me how to make *I-Ya-Tsu-Ya-Di-Su-Yi-Se-Lu*, also called Cherokee succotash. It is a simple recipe that we enjoyed as children, during the cool days of fall and winter.

I-Ya-Tsu-Ya-Di-Su-Yi-Se-Lu is hearty enough to serve as a soup meal with corn bread on the side or as a tasty side dish. Vegetarians, please feel free to omit meat (I do). I only provided the meat to make the recipe as close to authentic as possible. This recipe can be performed over an open fire as readily as it can be done indoors on the stove.

2 cups lima beans (frozen or
  dried)
1½ teaspoons sea salt, divided
4 cups corn, fresh from cob (or
  frozen if necessary)
1 medium onion (wild if possible)

1 tablespoon butter or bacon fat
1 teaspoon peppercorns
1 teaspoon sugar
Bear meat, ham hock, or turkey
  drumstick (optional)
1 cup cream (optional)

Wash dried limas and pick out undesirable beans or debris, if any. Put them in a pot of water (a cast-iron Dutch oven works well). Add 1 teaspoon sea salt. Bring to a boil. Cover and remove from heat for one hour (set a timer). Shuck corn. Put corn silk aside for tea or hair rinse. Cut corn kernels from ears with a sharp knife, following directions from above. Put corn kernels and corn milk aside in a large bowl. Finely mince a medium onion. Place butter or bacon fat in a cast-iron skillet over medium-high heat. Sprinkle with ½ teaspoon sea salt. Grind peppercorns and add (not traditional, but tasty all the same). Sprinkle 1 teaspoon sugar over onion and spices. Add corn, and cook till lightly browned. Once the one-hour timer goes off, add ingredients from skillet to the pot, along with the meat, if using. Simmer 2 hours or until meat is tender. (If omitting the meat, simmer

35 minutes to allow flavors to blend.) Stir in cream, if using. Simmer low, 15 minutes or so to warm thoroughly. Serve hot.

Thanks, Aunt Edith!

New Year's: January
Winter Spirit: Inspiration and Renewal

New Year's Eve is a time to look back on the previous year. We reflect on good times and bad, we mourn those we have lost as we make way for the new life ahead. New Year's Day is the time many of us choose to make resolutions for how to be a better person in the coming year. The New Year is a time when we can seek luck to have a prosperous, healthy, and abundant year. Traditionally we eat symbolic foods including black-eyed peas, white rice, stewed tomato, and collard greens.

HOPPIN' JOHN

1 pound black-eyed peas, dry
Olive oil (1½ tablespoons or
  spray)
1 large onion
1 green bell pepper
2 cloves garlic
Pinch sea salt

½ teaspoon freshly ground
  pepper
½ teaspoon cumin
Pinch dried cayenne pepper
5 cups chicken or vegetable
  broth, plus more as needed
2 cups chopped tomato

Soak a pound of black-eyed peas overnight in a bowl or follow quick-cooking directions on the package. Discard the water and rinse (this reduces the tendency for the beans to give gastric distress). Add oil to a Dutch oven, or use a stockpot if none is available. Set heat at medium. Mince onion, green pepper, and garlic cloves finely, keeping each separate. Sauté onion until translucent. Add green pepper, sauté 5 minutes, then stir in garlic and continue cooking. Add salt, pepper, and spices; stir to mix all ingredients well. Pour in broth, and stir well. Cover, and simmer on low for 30 minutes. Add chopped tomato, and cover again. Cook until beans are soft and tender. Test, and add more spices if desired.

STEWED TOMATO

3 cups chopped tomato
1 tablespoon white sugar
Pinch fine sea salt

¼ teaspoon ground white
  peppercorns
1 slice French bread
1 tablespoon unsalted butter

Add tomato to cast-iron or other pot. Turn heat to low. Add the sugar, salt, and pepper, and stir. Cube bread and add it and the butter. Cook gently 30 minutes.

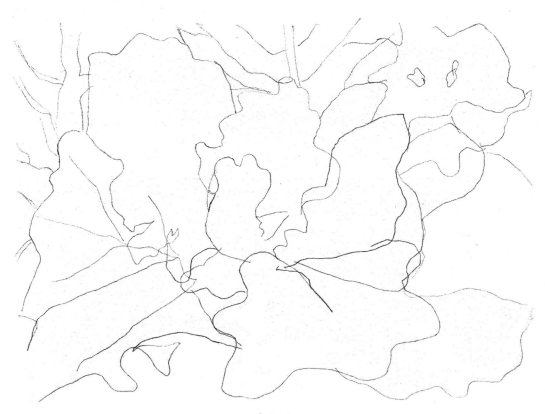

Collards

PLANT-BASED COLLARD GREENS

2 bunches of collard greens
(about 3 cups)
1 medium-sized yellow onion
3 cloves garlic peeled
Avocado oil
1½ teaspoon salt

1 teaspoon freshly cracked black
pepper
Sprinkle of red pepper flakes
(optional; to taste)
2 tablespoons champagne
vinegar, rice wine vinegar, or red
wine vinegar
1 to 1½ cup vegetable broth

Soak two bunches of collard greens in cool water in the sink if they have not been cleaned, to remove the sandy grit. Swish the greens around in the water with your hands to dislodge grit. Blot greens with a tea towel to remove some of their water. Tear or cut them as small as you like on a cutting board. Set aside. Mince onion. Crush garlic with the back of your cutting knife on a cutting board and mince. Heat some avocado oil in a Dutch oven or cast-iron skillet over medium heat. Add onion. Sautee until clear, fragrant and slightly caramelized. Add garlic. Sauté on medium low, for a minute or two (do not let brown). Sprinkle in salt, pepper, and red pepper flakes, if using, to taste. Gently add in the greens. Lightly pour in the vinegar of your choice, and toss greens in the vinegar. Pour in vegetable broth. Simmer on medium to medium-high, 15 to 20 minutes, stirring occasionally. Strain greens using a slotted spoon before serving. Serve hot.

Rice

Growing up on the East Coast, and with ancestry from North Carolina and Virginia, having rice regularly with meals was second nature. Little did I know as a youth of the steeped history of rice in my culture. Then, back in the 1990s, I happened upon the book *The Carolina Rice Kitchen* by Karen Hess. Through its pages, I learned that rice (*Oryza sativa*) is indeed a food of my soul—it's not just filler. Hess makes it clear that, while many of us connect rice only with Asia, especially China and Japan in the case of *O. sativa japonica*, rice has been cultivated since approximately 1500 BCE around the Senegambia and the Niger Delta.[8]

---

8 Karen Hess, *The Carolina Rice Kitchen: The African Connection* (Columbia: Univ. of South Carolina Press, 1992), 12.

It is uncertain how *O. sativa* was introduced, but they also had *O. breviligulata* and *O. barthii*, indigenous rices from the Senegal River, from the Nile, and from all the way south as far as Angola and Tanzania.[9] Black, indigenous Africans have a rich and full history with rice in Africa, from the indigenous types of rice to the domesticated cultivars. The Malay of Madagascar take our history back to 500 CE and stand to be an important historical source of rice on the Motherland.

Planters and colonizers were keen on enslaving the highly knowledgeable and adept rice farmers from sub-Saharan Africa. An area of Sierra Leone, referred to as the Windward Coast, was a preferred culling ground for rice-processing and rice-farming experts. The Windward Coast is also referred to as the Rice Coast.[10]

My ma's people include the great Wolof of the Wolof Empire, Gambia, and Angola. To stir the pot deeper yet, my mother's method for cooking rice is remarkable similar to this recipe from a Ghanaian diplomat named Dinah Ameley Ayensu. Ayensu shared this rice recipe in *The Art of West African Cooking*.[11]

MAMA'S RICE

2 cups water
1 cup Carolina Rice

2 teaspoons avocado oil or
olive oil
¼ teaspoon sea salt

For many, bread of one type or another is considered the staff of life. For me, growing up unknowingly food insecure, long-grain Carolina Rice was our staple food. Mostly, the humble but filling food was served as a side at dinner, on its own, or—cringe—topped with buttery spread to make it more palatable for us kids. For breakfast, we'd have it two ways, as a porridge with the buttery spread and—also very cringe-worthy—added sugar. My parents weren't shy about enriching their rice with Louisiana Hot Sauce, especially when pairing it with chicken. Sometimes my Daddy would add a tablespoon or two of the

---

9   Hess, *Carolina Rice Kitchen.*
10   Hess, *Carolina Rice Kitchen.*
11   Dinah Naa Ameley Ayensu, *The Art of West African Cooking* (Garden City, NY: Doubleday, 1972).

leftover plain rice from dinner to scrambled eggs; I still add rice to my eggs now and then.

Today, my family eats wild rice frequently (which is technically not rice, yet it is in the family of domesticated rice), and we eat brown rice, too. For a white rice option, basmati or jasmine rice is frequently the go-to. When we can get the true Carolina Rice of my youth, we cook it much as Ma did. Simply effective, we cook it a little something like this:

Rice cooker method: If using a rice cooker, which I highly recommend, use the manufacturer's measurements and directions.

Stove-top method: Add water to a medium-sized saucepan with a well-fitted top. Bring to a rolling boil. Add the oil and salt. Stir to mix well. Add the rice. Stir once and then not again. Boil 1 minute. Cover. Reduce heat to low. Simmer for 15 minutes or the time advised on your rice package. Turn off the stove. Let sit for 5 minutes. Uncover. Flake with a fork. Serve hot.

NOTE: It is possible to buy typically expensive wild rice in bulk for a better price at wholesalers like Costco. I enjoy Lundberg Organic Wild Rice. Organic brown rice and select types of white rice can be purchased in bulk up to 25 pounds, but you can also buy as little as 2 pounds. Buying in bulk is economically sound and earth-friendly. It is a comfort to have this filling staple on hand for food shortages, such as those caused by a crisis like COVID-19, or if you are on a tight budget. Red or black rice is also very tasty, especially when coconut oil is the fat used for cooking, as they have a more complex flavor profile, not to mention, they are a beautiful addition to the plate. Sadly, for the penny-pincher, they can be a budget-buster.

February 14th, Saint Valentine's Day: Making Way for Winter Romance

Saint Valentine's Day is a time to revel in the decadence of romance and love in its many different manifestations. Sweet-smelling flowers and comfort foods are featured treats, as are aphrodisiacs like chocolate, fresh fruit, and gifts of the sea. Shrouding ourselves in warmth and comfort provides a respite from winter, affording an opportunity to nourish the mind, body, and spirit. In the home spa, we tenderly care for dry skin, hair, and nails with herbs and natural oils at a fraction of the cost of a commercial spa.

The Rose (*Rosa* spp.)

No other plant is as intimately linked with love as the rose. I love my middle name so much, I continually use it. Not only is it connected to an incredibly medicinal and romantic flower, it also has family significance. My Great-Aunt Rose was my grandfather's beloved sister, a quiet, sweet, and gentle woman who reminded me of a flower caught up in a gentle wind. My Aunt Rose, on the same side of the family, was a shining spirit, basically without equal. She was my very generous and loving godmother. I have just taken a break to think of these beautiful and impactful ancestors, to really tap into the rose, and brought inside my Olivia rose and my Peace rose, which is a golden-yellow color and carries with it my wish for peacefulness in Chicago. When you are selecting healing roses, seek out the old-fashioned scented types such as those listed below, rather than the more neutral tea roses. Roses are beautiful, and like the lotus, they suggest female genitalia in the height of passion. The blush of the rose is often compared to the blush of a bride or a sexual partner during orgasm. In parts of Africa and the Middle East, holy temples are spiritually cleansed with the highly potent Bulgarian rosewater typically called rose hydrosol or simple rosewater. Rose hydrosol enhances the sacred environment.

A little-known fact is that roses are a systemic nervine—translation: they calm and soothe your nerves. Fresh roses, rosewater, rose otto (attar of roses), rose cream, and rose incense all cast a magical spell, binding love and romance. The following recipes feature high fragrance and the ubiquitous food of the gods—ingredients with a time-honored tradition in love magic cross-culturally.

Neroli Affirmations

After the flurry of holidays, sometimes there is a downturn in the mood by the time Valentine's Day rolls around. This is multiplied if you are single, on the verge of breakup, or widowed. These affirmations are useful healers for a variety of reasons. Are you sick of seeing and smelling roses this time of the year? Try neroli absolute or essential oil—it is a spiritual oil that builds confidence where it is lacking and cheers up the spirit. You can do this in three different ways, depending on what is available to you:

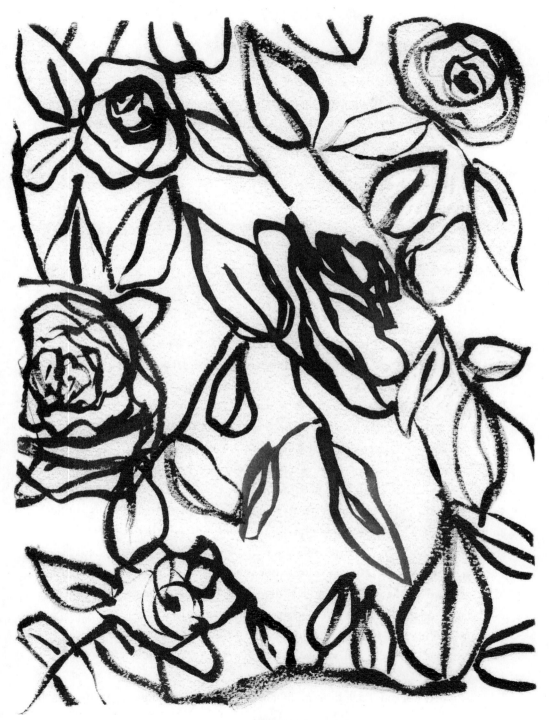

Olivia roses

- Place a bowl of fresh oranges you have carefully selected because they appeal to you on a piece of furniture or the sink near a mirror.
- Dab neroli oil (sparingly) on your pulse points (temples, wrists, back of the knees, etc.).
- Mist your face and hair with neroli hydrosol (also called orange flower water), then say each affirmation as you look in the mirror:
  - *I accept myself as I am.*
  - *I welcome the person I am becoming.*
  - *I surround myself with love.*
  - *I forgive myself for the mistakes I have made.*
  - *I forgive the harm brought to me by others.*
  - *I am ready to move forward.*

Ashe!

Romantic Flower Projects for Saint Valentine's Day

- Pink carnations suggest enduring friendship, warmth, and trust. They are inexpensive, even in the winter, and add a nice touch to a romantic dinner.
- Buy fragrant old-fashioned flowers of your favorite scent and color.
- Peel petals away from organic fragrant flowers (roses work well). Float these in a bath for two. Light vanilla-scented candles for a pleasant accent.
- Sprinkle rose petals on your mattress, under your bed, on your covers, in your closets, in your purse, and anywhere the compassionate spirit of the rose is desired.
- For a sexy bath, add ¼ cup rosewater to 1 cup milk. Stir in 8 drops jasmine absolute and 4 drops each lotus and patchouli oils. Mist your wet body (bodies) after a bath or shower with fragrant neroli hydrosol, also called orange flower water.
- Put a fragrant gardenia or lily in your hair before going out to a party or on a date.
- Mist your face and hair with lavender hydrosol before leaving home—especially if inhibitions and tension are coming between you and finding love.
- Set out 7 to 9 lit candles scented with a relaxing essential oil such as neroli, sandalwood, chamomile, or lavender, in the room where you will entertain your company.
- Old-fashioned stock and delphinium in blues, whites, and lavender are warming and invite a long, steady relationship.

SAINT VALENTINE'S DAY
LOVE POTION
AND MEDITATION

Collect yourself. Breathe deep and evenly. Focus on your intentions for love and healthy relationship as you collect the following ingredients:

2 cups high-quality dry red wine
2 slices orange
8-inch cinnamon stick
⅛ teaspoon allspice
2 cracked white cardamom pods
⅛ teaspoon ground ginger

Sterilized needle (to prick your
   finger)
Drop of your blood (optional,
   or blow into the mix with your
   healer's breath)

Take a cleansing breath (inhalation), and visualize your passion pouring out into the pot as you exhale. Your intention becomes the first ingredient. Pour wine into a pot. Cut orange slices in half and add them. Break cinnamon stick in half. Stir in spices and a drop or two of blood, if adding. Heat on medium low until warm but not boiling. Let cool slightly. Pour into glasses and drink with the intended.

Chocolate Soap

Some soapmakers, this one included, tend to get carried away with the chocolate soap theme, especially during the winter holidays. Using soap molds creatively adds even more fun. Molds used for chocolate making can easily be used to create soap. (Just pour the freshly made soap into chocolate molds as you would use any other mold.) Wholesale Supplies Plus produces heavenly scented chocolate fragrance oils that can be used alone or in combination with a variety of oils to carry through the chocolate theme. Orange, lemon, or cassia essential oils also work well with handmade cocoa butter products. Vanilla or coconut fragrance oils complement chocolate soap. Chocolate-colored soap poured into chocolate molds can then be put into heart-shaped or other traditional chocolate boxes as a novel Saint Valentine's treat.

HOW TO MAKE CHOCOLATE SOAP

4.5 ounces goat milk
10 ounces distilled water
5 ounces lye
12 ounces vegetable shortening
8 ounces tallow
12 ounces coconut oil

2 ounces unsweetened baker's
    chocolate
Soap or candy molds or
    rectangular Pyrex casserole
    dish
Vegetable cooking spray
1 ounce cocoa butter

Freeze milk overnight before soapmaking. Thaw milk in the morning by setting it out in the sink or countertop. Measure all ingredients on a scale. Put on goggles, apron, and plastic gloves for protection. Mix milk and water in a quart-sized Pyrex liquid measuring cup. Stir in lye using a stainless-steel spoon. Set aside.

Melt the shortening, tallow, coconut oil, and chocolate in a stainless-steel stockpot on medium. Remove from heat. Spray soap molds with the vegetable spray, and set aside. Melt cocoa butter in the microwave, on the stovetop, or in the oven. Set aside. Using a meat thermometer, take the temperature of the oils and the water/milk mixture (clean thermometer after it is used for the oils so it doesn't contaminate the water/milk mixture). When both sets of ingredients equal 120 degrees, slowly stir milk/water mixture into oils with the stainless-steel spoon. Continue to stir in a figure-8 motion. Chocolate soap is ready to pour into molds or dish when you drizzle a portion on top of the batch and it retains its shape—this is called trace. When soap reaches trace, stir in the melted cocoa butter, then pour the soap into the molds. Cover immediately with wool blankets. Do not disturb. After 24 hours, remove the blankets. Soap solidifies after 48 to 64 hours; when solid, remove from molds. If using a casserole dish, cut into 2-inch-by-3-inch bars that will resemble brownies. Set on shelves, away from direct heat or sunlight, for 4 to 6 weeks. Scrape residue off the bottom of each bar with a sharp knife; and use the knife to bevel the edges for a very neat look. Wrap in cellophane or put inside decorative boxes.

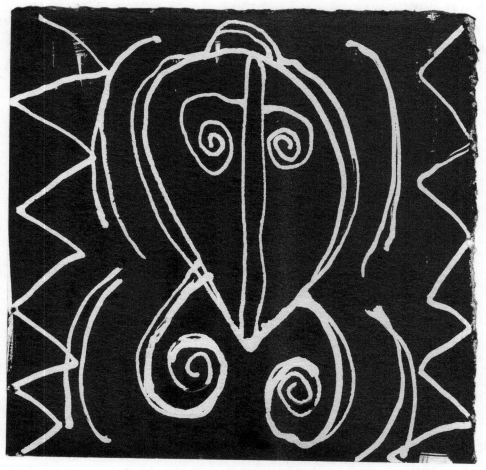

Odo Nnyew Fie Kwan: Love does not lose its way home. Those led by love always end up in the right place.

Spiritual Warmth, Good Health, and Immunity
Teatime

Winter is a time when we seek warmth in all of its variations—spiritual warmth, protection from the cold, and the nourishment of friendship and family. Some keenly feel the withdrawal from light, so much so that the nervous system is thrown off-balance and some folks suffer from depression. These special herbs and natural ingredients help us celebrate winter. Specific herbs can create warming ways of insulating the body and spirit from the harsh aspects of winter.

Making Tea

Tea is an herbal infusion or tisane. Sometimes tough herbs are decocted and taken as tea as well. Honey, lemon, and tea go together well. Milk (not cream) and honey are also pleasant accompaniments to full-bodied teas.

HOW TO MAKE A GOOD CUP OF TEA

To make a good cup of tea, you need patience.

Pour cold water into kettle. Boil the water, then turn off the heat. Pour some water into a clean teacup and let it sit 3 to 5 minutes. Pour this water out into the plugged kitchen sink to be used for washing up later. Add a tea bag or infuser with herbs inside (usually about 1 teaspoon herbs to 1 cup water) to the cup. Pour very hot water from the teakettle into the cup until it is three-quarters full. Steep at least 5 minutes, or longer for a stronger brew. Remove the tea bag or infuser. Drink as is or add what you prefer.

Black, Green, and Oolong Tea (*Camellia sinensis*)

Tea is one of the oldest natural remedies known to man. Legend has it that fresh leaves from *Camellia sinensis* fell from a tree and into the Chinese emperor's pot that was boiling water outside. He was intrigued by the smell, tasted it, and enjoying it immensely, so made it a regular habit. The type of tea the emperor made by mistake is called green tea since it was made from fresh leaves. Green tea is the strongest healing medicine, oolong is second, and black is third. Green tea contains antioxidants that are believed to be two hundred times stronger than vitamin E. Green tea protects the cells from carcinogens that can cause cancer—the substance responsible for this is catechins. Catechins lower cholesterol, metabolize fat, reduce blood pressure, regulate blood sugar, and have an antibacterial action. Green tea, and all tea for that matter, helps teeth and gums stay healthy. Green tea contains fluoride. Green tea helps with bronchial infections and mild respiratory ailments, as well as asthma and breathing difficulties. Black teas are fermented, creating numerous strong dark-colored teas. In China these teas are called oolongs, while in India the favorite tea is black Assam. There are more than three thousand varieties of tea created from *Camellia sinensis*.

Rooibos—a tea as good, or in some ways better, for the body is rooibos, which I discussed at length in chapter 8. When seeking antioxidants and a health tonic, reach for rooibos or green tea.

Roman chamomile (*Anthemis nobilis, Chamaemelum nobile*)

German chamomile (*Matricaria chamomilla, M. recutita*)—one of the most relaxing teas is made from perky yellow chamomile flowers. Chamomile tea reduces aches, strains, arthritis, and menstrual cramps. It helps reduce bladder infections and reduces the presence of *E. coli* in the bladder. Chamomile soothes the stomach and reduces vomiting. It is an all-purpose soother that calms, cools, and tranquilizes, helping you relax and sleep better. It calms the digestive tract and reduces abdominal pain, bloating, and gas.

With these excellent options to choose from, what could be better than a tea party?

Osayin Tea Party

What an excellent time of the year to invoke the deity we visited in chapter 4, orisha Osayin. This is customary during the wet growing season in Africa. Remember Osayin? The one who tried to hide all the herbal knowledge he possessed inside a gourd hung high in a tree so the other orishas wouldn't be able to use it. How the gourd fell down to earth, teaching us that herbal knowledge is not to be rarified but rather shared by all. Today, have an herbal tea party for your coven, friends, or family. Select some of the herbal kingdom's most powerful healing teas to share. Choose from one of the superb herbals listed above. Follow cooking directions on page 292. Use a special cup: handmade earthenware is the ideal choice as it speaks so well of the union of hand, fire, and earth. You will find these at arts and crafts fairs and specialty shops—unless you happen to make them yourself. After your tea is made, shake a gourd rattle over your guests' heads as you sing praise to each person:

I give this to you in good health
Blessings
Herbal knowledge is free
Blessings
Praise Osayin
Blessings
Praise Asase Yaa
Ashe!

Sweeten tea with honey if desired. Enjoy the fellowship of your circle on your feast day of Osayin.

Fragrant Woods

Quite naturally, as the days grow shorter, we gravitate toward the light. Here are a few suggestions for using smoldering wood to scent the winter home. Aromatic woods for the fire include cedar, eucalyptus, juniper, pine, cedar, apple, and balsam poplar. Most any herb can be added to a fire, particularly as it is almost dying out. Fragrant herbs for the fire include mugwort, lavender, juniper, sage, spearmint, rosemary, and lemon verbena.

Incense

Incense is a wonderful alternative to fires for those living in a home without a fireplace, and they can even be used in small, confined spaces such as apartments and dorm rooms—though good ventilation is required. There are incense recipes dispersed throughout the book; frankincense, myrrh, and a recipe for a release incense are included in this chapter. The following five ingredients are especially magical used alone or added to more elaborate incense blends.

Aloeswood—is the jewel of the East but something we here in the West might not be too familiar with. Take it from me, treat yourself; this is sultry, exotic, and unique. It is also a very relaxing wood. Aloeswood—or oud, as it is sometimes called—is one of the most sought-after aromatic woods on earth.

Cedarwood chips (*Cedrus libani, C.* spp.)—on the other side of the coin is the very common cedarwood. Cedarwood is sold at pet stores as bedding for small animals and is widely available (if you have a woodshop, you might even have your own). As an easily grown tree in the United States, cedar has been a highly touted aromatic wood used in sacred ceremonies by various Native American tribes for centuries. Cedar incense is quite complex, and it is a great spiritually cleansing smoke. The incense is said to cure head colds and the tendency to have bad dreams.

Cinnamon (*Cinnamomum verum, C. zeylanicum*)—usually sold in sticks made from quills of the inner bark, cinnamon burns easily and releases a spicy scent into the air. It is considered a protective smoke, capable of encouraging high spiritual vibrations and aiding healing.

Palo santo (*Bursera graveolens*)—many people in need of energy healing have fallen under the influence of misfortune. Incense from the mystical palo santo is useful for those individuals. Traced back to the Inca, it encourages deep relaxation. An energy healer whose ajna is opened and then stimulated by the ancient, woodsy smell of palo santo can cure those who suffer.

This incense is typically used in South America, growing readily on the coasts and in forests of Peru. Healers use it in a practice called sahumerio (fumigation). Sahumerio goes back to the rites and ceremonies of the Inca. Containing age-old wisdom from thousands of years ago, its fumes and smoke capture and ground negative energy. It is returned to the universe transformed into healing light. Even unlit, as a sacred object placed where you choose, aromatic palo santo activates astral body. Its scent opens ajna (also called the Third Eye, ajna is the 6th chakra). Stimulation of the ajna is provided by incense trees like palo santo. With these portals opened by palo santo, gifts of prosperity and good fortune flood in; healing energy takes hold.

Akin to the Native American smudge stick, palo santo incense is used primarily for cleansing and clearing. By working on all the physical and astral components of the body, this incense balances chakra energy, enabling peace and luck to prevail.

You'll burn it like a smudge stick, smoldering not burning. Hold it at a forty-degree angle away from your body. Light it, then let the fire die out. Smoke released from its smoldering works healing magick on both of you.

Sandalwood (*Santalum album*)—though sandalwood hails from India, the three-hundred-year-old Baieido Company from Japan makes choice incense from sandalwood chips. (For more see chapter 9.) Sandalwood is considered an aphrodisiac that builds self-confidence and generates well-being within the environment. Sandalwood blends well with any of the incense herbs listed in this section and with frankincense and myrrh.

These woods are sold already prepared as stick or cone incense or sometimes loose. Mix any three of these and burn on a white-hot bamboo charcoal that is placed on a fireproof burner. You can also add pinches of these natural incenses to a wood-burning fire. Make sure you have good ventilation for whichever way you decide to use incense.

Spiritual Essential Oils, Floral Waters, and Absolutes

Full submission to the home, community, and family is greatly enhanced by herbs and deities. The following herbs have strong spiritual energy; many of them assist with the prayer and invocation of specific goddesses. Here are a few useful herbs, flowers, and resins with qualities that enhance spiritual communion during the winter:

Carnation absolute (*Dianthus caryophyllus*)—purportedly the actual fragrance of angels, fresh carnations or carnation absolute encourages friendship, nurtures relationships, and creates an inviting atmosphere. Carnations are useful during tarot card readings and other forms of divination as the scent encourages prophetic dreams and brings us to a higher plane than where we normally exist. Only 1 drop of carnation absolute should be added to the bath, dream pillow, sachet, potpourri, or other botanical as it is very potent.

Frankincense (*Boswellia sacra, B.* spp.)—a symbol of divinity, frankincense is considered sacred incense. It is often utilized for meditation, prayer, invocation, and healing. Frankincense is considered a protective resin and it dispels fear. Try a frankincense smoke bath outdoors. Burn a few resins at a time on a charcoal block on a fireproof surface; pull the smoke overhead with your hands.

Jasmine (*Jasminum officinale*)—a high-frequency, sweet, romantic scent that eases anxiety and aids sleep, jasmine is one of the ewe (herbs) of Yemaya, thus it is thought of as a maternal, kind, caring, and instructive herb that is great for dreaming and vision quests. Try 1 teaspoon dried flowers to 1 cup very hot water, sweetened with honey, as a bedtime tea. Jasmine is a wonderful addition to dream pillows, and it can be used as a scent for powders, candles, sachets, or food for a mojo bag.

Lavender—a hard worker, it calms and balances. Lavender is considered a sexual aphrodisiac (used abundantly in the nonbinary and LGBTQ+ community) by Hoodoos and an anaphrodisiac (reducing sexual desire, inspiring chastity) by early Western herbalists. Lavender soothes and comforts. Fill a spray bottle with lavender water, and use it to charge altar space or your home or work environment, or spray it on your hair, face, and body to revive your spirit. The essential oil can be used externally, neat. Lavender is a wonderful scent for handmade furniture polish and as a spiritual floor wash.

Lemongrass (*Cymbopogon citratus, C. flexuosus*)—an energizing spirit lifter. Burn lemongrass with lavender, sandalwood, and cedar chips or with crushed frankincense and myrrh. Add ½ teaspoon lemongrass to a bucket of soapy water, and use it as a spiritual floor wash or house cleanser.

Lotus (*Nelumbo nucifera*)—considered a representative of the divinely feminine and as the embodiment of Tehuti in Egyptian tradition. The scent is moist and watery, suggestive of the fecundity of the Great Earth Mother. Lotus oil comes from blue, white, and pink flowers, each with a distinctive scent. Blue or white is great for an introduction to lotus. Pink lotus flowers represent Lakshmi Devi, goddess of prosperity in Hinduism. Dab lotus oil onto pulse points or chakras or add a few drops to the bath. It is a very sensual, unusual oil.

Myrrh (*Commiphora erythraea*)—break off about ½ teaspoon myrrh from a larger block; it breaks easily with a mallet. Burn the myrrh on a charcoal block in the same manner as frankincense—myrrh and frankincense are usually combined for a more spiritually balancing blend, with two parts frankincense to one part myrrh because of its high strength. Combined myrrh and frankincense represent Yoruba orishas Egungun-Oya, arbitrators of destiny and fate, as well as facilitators of communication with ancestors. Add 3 to 4 drops myrrh to a bath, or use it neat, dabbed on the pulse points or chakras. Please note that myrrh is not for use by pregnant women.

Rose otto (*Rosa damascena*)—whatever you need—calm, balance, stimulation, an aphrodisiac, cooling off after an argument—rose otto, or attar of roses, can help. Bulgarian roses are widely available in East Indian shops and health food stores, prepared as a rosewater that can be put into a spray bottle. Rosewater is considered cleansing, a blessing oil that also purifies the environment. Rose otto is very expensive but is also very powerful—a few drops will do the trick! Add 2 drops to a full bath, dream pillow, sachet, or mojo bag. Roses are associated with a variety of love goddesses including the orisha Oshun and Greek goddess Aphrodite. White roses are associated with the tears of the Roman goddess Venus. Pink roses suggest the perfume of Erzulie Freda in Haitian Vodou. Please note that pregnant women should avoid the use of rose otto.

Sandalwood (*Santalum album*)—the mellow scent of sandalwood eases inhibitions, builds self-confidence, induces a calm, sedate mood, and can assist in achieving a meditative state. Sandalwood is considered an aphrodisiac; fittingly it is also a ewe (herb) of orisha Oshun. Wonderful applied to the body as a massage (diluted with sweet almond oil in a ratio of ½ teaspoon sandalwood to 8 ounces oil), it can also be applied to pulse points or chakras neat before going out or at bedtime. Baieido Sandalwood Incense is a high grade and fine cut suitable for mixing with other incense ingredients or burning on a charcoal block alone.

Bugs Running Interference

One of the major drawbacks to winter is the profusion of germs passing from one person to the next, sparking the likes of COVID-19 and similar illnesses, colds, and various strains of influenza. To make matters worse, African Americans are disproportionately afflicted by upper respiratory illnesses like asthma and bronchitis, as well as compromised immune systems. The following herbs allow you to tap into the healing energy of the earth's plants and trees to fight ailments that strike frequently during winter. These herbs and natural ingredients have a history of helping us build immunity.

Camphor Tree (*Cinnamomum camphora*)

Camphor leaves have a clean-smelling scent reminiscent of mothballs. Camphor is used medicinally, particular in Chinese medicine, where it is called Zhang Nao. The Chinese prize this substance as a treatment for heart ailments and circulatory problems and as a digestive. Camphor is used as a sedative and calming agent and to treat convulsions, hysteria, and insomnia. In the West, we have concentrated on using camphor to treat the discomforts of cold and flu, upper respiratory ailments, rheumatism, muscle pains, and body aches. Camphorated oil can be made by adding a few drops of the essential oil to 3 tablespoons melted aloe butter, shea butter, or mango butter. You can also add a drop or so of camphor oil to a handkerchief and inhale the scent to clear nasal passages and sinuses. Likewise with eucalyptus, described below.

Wild Camphor Tree (*Tarchonanthus camphoratus*)

Several South African companies sell bush teas (wildcrafted, organic indigenous herbs) internationally. Wild camphor tree offers many benefits. The South African Khoisan people, whom I discussed in part II, use wild camphor for its soothing qualities. Dried leaves are used in ceremonies to anoint the body during rituals. The leaves and seeds are used to fumigate. Camphor smoke treats rheumatism, headache, and insomnia. The tea relieves stomach ailments, asthma, anxiety, and heartburn. The leaves contain an insecticide used to deter lice and external parasites.

Echinacea (*Echinacea angustifolia*)

Echinacea roots, flowers, and stems have been used traditionally as an antiseptic and blood purifier, as well as for eczema, acne, and boils. Echinacea is also a digestion aid but today it is used largely as an immunity booster. There are plenty of teas available containing echinacea, but you can also easily grow it and take a tiny bit of the root up in the spring to make your own decoction. See page 101 for directions for preparing roots and for directions on how to make a decoction.

Eucalyptus (*Eucalyptus* spp.)

The leaves of the eucalyptus tree are antiseptic. Australian Aborigines brew them extensively to soothe coughs and colds. The essential oils are also antiseptic and provide antiviral actions as well. Tasmanian blue eucalyptus is used as an inhalant for tuberculosis and upper respiratory complaints. This oil can also be dispersed through the air using a pot of simmering water or a vaporizer.

Lemon and peppermint eucalyptus (*E. citriodora, E. dives*) are also useful in the treatment of asthma, colds, and fever; lemon eucalyptus is an antifungal. Peppermint eucalyptus is a pain reducer useful for flu.

To enjoy the healing medicine of eucalyptus, simply hang a bunch of it on the showerhead. Tie with hemp string to affix. Steaming hot water releases the essential oils contained in the eucalyptus leaf.

Flaxseed

Flaxseed boosts fiber intake and contains important phytonutrients. It is a natural source of fiber, trace vitamins, minerals, amino acids, omega-3, lignans, and phytonutrients. One tablespoon is the usual amount used, and that contains seventy calories. Look for organic flaxseed and buy seeds whole. Grind with a mortar and pestle or with a coffee grinder until fine. Store ground and whole seeds, as well as the oil, in the refrigerator. To use: sprinkle this onto salads, main dishes, oatmeal, or other nutritious cereal. Take oil orally 1 teaspoon a day, or add to salad dressing. Brewing and drinking flaxseed as a tea adds regularity. You can also try adding flaxseed to yogurt or juice.

Garlic (Allium sativum)

Garlic is a digestive aid that clarifies the liver and gall bladder. It is known to reduce blood pressure and help with circulatory problems. Garlic juice and supplements are used as an expectorant and to treat stomach flu. Those with chronic bronchitis and compromised immune systems can utilize garlic raw in salads, minced and sweetened with honey, or as a tea. For the hardy, eat garlic whole or mince and add it to water and drink immediately. This gives a buzz of energy, which is quite nice when you are feeling worn down.

Ginger (Zingiber officinale)

Ginger can be infused to make tea, to be served hot or iced with lemon. Cooking with grated or dried ginger (adding ½ to 1 teaspoon depending on the size of the meal) adds zest and warmth to just about any dish. Ginger is warming and anticatarrhal, and is a tonic, a detoxifier, and a digestive aid. It speeds elimination and lowers cholesterol and blood pressure.

Hyssop (Hyssopus officinalis)

Hyssop is a strong herb that is ideal for treating winter ailments. Hyssop helps with stomachache from overeating or indigestion. It is good for sore throats, breast and lung problems, coughs, colds, nose and throat infections, mucus congestion, gas, and catarrh.

Hyssop should be used sparingly and not for extended periods; ½ to 1½ cups per day for 3 to 4 days per month should be the limit. To prepare, steep 1 teaspoon hyssop in ½ cup boiled water.

Lemon (*Citrus limonum*)

Lemons are highly touted by the Gullah and Hoodoos. The Gullah use lemon in herbal teas as a natural remedy. Lemon is often paired with herbal tea and honey to treat the symptoms of cold or flu. It can also be paired with honey and taken by the spoonful for sore throats and coughs—the two enhance the efficacy of herbal teas when treating cold and flu. I suggest 1 teaspoon of your favorite honey mixed with ½ teaspoon lemon juice for a sore throat—take as needed.

Life Everlasting, Also Called Rabbit's Tobacco (*Gnaphalium polycephalum*)

The bright-yellow flowers of the life everlasting plant address body, mind, and spirit wellness, just as the name implies. It is popular in many different types of folk medicine including Hoodoo.

Here are some ways it can be used:

- Infuse the flowers in hot water to make a tonic that deters illness.
- Life everlasting tea with fresh lemon juice is a Gullah treatment for colds and fever.
- Hoodoos place life everlasting inside mojo bags as a good health charm.

Mullein (*Verbascum thapsus*)

Mullein is a gentle treatment for coughs, colds lung weakness, asthma, chronic cough, and bronchitis; it is calming and soothing to the lungs, and bronchial tubes. Mullein contains vitamins and flavonoids as well as saponins that cleanse the body. To create mullein tea, add 1 teaspoon herb to 1 cup boiled water. Strain, and flavor if desired with lemon and honey.

Onion (*Allium cepa*)

Onion is a relative of garlic and is useful in much the same way. Use raw or juiced onion to treat cough or stomachache, as a tonic, for antiseptic purposes, and to reduce blood pressure and increase virility. Some people in the Caribbean grate onion, soak it in a cup of water, then sip the water all day to reduce weight. To enhance its efficacy, improve the taste, and boost immunity, lemon and honey can be added to the onion water. Add thinly sliced raw Vidalia onion to salads or sandwiches. Make it a habit to season your food using minced onion as the first ingredient that you sauté. Sauté using virgin olive oil—this is tasty and heart healthy, and reduces the need for large amounts of salt.

Peppermint (*Mentha piperita*)

Peppermint was once considered a panacea—a cure-all for just about every known discomfort. Peppermint tea works as a decongestant when inhaled from a pot of simmering water. Just put a towel overhead to form a tent (being careful not to allow it to touch the flames below) and inhale the aromatic peppermint. This will help clear the nasal passages and chest. Inhaling peppermint is also a treatment for both laryngitis and bronchitis. In England, peppermint tea is consumed at the onset of a cold to lessen its severity and length. Putting a couple of tea bags inside a washcloth works as a compress to relieve headache and body pain associated with influenza. Its ability to reduce pain also makes it useful as a mouthwash for toothache, gum disease, and cavities. Peppermint also soothes the nerves and lifts mild depression, which can strike due to illness or light deprivation. Peppermint tea is made from the dried herb in the same way as mullein (see above).

Rum

In the book *Jamaican Culture and International Folklore*, Jamaican author Claudette V. Copney shares a variety of herbal remedies featuring bay leaf laurel herb prepared as rum:

* For flu: rub down person with bay rum to draw out fever; stay under the covers.
* For headache: pour bay rum on a small face cloth and inhale as needed.
* For toning internal organs (cure-all): add 1 shot of bay rum to coffee or tea any time of day.[12]

Elders

In African society and other indigenous cultures, community is vital. At the center of community and family life is the elder. Elders are celebrated for their wisdom and are seen as

---

12 Claudette V. Copney, *Jamaican Culture and International Folklore, Superstitions, Beliefs, Dreams, Proverbs, and Remedies* (Edinburgh: Pentland Press, 1998).

reservoirs of information regarding families and the culture at large. We could learn much from following the lead of our ancestors in Africa.

Winter is an especially important time to stay in close communication with elders in temperate zones. Elderly people suffer greatly from ailments that young people recover from quite easily, like colds and the flu. It is important to check in with family members who are seniors, and it is a very nice gesture to call on elderly neighbors.

In this chapter devoted to winter, there is a plethora of ideas for nurturing the health of the elders, from immunity boosters to foot soaks and massage. If you don't have time for these things, a simple cup of peppermint tea or ginger beverage would do a great deal to revitalize the spirits of your elders. This section features information and recipes geared toward the health of elders. Herbal massage, tonics, memory boosters, home spas, sleep aids, and a fun group project are included.

Elder Tree (Sambucus nigra)

The elder tree has much to offer seniors in the community, as the trees symbolize stability and wisdom. Infusion of elder flowers promotes perspiration and treats rheumatic complaints when used as an oil infusion, ointment, or salve. Elder flowers ease depression and are a relaxant and treatment for puffy eyes and rheumatism.

ELDER RITUAL

Elder trees are imbued with many mysteries connected with death, resurrection, and rebirth. The glyph of elder means, "I am a wave of the sea. On the boundless sea, I was set adrift. All these things shall pass away but the soul and spirit shall remain."

Steep 1 cup elder flowers in 4 cups water. Dip two cotton squares in elder tea, put them in a bowl, and then place the bowl in the freezer. Strain 1 cup of infusion, and set it aside. Pour remaining tea with flowers into a basin. Have your elder put her feet up, relax, and drink tea (with honey and lemon if desired). Test the temperature of the elder infusion in the basin; when it is not too hot, add 1 teaspoon lavender buds. Have your elder place her feet into the floral infusion. Then put the cotton squares on her eyes. Let her relax as long as she'd like, then gently towel-dry her feet and have a pair of comfortable slippers waiting to complete the spa.

Salt

Salt, as the essence of the sea, is a wonderful substance, symbolic of life, and an enhancement for our lives during the coldest days of winter.

Dead Sea Salt

Dead Sea salt is a natural substance from Israel, used to encourage relaxation and reduce tension, body aches, and headache when used in a bath. Salt is associated with spiritual cleansing, nurturance, and the Mothers of the Sea.

Epsom Salts

Epsom salt is recommended for relaxing strained or bruised muscles. The combination of Dead Sea and Epsom salts can help the winter spirit reach a relaxed state. Salts are believed to be rejuvenating to the overworked body, mind, and spirit.

Sea Kelp, Also Called Bladder Wrack (Fucus vesiculosus)

Used magically in the following bath salt, sea kelp works with the spirits of the ocean and is a protective healing plant. Sea kelp encourages positive vibrations, psychic abilities, and prosperity. It also contains important vitamins and minerals for skin care.

QUEEN MOTHER'S ELDER BATH SALT

2 cups Epsom salt
2 cups coarse Dead Sea salt
2 cups fine sea salt
½ cup sea kelp

1 teaspoon chamomile essential oil
1 teaspoon lavender essential oil
Large glass or metal screw-top container

Put the three kinds of salt and the kelp into a bowl. Sprinkle with the essential oils. Stir, then pour into the container. Shake, then let rest 48 hours. Use 1 to 2 cups per bath. Soak for 20 minutes or more.

Feel-Good Rituals and Elements

To the Yoruba people of Nigeria and other followers of Ifá, Yemaya-Olokun is an orisha that embodies the spirit of creation. This spirit lives in natural bodies of water. She is thought of as the Great Mother or Cosmic Womb. This powerful mother figure is beloved by many for her capacity for deep understanding and generosity.

To invoke the spirit of Yemaya-Olokun, try this spirited bathroom ritual. Create an altar on your bathroom window ledge, table, or tub as follows:

- Clean the designated surface (ledge, table, or tub) by lightly brushing it with a feather.
- Lay down a white satin or white silk cloth.
- Arrange cowries and conch shells (or other available seashells) on the cloth.
- Put a rock or fish fossil in the center of the shells.
- Next to the circle of shells, put a glass of vodka, brandy, or rum surrounded by coins in the directions of north, south, east, and west.
- Dip a crystal or semiprecious stone into the spirit glass and then set it on top of the central rock (or fossil).
- Set out a few tropical leafy green plants or ferns.
- Light frankincense or myrrh incense or burn tobacco or a blue candle.
- Add bath salts under running water in the plugged bathtub.
- Relax and enjoy!

Black Cocoa Butter Body Bliss Treat

I love this silky treat for achy muscles around the back, shoulders, and wrist joint areas. You know, the type of pain we get from using the computer keyboard and gazing at the monitor a little too long? This treatment is simply delightful.

Warm up the sore area using any of these methods:

- Fill a hot water bottle with boiling or very hot water and seal tightly—careful not to scald yourself.
- Warm a flax-filled body pillow in the microwave for the recommended amount of time. (Mitts for sore hands and booties for tired feet are also available.)
- Apply a warm heating pad to the area.

Have your partner or a friend scoop out some cocoa butter and warm it by pressing it together in their hands until it is melted. Remove heat source (selected from above). Your partner can then apply the melted cocoa butter directly to the painful area, massaging until you feel your tight muscles released.

Arnica (Arnica montana), Also Called Leopard's Bane

For those of you familiar with my daughter Olivia and my botanica, SRB Botanica, you will recognize the name and perhaps the wonder of the arnica-based salve Salve-ation, which Olivia developed.

As I mentioned on page 32, your herbs will show up for you in your life. For Olivia, as a stuntwoman and body double, pain comes with the job. To assuage the pain, arnica has been there for her, and through her product, she shares pain reduction with the general public. Arnica is well respected as a treatment for pain, rheumatism, sore muscles, and joints. It is typically extracted in oil and used as a warming massage. It assists with wound healing, phlebitis, inflammation, burns, and swelling from broken bones; and I recently personally discovered that it soothes chapped lips.

How to use: to make arnica oil, fill a sterile jar loosely with arnica flowers, then cover with safflower, sweet almond, grapeseed, or olive oil. Cap, then store away from direct sunlight for 6 to 8 weeks. Swirl daily to release arnica into the oil.

This member of the herbaceous sunflower family should not be used too long, not be applied to broken skin, nor should it be taken orally. It is a subcutaneous herb, meaning it is used on the skin.

Foraha (Calophyllum inophyllum), Also Called Tamanu

Foraha is a dark-green oil with a thick and waxy consistency. This oil has a wide array of medicinal qualities, including its analgesic, anti-inflammatory, and antibiotic capabilities.

Foraha is useful in the treatment of wounds, eczema, burns, insect bites, herpes, varicose veins, and scars, and it makes a nutritious face oil. Revered for its ability to regenerate cell growth, foraha oil is also a treatment for fragile or broken capillaries.

How to use: foraha oil is great for massaging sore muscles and aching feet, legs, or joints. It has a strongly nutty smell, which can be counteracted by adding a few drops of lavender, clary sage, or sandalwood essential oil; a single drop of rose otto or neroli would also mask the nutty smell. Each of these essential oils conditions the skin and is generally relaxing as well.

Mugwort (Artemisia vulgaris)

Mugwort is associated with the elder wisdom of the crone. Mugwort is a hardy plant with feathery leaves that spreads quickly and can pop up anywhere. Mugwort is used as a bath to treat rheumatism, fatigue, and gout. This herb is harmful in high doses.

How to use: Steep 1 teaspoon herb in ½ cup water and sip throughout the day. (Limit to ½ cup daily.)

Tonic Teas

Earlier in this chapter, numerous herbs were presented to calm, soothe, comfort, boost immunity, and fight illnesses. The following herbs are considered systemic tonics. They have been used historically to boost memory as well.

Ginkgo (*Ginkgo biloba*)—at two hundred million years old, ginkgo is the oldest tree in the world. Ginkgo leaves are associated with longevity and good health as well as memory. Ginkgo facilitates good circulation. Proper circulation helps concentration, which in turn supports the function of memory. Ginkgo tea or extracts can also be used to reduce headache, maintain balance and equilibrium, reduce strokes, and assist with hearing.

Rosemary (*Rosmarinus officinalis*)—like ginkgo, rosemary is a systemic tonic for the heart and mind. Rosemary is associated with love and remembrance. This herb helps blood circulate efficiently, facilitating concentration and helping memory. Rosemary relaxes nerves, though it is also a tonic to the whole system. It contains a substance called rosmarinic acid, which has an antiviral and antimicrobial function in the body. Rosemary aids healing from upper respiratory ailments like bronchitis and generally speeds recovery from numerous complaints because of its high level of antioxidants. The tea also darkens gray hair.

Sage (*Salvia officinalis*)—sage has many of the same properties as rosemary. It has been highly regarded throughout history as a tonic, an aid to longevity, and a stimulant to the memory. This herb is useful to women going through menopause and those with fevers, as it reduces perspiration. Sage tea soothes the nerves, curtails trembling, and eases mild depression.

Sage tea, like rosemary, can be applied to the hair as a darkening rinse. The two herbs darken hair slowly through a staining process resulting from the tannins they contain.

How to use: Steep 1 teaspoon herb in ½ cup water. Limit use to 1 cup a day and then only use occasionally, not on a daily basis. Excessive use of sage is dangerous and potentially toxic.

Winter Dreaming

Let's face it: if possible, we nap and turn in earlier during winter. That is, if we are allowed to follow the circadian rhythms. Dreams are potent ways of bridging the world of humans with that of the ancestral spirits, and many indigenous African cultures, including African Americans, pay serious attention to dreams. When I was growing up, the oracles in the family were my maternal grandmother and my baby sister. When they had a dream that seemed to offer to tell us something significant, which was quite often, we all sat down to listen and then figure out the meaning within the dream. Dream books are another tool that was heavily utilized not only by my family, but in the Black community. We made numerological correlations with the important features of the dream and then parlayed that into potential abundance by playing that particular number in betting games akin to but not the same as the lottery. "Numbers" dream books and oracular interpretations of dreams was one of my early introductions into the other world.

Dream Pillow

Dream pillows, such as the one described below, deter insomnia and encourage fascinating dreams. You will notice that this dream pillow includes the very evocative Spanish moss, which is at home on many Southern trees. Spanish moss is a vessel, a tight one at that, both physically and metaphysically. It will hold scent as well as it holds intent.

This is designed as a group project for four or up to eight participants. If you are working on your own, store extra pillows in an airtight container or ziplock bag until ready to use.

MAKING DREAM PILLOWS

Handful each of the following herbs:
dried lemon verbena leaves
dried rose petals
dried chamomile flowers
dried French lavender buds
dried bay
dried mullein
dried Spanish moss
dried hops

⅛ teaspoon chamomile essential oil
½ teaspoon French lavender essential oil
6 drops attar of roses (or ½ teaspoon rose fragrance oil)
2 teaspoons orris root powder

Crumble the lemon verbena leaves, rose petals, chamomile flowers, lavender buds, bay, and mullein into a large bowl until fine. Tear Spanish moss into 1-inch pieces. Add hops (please note that this is an allergen; see below). Sprinkle oils over bruised herbs. Stir in orris root powder. Mature by placing in a dark jar away from direct light. Shake daily for 4 to 6 weeks. While waiting for mixture to mellow, each participant should make a small dream pillowcase using gingham, linen, hemp, or fabric scrap. Use two 9-inch squares of fabric and cotton thread. This particular dream pillow is designed for strength, restful and deep sleep, and prophetic dreams.

NOTE: Allergy-sensitive individuals should wear a dust mask to complete this project.

Dream-Telling Circle

A dream pillow can be a powerful tool for observing midwinter, particularly for seniors. Bring a small group of people together to make the pillow; a week or two later, meet again to discuss dreams inspired by the dream pillows.

If this is not possible, have those around you write down their dreams and put them into a collective jar. The following year during midwinter, have a special dinner and go through the dream jar, sharing and interpreting each other's dreams.

Examining dreams is an age-old way of storytelling, connecting, and remembering those who have passed beyond. Dream-telling is a strong African tradition that has survived to the present day.

PLEASANT DREAM TEA

Enjoy a good night's sleep using herbs and flowers to brew tea.

Select from the following dried herbs in any combination:

jasmine flower	catnip
hops[13]	peppermint
lavender	valerian
chamomile	

Add 2 teaspoons herb to a strainer, and set aside. Boil water. Pour ½ cup boiling water into a cup (without herbs). Heat cup 3 minutes, then pour out water. Add the strainer to the cup. Pour hot water over herbs, cover, and steep 10 minutes. Add honey and milk or lemon if desired.

---

13 Avoid hops if you are recovering from addictions; it acts as a catalyst for some people.

JAMAICAN RUM TODDY

1 cup milk
1 cardamom pod

1 shot Jamaican rum

Heat 1 cup milk with one crushed cardamom pod; when milk is very hot, remove cardamom pod. Add 1 shot of Jamaican rum, and enjoy.

Death, Release, and Remembrance

Death becomes a reality during the winter. The landscape, colors, and even the temperature are all suggestive of death. Death has positive aspects. For example, decomposing matter becomes nourishing mulch for new plants, as I discussed earlier in the case of neem leaves. Death makes way for the birth of the new, both physically and metaphysically; consider the story of Jesus Christ. Each New Year, we celebrate the death of old times and old ways that have a negative effect on our lives. Death, as embodied by winter, offers a chance for renewal, growth, and change. Even inclement weather, the phenomenon that we dread and curse, plays an important role, as it gives us no choice but to slow down, pause, and think about our lives.

For those of us who have lost people who are dear, death can be a harsh reality—a barrier that we wish to cross. Elders keenly feel this relationship with death, as often their friends and loved ones have passed on. Following is an incense made with a combination of herbs with magical qualities designed to address all the issues that winter stirs.

RELEASE INCENSE

5 bay leaves
3 anise stars
2 small cinnamon sticks or ¼ cup
    cinnamon chips
Handful each of dried uvaursi,
    mint leaves, rosemary, and
    chamomile
3 chunks myrrh

7 tears frankincense
⅛ teaspoon each myrrh, bay, and
    ylang ylang essential oils
Aquamarine and tourmaline
    (stone or bead)
Mortar and pestle or coffee
    grinder

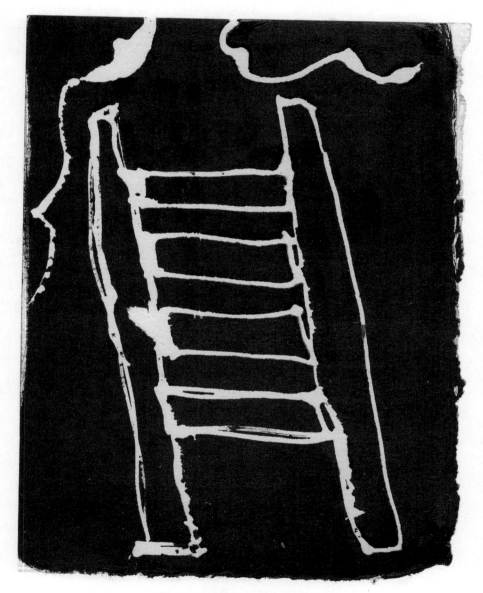

Owuo Atwedee: Ladder of Death
Meaning: Death is certain and universal

Using a mortar and pestle or coffee grinder, pulverize bay, anise, and cinnamon into a coarse powder. Transfer to a bowl. To release essential oils from the following herbs, pulverize them using a mortar and pestle: uvaursi, mint, rosemary, and chamomile. Add these to the bowl. Grind myrrh and frankincense, then add them to the bowl, and stir. Sprinkle the essential oils over all ingredients, then mix well. Place mixture and stones into a capped container. Shake daily for one week.

Burn the Release Incense in a large seashell or on top of a stone, or sprinkle a pinch of the incense on a hot charcoal. Replace as needed. Release grief, sorrow, despair, or communications to the spirits into the smoke.

REMEMBRANCE GARLAND

Garlands are an age-old symbol of winter that capture the magic of the season.

Cranberries
Cinnamon stick
Allspice
Bay leaves
Orange peels

Florida water or Kananga water
(or plain water if these are
unavailable)
Waxed linen or hemp string
cockscomb
dried lemon slices

Soak cranberries, cinnamon, allspice, bay leaves, and orange peels overnight in Florida water or Kananga water (or substitute plain water if specialty waters are unavailable). The next day, cut a suitable length of waxed linen or hemp string for the welcoming area of your home. Begin the strand and end it with cranberries, and create your own pattern with the remaining botanicals. A remembrance garland is a fragrant invitation for your ancestors and departed loved ones.

CHAPTER 13

Spring into Ritual

RAIN, THUNDER, THE WATER ELEMENT, AND FLOWERS

East: The Advent of Spring

Spring is the season that shows our ability to survive the toughness of winter. The Adinkra symbol *aya* ("fern") aligns with the notion of this type of survival perfectly because the fern is a plant that demonstrates many survival instincts. Aya is a reflection on grit, endurance, stick-to-itiveness, will, resourcefulness, and endurance. The snow and ice of the northern spirit has been shoveled, melted, and broken. Now we look eastward to the rising of the sun.

In Chicagoland this is a lovely time of the year, though like many other places near it in the Midwest, we must be patient until it decides to reward us with its appearance. I use the word *lovely* because we are greeted with blooming trees and bushes heavy with blossoms, fragrant as they are breathtakingly beautiful, in shades of white, lavender, pink, and strong yellows.

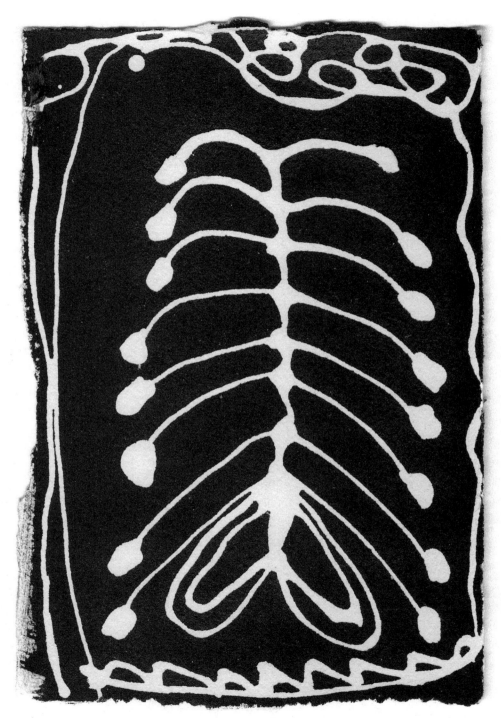

Aya: Fern
Meaning: I have endured many difficulties and outlasted much difficulty

Spring Solstice Ritual and Ceremony: *Welcoming Spring with the Goddesses*

The beginning of spring is called variously Ostara, Vernal Equinox, and Spring Solstice. Spring is that special time of the year focused on awakening, new beginnings, growth, development, and balance. For many embarking on the journey into the womb, new feelings are stirred to life that once laid as dormant as bulbs planted in the fall.

Forced Bulbs

One of the most cheerful sights after a long, cold, white winter are the colorful bulbs of spring. Some people find that growing these indoors, before the season, brings spring cheer into the home before these plants could thrive outdoors. The technique called "forcing" is one of the easiest yet most pleasurable activities for spring plant lovers. The easier types of bulbs to get to bloom indoors, or force, are amaryllis, which you will find a proliferation of around Christmastime, Yule, and Kwanzaa, as well as paperwhite lilies with their delicate appearance. They are almost exclusively "forced," thus they typically come with directions and sometimes ready to go in a pot. With a little more patience, you can also force narcissus, daffodils, hyacinth, and even tulips.

Choose a shallow terra-cotta pot (I usually use the clay tray for an extra-large terra-cotta pot). Cover the bottom with river rocks or pea gravel for good drainage. Fill this with potting soil. Add vermiculite to lighten the soil. Gently press bulbs into the soil. Set the pot in a sunny area, and water it. As green appears, continue to water. In a few weeks you will have a lovely, aromatic blooming bouquet.

Naturally Colored Eggs

Eggs are used in prosperity, abundance, crossroads, and fertility rites, as they are associated with spring. There are so many natural dyes available and they enhance the magical nature of eggs. I encourage experimentation with natural teas to enhance the natural beauty inherent in the promise of eggs.

CRACKLED AND TEA-STAINED EGGS

I recommend using one of the eggs in an abundance spell. To make the tea-stained crackled egg, first gather the ingredients.

3 tea bags (rose hips yield a soft red; currant and blueberry yield soft purples; black tea makes tan)

24 ounces water
6 eggs

Put eggs in 16 ounces cold water in a pot. Set heat to medium high. Boil 20 minutes. Put cup of fresh water on in a kettle separately. Make tea. Let steep 15 minutes. Tap each egg lightly to crack its surface. Put eggs in a bowl with tea. Soak overnight. In the morning, remove eggs from the tea, blot excess tea, and display as desired.

Isis Snake Divination

Spring is a time of nature revelation and discovery. Just as plants peek out of the ground, so do snakes and other creatures that have rested over the winter. March is the time of Isis, Moon Mother and Mother of the Sea. Snakes are one of her symbols. This ritual respectfully conjures her symbolic reptile and pays tribute to her while invoking her spirit.

- Draw a bath.
- Add ¼ cup Epsom salt, ¼ cup coarse salt, and ¼ cup fine Dead Sea salt.
- Put on a piece of moonstone (e.g., a ring, necklace, bracelet, or anklet).
- Light a blue candle and place it on a fireproof container near the bathtub.
- Bring a crystal ball with you into the bath.
- Gaze at the candle as you breathe deeply and very slowly, until you are very relaxed. Realize that you are bathing in the smoke of Isis.
- Call her name quietly but deliberately, drawing it out slowly like a snake's hiss, I-*sisss*, I-*sisss*, I-*sisss*. Breathe in, and with the exhale, whisper I-*sisss* for about five minutes.
- Lift crystal ball into the air once you feel the spirit of Isis within the room. Hold the ball in front of the candle flame. See what is in store as you divine by scrying both fire and crystal.

Mmilika e ji-asa ife
Na ejiro ife asa mmili.
—*John Anenechukwu Umeh*

Translation: "Water is used in cleansing things, but nothing is used in cleansing water."

Rain

Here is a goddess who is believed to have come to the earth in the opposite region of Africa from Goddess Isis's homeland—South Africa. I have been into DNA ancestry for many years before it was widely known and popular. Recently, I learned more definitively about my tribal affiliations. I am quite very Nigerian, and in fact, I have cousins still there from the Igbo tribe. The Igbo are from the Southeastern part of Nigeria, and some also live in Southern Africa. Whereas, at first, I wondered about my place in this incredible constellation of groups of people, my fascination with goddesses and beliefs from this part of the world makes more sense now.

Goddesses seem mythic, divine—often outside the realm of mere mortals—yet in parts of Southern Africa, there is the belief that certain rain goddesses come down to earth to inhabit the bodies of queens. This segment explores Mujaji, the goddess whose lineage continues to the present day. Before we get to our work, here is a snapshot of Mujaji's homeland. It's always best to have some understanding of a goddess before invoking her energy.

Mujaji is a sacred leader, goddess in the flesh of the Shona. Shona are people from Southern Africa who speak Bantu-based languages called ChiShona. Mujaji is the goddess of fertility, sustenance, cycles, and life itself, hailing from a distinctive line of rainmakers beginning with Mambo Monomotapa. Mujaji I, daughter of Mugede, was the first of these goddesses. She came to live on earth around 1800. Mugede fathered Mujaji II too, so this rain queen was both daughter and stepsister to Mujaji I, and so it has gone for many generations. Mujaji's exploits are legendary. Leaders including Sochangane of Gazaland, Shaka of the Zulu (whom you have probably heard of), and Moshweshwe of the Sotho, all appealed to Mujaji I for rain. During numerous African wars, Mujaji's reputation saved her people.

Mujaji is immortal and relatively inaccessible. She is at the center of life, as only she possesses the power to create rain, change seasons, or inflict society with droughts or floods. If

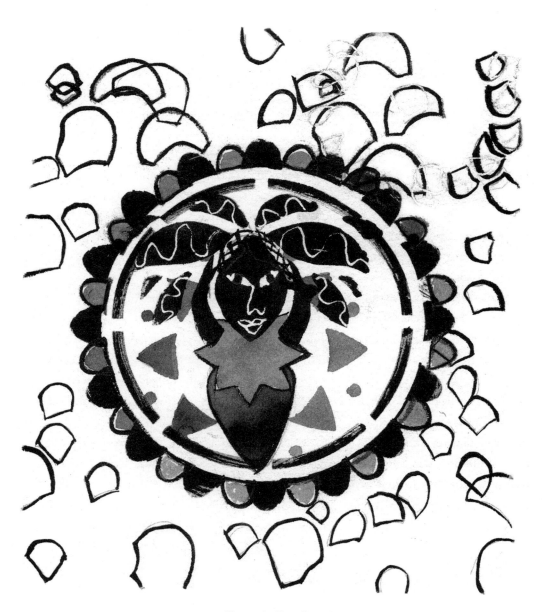

Mujaji, the Rain Queen

she is angry, there is no rain, which leads to horrendous droughts. Constant care, respect, and vigilance to her honor are required year-round to assure her continued assistance.

The Mujaji rain queens continue to be with us through myth and legend. Her contemporary descendants have no military power but still yield spiritual influence within their community because of their ability to conjure rain. With the major seasons in Africa being the wet and the dry, there is a great deal of emphasis in conjuring life-sustaining rain in dry times. John Anenechukwu Umeh, author of *After God Is Dibia*, gives a comprehensive view into the many magical uses of the water element by West Africa's Igbo people with the following three examples:

- *Igba ogogo mmili* is "dancing waters"—since *ogogo* is an excitedly playful washing of one's body during a rain shower, without collecting the rain into any vessel or container.
- *Mmili uji osisi* is water gathered from natural bowls or depressions or holes in trees.
- *Mmili akwukwo osisi* is water gathered by plant and tree leaves.[1]

Collecting the Essence of Mujaji

Try some of these Igbo methods of interacting with the rain when you feel that your ideas are stale and lack creativity. Of course, those of you desiring physical fertility to bear children can also benefit from this engagement. To do your own *Igba ogogo mmili* bath, take a wash outdoors during a rain shower, nude if possible. Try gathering water from inside burls and other depressions in the surfaces of trees.

---

1   John Anenechukwu Umeh, *After God Is Dibia: Igbo Cosmology, Divination, and Sacred Science in Nigeria* (London: Karnak House, 1997).

Get In the Water

Instead of hiding out from rain, sulking, or complaining about it, shift your focus to the gift of rain. Without rain, life as we know it would most likely cease to exist. Get into rain, literally. Here are some ways to enjoy the rain and use it in your life:

- Rainwater is easy to collect on the ground. Collection from a rural environment, or at the very least away from excessive traffic or from under eaves, is best. Place multiple containers outside for greater quantity. Fresh rainwater is best, but you can store rainwater in the fridge for a few days if necessary.
- Lightning water is collected from a thunderstorm. Lightning water is believed to bring dramatic changes to situations and can also bring an air of spontaneity or even capriciousness. Lightning water is associated with Yoruba orishas Shango and Oya.
- Use rainwater to bless your besom before spiritual cleansing and clearings, during the creation of a circle, or to bless a new grimoire.
- Use rainwater to charge or renew crystals, rocks, and minerals. Once they are cleansed, clear stones again with sun and moonlight.
- Record the sounds of rain or a thunderstorm. Play earth sounds during rites or ceremonies involving new beginnings, to generate ideas or to relax or meditate. High-quality natural sound CDs or cassettes can also be purchased.

ESSENCE OF HARA KE

This elixir continues to engage the spirit of rain goddesses. This is a type of potpourri I use to bless my home and that of others under the inspiration of gods and goddesses. Since Hara Ke is one of the African rain goddesses, choose a rainy day in early spring to create her floral essence potpourri. This is designed to promote creativity, new beginnings, and fertility. Reflect on the revelation of one of these three facets of rain. Choose the one you desire the most in your home. Focus with great intention as you craft this blend.

4 cups dried pink rose petals
mixed with whole dried
rosebuds
2 cups blue lavender
½ cup cut and sifted lemongrass
½ cup pine needles
1 cup dried lime slices
5 to 6 dried pomegranates
1 cup dried orange slices
¼ teaspoon neroli essential oil
⅛ teaspoon jasmine absolute
⅛ teaspoon tuberose absolute
⅛ teaspoon attar of roses

¼ teaspoon eucalyptus
essential oil
¼ teaspoon patchouli essential oil
⅛ teaspoon vetiver essential oil
½ teaspoon pure sandalwood
essential oil
½ cup Queen Elizabeth root
powder
5 cardamom pods, ground
2 nutmegs, ground
4 tablespoons ground
cinnamon stick

Put the rose petals, rosebuds, lavender, lemongrass, pine needles, lime slices, pomegranates, and orange slices into a very large container (e.g., an extra-large mixing bowl or stockpot). Mix all the absolutes and oils in a separate nonreactive bowl such as Pyrex or stainless steel. Blend oils with a stirring rod if you have one, or swirl. Take a moment to inhale this complex blend of scents and listen to the rain as you focus on your intentions. Mix the Queen Elizabeth root, cardamom, nutmeg, and cinnamon together in a separate mixing bowl. Pour the oils over the botanical blend, and mix. Shake on the powdered spices mix. Stir all together. Put in a plastic container with an airtight lid. Let mature for 4 to 6 weeks away from the direct sunlight, and then it will be ready to use. Try the Hara Ke ritual (see below) once it is mature.

Hara Ke Ritual

I remember seeing my godmother mist the tips of her broom with hydrosols like rose or lavender waters. You may have observed your elders doing this as well. It is always wise to observe the elders because many of their daily rites continue to have practical applications. The one I saw aids home cleaning with a broom since the wet bristles hold dust more readily than dry. I also realize that natural water, fresh from a rain or thunderstorm, has a power all its own. You can refresh the energy in the home through the judicious use of this type of natural force.

- Take your special broom outside.
- Tilt it upward so raindrops wet the broom's bristles from the top.
- Keep broom or besom upright until you get to the area you intend to ritualistically sweep. For example, sweep the bathroom floor with the rainwater-kissed broom. When you are finished, toss small bits of Essence of Hara Ke into the bathtub and under throw rugs. When you place the essence under rugs, footsteps release the energy and allow you to engage in the foot track magic of the Hoodoo.
- As an auxiliary step, put a small closed jar of Essence of Hara Ke near the bathtub. Open the jar while enjoying a soothing bath. Pull energy down from the heavens, like rain pelting the thirsty Earth Mother, so shall you be replenished. (Close jar after ritual.)

Rain Season Ceremony

Here is a third way to work the rain:

- Bring a bowl with a floating candleholder outdoors on an evening of heavy rains during the new or waning moon.
- Leave this out overnight in a safe location to collect rainwater.
- Go outside at dusk the next evening wearing all white. (If it is still raining, bring the candle bowl inside to conduct the ritual.)
- Focus on your intentions, then place three small lit white or pink floating flower candles inside the bowl of rainwater using your dominant hand.

- Face west.
- Recite as you continue to focus on the floating candles:

> As rain comes from the sky
> Show me the reasons to try
> Drops of the rain goddesses, fresh as morning dew
> Cleanse, renew
> Sweet Mujaji, make everything in my sight
> Bright, fresh, and sparkling like you.

- Recite this three times, building intensity with each invocation.
- Gaze at the fire as you visualize a successful transformation.
- Use some of the rainwater on your fingers to snuff each candle.
- Lift your hands high in the air.
- As the smoke is released toward the night sky, chant:

> So it is written, so it will be done!

- Gently blow the smoke so that it will carry your messages forward.
- Like the rain from above, let your energy, passion, and creativity flow.

Remember to look forward to rain, welcome it, and use it in your magical workings. Thank the Mujaji goddesses of the rain daily for the gifts they bestow upon the earth.

Thunder Orisha Invocation

Whereas we can have a tendency to shrink away from rain, thunder invokes fear. In Ifá there is an important orisha and cult dedicated to working thunder. Shango is the magnetic warrior deity with a large personality. His tremendous inner energy force raises thunder. He is noble, elegant, protective, and tricky. To engage the positive aspects of this deity, go outside where there are plenty of trees—his element.

- Face northeast, as it is his direction.
- Burn his favorite incense—frankincense tears—in a censer, careful to use fireproof protective surfaces.
- Spread cayenne peppers, hibiscus flowers, and bay leaves around the circumference of a tree that has some of Shango's characteristics.
- Keep your head low; defer to this spirit.
- Walk away backward, as quickly as possible without falling, until you are well away from the tree.

Up Pops the Mushrooms

With all the rain previously described, there's something else lurking about, waiting to spring forth and catch your attention—mushrooms! Foraging for wild mushrooms is a favorite pastime for many. Growing up in England, it was a favorite pastime for my husband in his youth. Here in Illinois, where we live, you can collect morels in April, yet other delightfully wholesome mushrooms such as hen of the woods, lion's mane, chanterelles, chicken of the woods, pheasant backs, and even the more commonly known oysters, all become available and await your foraging baskets.

We discussed ecosystems at length in part II, and wild mushrooms have a significant role in the native ecosystems in many lands. I have grown shiitake mushrooms and found it to be inexpensive, pleasurable, safe, and fun. As a longtime vegetarian, I make mushrooms a large part of my diet. In some ways, because of their umami, texture, and flavors, they are my preferred meat substitute; a portabella mushroom, slapped on the grill, is hard to beat as a veggie burger—and it's low-cal to boot.

Mushrooms are stepping out of the undergrowth of trees and into the limelight as a superfood. For decades, I have recommended that many people utilize the active compounds in reishi among other types of mushrooms, as they fight serious illnesses like cancer, HIV, and AIDS.

I recommend adding a pulverized blend of your own creation; if not, try a blend of as many as ten prepackaged powdered mushroom species added to your oatmeal, 7- or 9-grain hot cereal, steel-cut oats, millet, grits, or whatever hot cereal you're into. Typically, the packaged types contain a scoop that dispenses about 2.6 grams. You can also add this to your coffee, matcha, smoothie, juice, or soup.

For what reasons beyond taste would you engage with these fungi? Well, according to UCLA Health:

- The macronutrients in mushrooms help support your immune system.
- Cremini and portabella, two easy-to-obtain mushrooms, contain a healthy amount of selenium, which prevents cell damage.
- Maitake mushrooms are rich in vitamin D and help grow cells, reduce inflammation, and raise your immunity.
- Shiitakes help formulate red blood cells, DNA, and protein with their richness in vitamin B_6.
- As a healer, I'm crazy about reishi mushrooms. They work on your nervous system in several ways, making you feel more relaxed; but when needed they will energize you, and they fight against insomnia. Reishi are useful to deter hypertension and to positively impact kidney and liver disease; they work with your body to reduce cholesterol and can lessen cardiovascular disease. They have been used to support people through chemotherapy treatment for cancer, and they soothe the respiratory system and ailments such as flu and COVID-19.[2]

---

2   "7 Health Benefits of Mushrooms," UCLA Health, January 24, 2022, https://www.UCLAHealth.org/news/7-health-benefits-of-mushrooms.

First Week of April
Seed Moon Bird Ritual

Now that you have engaged the rain and thunder, don't forget about the area's wildlife; this is vital year-round. Just about any place you live has birds; if not, something is seriously wrong. Birds are magical, and they also have needs like all the earth's creatures. Together you can assist one another. This spell works like a charm. Celebrate the Seed Moon by planting seeds of positive energy for greater abundance.

- Go out under the light of the Seed Moon, dig a shallow hole, and bury all your pocket change.
- Draw a symbol of love or peace out of wild birdseed. Leave them out for forty-eight hours.
- At the end of this period, most of your seed and symbol will have been consumed and spread elsewhere, bringing your wish for peace and love along with the seed. In the morning, plant a few sunflower seeds on this spot. During the growing season, birds and butterflies will continue to grow and spread your message of love and peace.
- A year later your change abundance should flow back your way. Look for your change; most likely it will have doubled.

Spring Break Traveler's Spell

When once it was rare, today it is increasingly more feasible for people to take a spring break of one kind or another. If your journey crosses water, try this helpful spell for a bon voyage.

On the day of Mercury during the waxing cycle of the moon, it is the time to undertake a spell dedicated to successful travel by engaging the herb of seafarers, Irish moss. Irish moss assures prosperity and abundance in all your work. Gracefully use dried Irish moss, knowing that it comes from the depths of our sea mothers.

- Crumble it finely over a bowl. Think: *Safe by day, full at night,* and repeat this as a mental mantra.
- Set the bowl out under the moonlight overnight.

- Afterward, tuck some of this moss into your suitcase and a piece in each shoe.
- Each night visualize waves of prosperity rolling toward you from the sea.

Hold the thought steadily, think of it frequently, and prosperity as well as safe travels shall be yours!

Parcels of History: A Reflection

Hundreds of years ago, long before we were firmly rooted in the African diaspora, our ancestors, by and large women, had a vision and it involved seeds. We are discussing planting season here, and we are about to move on to other modalities for working with plants. Take note as you settle into this important thought. Our ancestors brought a variety of seeds here to the Americas and beyond to sustain them. How so? They wove them into their hair—and who would think of that except for an ingenious group of thinkers? Cornrows can be simple or elaborate; within both styles, there is the capacity to hide secrets—even the seeds of our soul food. You shall see, as you read on, that there are many ways nature can entwine with us in everyday life, meaningful ways that may at times be sacred. Here is something you might not have considered.

Spring Tonic: Inner and Outer Beauty

Now here is something you don't see every day: a tonic that revitalizes energy and perks up weather-beaten hair—all in one. This spring tonic enhances hair color, bringing gray from dingy to golden, and does the same for your spirit. It brings depth to dark-brown and black hair, lifts mood, relaxes anxiety, cleanses internally, is a uterine tonic, gently stabilizes hormonal upsets, and boosts immunity.

Contains: dried, cut, and sifted oat straw, pau d'arco, black tea, lavender, bay leaves, parsley, chickweed, calendula, rosemary, sage, and marshmallow root.

How to use on hair: add 2 tablespoons to 4 cups of water. Bring to a boil.

Cover, and reduce heat to low. Infuse 20 minutes. Let cool, and strain well. Pour over your hair. Then rinse lightly with cool water.

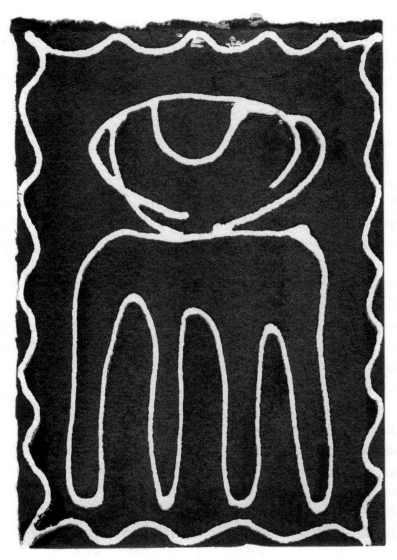

Duafe: The Wooden Comb
Meaning: Duafe symbolizes patience, prudence, sweetness, love, and nurturing

Loud and Proud: Black Hairdos

Curly hair is beautiful; it is also very complex. Sometimes we treat it forcefully, especially in an attempt to detangle, but ultimately this is the wrong approach. Curly hair has a complicated hair shaft; pull out a strand and examine it. I'm sure you will find variation in the width of the strand—at points it is quite thick, while in other areas it is thinner. The irregularity in the hair shaft, especially at the thin points, makes it more likely to break if stressed than straight hair.

Herbs and Curly Hair: A Caveat

In addition to the five saponin-rich natural shampoo herbs discussed below, other herbs can be added too, for various effects. One thing to remember, though, is that most herbs are astringent (drying). Many herbs popularly used for hair care are well suited to straight, oily hair, but may challenge curly or kinky hair; this includes the popular hair herbs rosemary, sage, horsetail, and nettles. Second, although herbs are natural, they can still be irritating and drying and can even cause a rash. Add herbs judiciously, one at a time, testing for allergic reactions. If your hair is described as coarse, kinky, nappy, or very thick, pay special attention to these warnings. Typically, these types of hair tend to be dry. You may benefit from the addition of a teaspoon or two of olive oil, hempseed oil, neem oil, jojoba (a wax), or melted shea or mango butter when adding extra herbs. Herbs that release plant mucilage—burdock root, marshmallow root, slippery elm, and emollient comfrey—retain moisture. If you suffer from frizziness and want to define your curls, add 1 teaspoon vegetable glycerin or aloe to the recipes. Herbs used historically in natural shampoos include rosemary, sage, and walnut hulls for brunette or black hair; chamomile, calendula, and mullein for blond or light-brown hair; and rose hips, henna, hibiscus flowers, and cinnamon for red, auburn, or burgundy hair. Nettles, horsetail, and sea kelp strengthen hair and encourage growth. Chamomile, comfrey, and catmint soothe scalp irritation. Tea tree, garlic, onion, and neem are used as antibacterial, antifungal agents to deter scalp disorders and infections. Hops (one of the main herbs in beer, which is why beer rinses have been used for hundreds of years) and chamomile add body and thickness.

Saponins

Shampoo was not always formulated by chemists or in the factory; this is a very new approach that came into vogue during the late nineteenth and early twentieth centuries. Saponins are nature's sudsing agents, and they are found in herbs. Saponin-rich herbs come from specific fruit trees, roots, flowers, and mineral-packed weeds.

Make Your Own Botanical Shampoo

Most herbs do not produce frothy lather—and who needs it anyway? The idea, particularly with curly hair, is to cleanse gently without stripping hair of sebum (natural oils). Listed below are some of nature's better cleansers:

Lamb's-quarter (*Chenopodium album*)—a common North American and European weed, probably already lurking about in your garden, ready for harvest, lends mild cleansing action.

Papaya leaf (*Carica papaya*)—from the pawpaw tree, papaya leaf releases gentle cleansers when infused in hot water.

Soapbark tree (*Quillaja saponaria*)—the bark, as it sounds, contains enough saponin to provide a good soap, useful as a shampoo. Barks need to be decocted, rather than infused.

Soapwort (*Saponaria officinalis*)—this weed has been used for cleansing hair, the body, and fine textiles for centuries. Some museum preparators continue to use soapwort to cleanse ancient textiles. This attests to soapwort's mild, nurturing nature. To make soapwort shampoo or lingerie wash, infuse 1 cup soapwort in 2 cups water, covered, for 20 minutes.

Yucca (*Yucca glauca, Y. baccata, Y. angustifolia*)—also called soaproot and amole. Used in traditional rituals and rite of passage ceremonies in Mexico, by the Hopi, and a few other Southwest Indians, yucca is also used to deter dandruff, baldness, and thinning hair. Yucca needs to be pulverized and soaked before using.

Yucca—and sometimes its relatives from the *Agave* spp., such as *Agave lechuguilla*—are used to make shampoo, soap, and clothing detergent. To prepare, peel a young root so that only the white inside remains. Pound this white interior in a large mortar and pestle, with a mallet, or with a hammer until it is mashed. Put the bruised root inside a piece of muslin. Tie shut with a rubber band or piece of natural cotton string. Place in hot water. Work the root between your hands until the soapy substance is released into the water. Use this liquid to spiritually and physically cleanse your hair.

Why Bother?

Of course, you and I know that it is easy to run out to the local shops and choose from a wide array of shampoos, so why bother making your own? Here are some of the reasons:

Connection—many people enjoy direct engagement with herbs, feeling that they benefit spirituality from contact with nature.

Avoiding chemicals—other people do not trust the plethora of chemicals used in shampoo formulas—these "do-it-yourself" types prefer to make their own from scratch.

Ecology and sustainability—some people want to participate in the natural ecology around them in a positive way. They would never use weed killer, for example, to kill lamb's-quarter; instead, they use the prolific weed for its nutrients in hair care formulas and in other holistic ways. Abundant leaves from the papaya tree can be used, rather than simply disposed of, when they fall from the tree. Making shampoo offers opportunities to reuse and recycle old squeeze-top bottles rather than discarding them. Homemade herbal brews bring satisfaction from growing, harvesting, and then using your own organic ingredients.

Ancient traditions—Mexican and Southwest Indian peoples—notably, the Hopi—have long used yucca as an important element in beauty, rites of passage, and ceremonies during prenuptial rites. Some people feel that they too can benefit from these ancient traditions. Yucca is ideal for the rich brown and black wavy, thick hair prevalent in Middle Eastern, African, Southern European, Native American, and Latino cultures. Soapwort and soap-bark have also been used historically. The two "soap" herbs, along with lamb's-quarter and papaya leaf, are gentle and effective cleansers, well suited to the delicate curly, kinky, or nappy hair that people from various ethnic groups have.

Essential Oils for Healthy Hair

Essential oils are organic ingredients that accentuate the effects of prepared shampoos. These precious oils are the condensed essences of plants, prepared as an oil. Aromatic botanical oils are regaining the popularity they enjoyed historically in early civilizations. They are well respected for their ability to address a variety of issues, such as dull, dry, and thinning hair, as well as itchy or irritated scalp—these are aromatherapeutic benefits. The scents of essential oils provide a therapy of their own, sometimes referred to as aromachology because they affect our psychological makeup and mood. Since essential oils are highly concentrated, only a few drops are necessary to achieve great results. This table on the next page, inspired by *The Complete Book of Essential Oils and Aromatherapy* by esteemed aromatherapist Dr. Valerie Ann Worwood,[3] illustrates the suitability of essential oils for various types of hair.

Hydrosols

Aromatherapist Jeanne Rose of the Aromatic Plant Project coined the term *hydrosol*, though they are also referred to as floral waters. Hydrosols are the essences of fragrant plants extracted and preserved in distilled water. The three most popular hydrosols are:

Rose (also referred to as rosewater)—astringent, energizing, calming, fragrant

Neroli (also called orange flower water)—uplifting, hydrating, mellow

Lavender (also called lavender water)—moisturizing, balancing, unisex

Hydrosols are the lightest natural hair spray/moisturizer available. They work like a charm with Afros and other curly dos, especially when the emphasis is on enhancing natural curl, not controlling it. You can use them to replace some or all of the plain water used to create herbal shampoo, as in the recipe on p. 336.

---

3   Valerie Ann Worwood, *The Complete Book of Essential Oils and Aromatherapy* (Novato, CA: New World Library, 2016).

Essential Oil for Hair Table

Essential oils	Normal Hair	Dry Hair	Oily Hair	Fragile Hair
Birch (*Betula lenta*)		X	X	
Carrot (*Daucus carota*)	X			X
Clary sage (*Salvia sclarea*)				X
Lavender (*Lavandula angustifolia, L. officinalis*)	X	X	X	
Lemon eucalyptus (*Eucalyptus citriodora*)	X		X	
Neroli (*Citrus bigaradia, C. aurantium*)	X			
Parsley (*Petroselinum sativum*)	X	X		X
Patchouli (*Pogostemon patchouli*)	X			
Peppermint (*Mentha piperita*)	X			
Rosemary (*Rosmarinus officinalis*)	X	X	X	
Sandalwood (*Santalum album*)		X		X
Tea tree (*Melaleuca alternifolia*)	X		X	X
Yarrow (*Achillea millefolium*)			X	X

RELAXING RHASSOUL SHAMPOO

¼ cup Moroccan rhassoul mud
½ cup rosewater
½ cup orange flower water

7 drops neroli essential oil
5 drops sandalwood essential oil
3 drops patchouli essential oil

Put rhassoul mud in a nonreactive bowl (Pyrex or stainless steel). Slowly whisk in rosewater and orange water. Drop in essential oils. Whisk until smooth. Cover hair with the shampoo and massage gently. Cover with a plastic cap, leave on 15 to 30 minutes, then rinse well.

Shortcuts
Doctoring

With our busy lives, many people simply do not have the time to make personal care products themselves. If you fit into this group, yet want to add your own unique touches, doctoring is the right method for you. Doctoring is old slang for taking something that already exists and adding your own personal touches. Suggestions follow.

Castile soap—Castile soap is highly touted in homemade shampoo recipes. Castile soap is made from shredded olive oil soap, dissolved in water. It is widely available from health food stores and natural product suppliers.

Shampoo base—A popular option for those pressed for time is to purchase prepared shampoo bases that are unscented, natural, or organic and then add essential oils.

Tip: Add 8 to 16 drops (total) essential oils (refer to the table on p. 335 for options) to 2 cups shampoo base. If shampoo base is unavailable, try unscented baby shampoo.

Nutrients—You can also add ¼ cup dried, ground sea kelp or seaweed to emulsify (thicken) shampoo and add nourishment.

Dairy products, buttermilk, full-fat "real" mayonnaise, sour cream, or whole cream are natural softening ingredients that hydrate and help detangle; pick one and add ¼ cup to strained, scented shampoo brew. Refrigerate unused portion. Use within a week. Eggs have already been discussed; they are useful because they add body, shine, and protein. Always use at room temperature. Separate the egg and use only the yolk for hair (it's easier to rinse out).

The great part about making your own hair care products is that you can experiment with the ingredients, adjusting them until they are perfectly suited to your hair texture. By tailoring the essential oils, you can create an alluring scent that is unique. Creating shampoo in bulk is economic, wholesome, and relaxing.

Locs: A Journey of Personal Transformation

Not long ago, the main places you would see locs (sometimes called dreadlocks) was in Africa or the Caribbean, particular Jamaica. For the Rastafarians of Jamaica, the Shaivas (devotees to Shiva) and Vaishnavas (devotees to Vishnu) of India, and numerous clans in Africa, including the Turkana, Maasai, Samburu of Kenya, Himba of Namibia, Fulani of Senegal, and the Baye Fall (Black Muslims), locked hair is not a hairstyle, it is a reflection of a way of life, grounded by culture, tradition, and most of all spirituality. Just as many different cultures have hair-locking traditions, so too does this distinctive way of wearing the hair have diverse names including natty dreads (Rastafarians); ndiagne (Senegalese; meaning "strong hair"), and jatta (gurus of India).

Many people of Jamaican and African heritage have migrated and now live on the East Coast in and around New York City. It is in New York that locked hair took a hold on popular culture, transcending its traditional connection to spirituality and faith to become a cultural statement with all people. Acclaimed author Alice Walker has worn locs for many years, and so have other artists including Bob Marley and Whoopi Goldberg.

In the beautiful book *Dreads*, Francesco Mastalia and Alfonse Pagano[4] interviewed people from around the world about why their hair is worn in what they call dreadlocks. (Today, most people reject the combination of terms *dread* and *lock* because it has negative connotations, particularly because of the word *dread*, which evokes fear.) As might be expected, there was a wide range of reasons—from strong faith-based cultural tradition, to easy grooming, to attraction, to the style, and everything in between.

---

4   Francesco Mastalia and Alfonse Pagano, *Dreads* (New York: Artisan, 1999).

Decisions, Decisions

There are various schools of thought within the curly-topped community. Some folks long for straight hair and lean toward the tools, chemicals, and techniques that will give the desired effect. Others absolutely adore their curly locks and wouldn't have their hair any other way. These folks seek out products and techniques that will accentuate their curls or leave their hair to do what it will. Still others like their naturally curly hair but wish for an easier grooming regimen. For those individuals looking for relatively easy grooming and a natural look that is a throwback to Africa, or who seek connection to earth-based spiritual wisdom from around the world, locs are an ideal choice.

Many people, including myself, enjoy naturally curly hair but find a variety of challenges as well as opportunities with our curly locks. Issues include the expense of products that promise to manage, enhance, or accentuate curly hair but often fall short. Curly hair, particularly of the densely coiled nature of African-descended people, is very resistant to change so we investigate what it is it naturally wants to do. While there are many excellent products on the market, many of which are discussed on websites like www.naturallycurly .com, African curls tend to have a mind of their own. Our curls naturally coil around each other, producing awesome ringlets and sometimes tangles. We are not alone in this phenomenon; people of various ethnicities have tightly curled hair.

Many of us spend hours, and indeed years, as well as thousands of dollars to manage or prevent tangles. If we keep our hair short, it is lovely and generally manageable. This is an ideal situation for tightly curled hair. The tangles of shorter hair are easier to manage, but they can become quite a bit more challenging with longer hair. The battle of the tangles, or as we typically call them, naps, leads to breakage. Long nappy hair that is tightly curled often becomes uneven, damaged, and ultimately frustrating. For individuals with tightly curled hair that tends to tangle, snarl, or nap up, locs are an ideal choice, particularly if you also desire longer hair.

Grooming with Spirit, Purpose, and Patience

Patience is an issue that arises even for those with ideal hair for locs, which would be hair that is tightly curled without any chemical straighteners. For these individuals, locs can take at least six months to become permanent; for those with looser curls or wavy hair, it could take two years. If you can be mindful and focus on the end result, this time will be part of a larger metamorphosis, a change within that allows change to occur at its own rate.

Some people will find yoga and meditation especially helpful as well because they encourage a focus within rather than on outward appearance.

Social and Psychological Implications

The appearance of locked hair evokes a wide variety of responses. Some people find locs suggestive of the counterculture or to be radically different from their personal orientation. If these people exert control over your life—perhaps your parents, administrators, advisors, or a boss at work—you will need to enter a meaningful conversation during your transformation. Sometimes there are so many issues that go much deeper than hair that a conversation may have been long overdue. Talking can help strengthen and develop stronger ties. You will need to weigh your priorities, and if it turns out that your priority is the locked hair and those around you strongly reject the idea, you will need to evaluate how to proceed.

The Nitty-Gritty

Once you decide to loc your hair, you will of course need more than anything to be patient. I started my locs—or rather, they started themselves—approximately a year ago. They are still not all the way locked because my curls are loose. I twist them regularly but not fanatically, and I see a loctician when possible. A good loctician is indispensable, especially early on in the process when the locs are being established. She will clean your scalp well, condition your hair, repart your hair, and carefully twist or roll the hair. Having a skilled loctician is a great way of keeping a very neat look.

One of the most highly recommended technical books for those trying to establish locs is *Plaited Glory: For Colored Girls Who've Considered Braids, Locks, and Twists* by Lonnice Brittenum Bonner.[5] Another popular book, *No Lye: The African American Woman's Guide to Natural Hair Care* by Tulani Kinard,[6] gives practical advice for beginning locs naturally. Kinard advises readers to part the hair evenly in small pieces of about ½ inch and to either palm-roll, twist, or braid each segment tightly. These twists or braids should be left alone for at least one month. After this time period, the hair can be washed, with an emphasis on cleansing the scalp, rather than the hair itself. Some people cleanse their scalp with

---

5   Lonnice Brittenum Bonner, *Plaited Glory: For Colored Girls Who've Considered Braids, Locks, and Twists* (New York: Three Rivers Press, 1996).
6   Tulani Kinard, *No Lye: The African American Woman's Guide to Natural Hair Care* (New York: St. Martin's Press, 1997).

natural herbs like a witch hazel tincture in between shampoos to feel fresher. After about one month, the hair is shampooed, rerolled or twisted, held down with hair clips, and dried under a hair dryer or naturally in sunlight. This is repeated for many months until the hair is permanently locked. According to Kinard, the ideal method is for a hollow core to form at the center of each loc and for the hair to be encouraged to curl around this core. This allows light and airy locs, which move freely and have a natural sheen and which are also easy to clean. The problem with quick-and-easy methods, particularly those promoted for use on straighter hair, is that the hair gets irreparably dirty, and when using grease or wax, the locs actually become dirt magnets. Moreover, there is not a natural, light, and airy hollow core to the hair; it is simply clumped together and can be quite unattractive.

I am a do-it-yourself type. I had been wearing two-stranded twists for about three years, and when they started to lock up I embraced the possibility of physical transformation. Eventually, I did seek out the expertise of several locticians, and I was grateful to have some of the messy areas sorted out. You can find a loctician in most major cities, and typically they advertise as "natural hair care salons." There are numerous products available to help manage your locs, though it is a personal choice, just like the decision whether or not to consult a loctician. Generally, less is more with locs. My loctician, who is an Igbo person from Nigeria, even warns against naturally oily ingredients like shea butter or lanolin for loc maintenance because they weigh down the locs and attract dirt.

Essential tools:
- A rat-tailed comb to part and roll the hair
- A light, clear shampoo such as Johnson and Johnson baby shampoo or a salon brand containing essential oils like lavender or chamomile
- A natural conditioner, either homemade or from a manufacturer, that promotes natural essential oils, for example Aveda or African Root Stimulator
- A water-based gel (that obviously does not contain heavy waxes or oils); I suggest that you create your own: simply use pure aloe vera gel, applied in dime-size portions
- Patience, patience, patience

Remember it's not the destination, even with locs, but the journey itself that can lead to personal transformation.

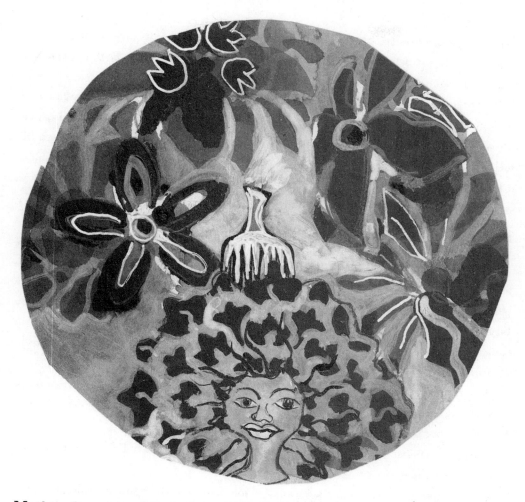

Mother-Daughter María Lionza Natural Hair Ritual

There is a deity with millions of devotees that some are unaware of. This deity combines indigenous African, indigenous South American, and Abrahamic beliefs in the form of Catholicism. I'm speaking of María Lionza, and her religion is *Marialionceros*. I am invoking her energy with this ritual because she is the Queen of Nature. All that is natural yet unruly in nature and elsewhere falls under her auspices. She loves nature and those things that are natural because that is her entire being. She was first a human, before she was eaten by a gigantic anaconda and became part of Sorte Mountain. During her time as a human, she had a daughter, and the two are sometimes celebrated together. María Lionza is a green-eyed indigenous woman, whereas her daughter, who some believe is Elvira, daughter from a conquistador, is believed to be the first mestiza. She is brown-eyed. Both are beautiful and close to one another in spirit and purpose.

Keeping the powerful duo in mind, I want to share my story and how I came to work with my daughter's hair. First of all, I grew up as a "tender-headed" child. Like many people with thick, tightly curled, easily tangled hair that has a tendency to grow long, I readily feel pain when my hair is combed, and I am not shy about letting everyone know about it. The word *ouch*, followed by a flood of tears, was synonymous with hair-washing time and with being tender-headed during my youth.

Today, as an herbalist and aromatherapist, I have discovered numerous ways of easing pain naturally. You can employ and engage the powers of María Lionza and her daughter as you set yourself up for this ritual. Mother and daughter benefit from bonding, trust, affection, and sharing, especially since something like the combing of curly hair can spark pain. The María Lionza ritual shared here is useful for those who are African-descended, biracial children, and anyone with tightly curled hair.

Soothing Ritual

- Put on a melodic playlist: María Lionza would be pleased with tropical bird sounds, what is called "jungle" or "forest" music, rhythmic djembe drumming, and all primal and outdoor sounds.
- Warm ¼ cup or so sweet almond, jojoba, or avocado oil or shea butter on the stovetop or in the microwave.
- Have the child sit on a zafu or zabuton (Zen meditation pillow.) These types work especially well, though any pillow will do.
- Retrieve oil from microwave or stovetop. Add 3 drops lavender, sandalwood, or chamomile essential oil or 1 drop rose otto—to accentuate the relaxing nature of the oil. Situate yourself so that your child is between your knees on her pillow. Dip fingers into the oil and gently massage it into the entire scalp.
- Put on a cap or wrap her hair in cellophane. Wrap again in a large towel. Have the child lie down on the pillow and listen to the natural sounds for 20 minutes.
- While the child is relaxing, light an incense of either sacred frankincense and sandalwood or another pleasing scent; place it in a censer or fireproof holder.

- Shampoo hair using a gentle shampoo, perhaps one made solely out of soapwort roots and leaves, or use a homemade shampoo and conditioning bar or your preferred herbal cleansing routine; towel-dry (non-terry cloth so as not to further disrupt hair).
- Put a clean, dry towel around her neck; apply an herbal mucilage gel to her hair—perhaps flaxseed, aloe vera, okra, or a marshmallow gel—one small portion at a time.
- Mist her face and hair again, this time using lavender water or rosewater. Mist your face as well; repeat when you encounter knotted hair.
- Separate wet hair with an Afro pick; mist as needed. Style, using the widest comb available.
- Take slow, deep breaths as you work, and reflect upon the image of the beautiful María Lionza and her daughter, if they are available to you. Know that she tames and soothes all the nerves.

Gentle Styling Ideas

The blessing of kinky and curly hair is the numerous styling options. Mom[7] or another caretaker can allow individuality and creativity to shine. Each style becomes a makeover and an adventure. Here are a few options that are easy for you, gentle to children's scalps, and well suited to curly hair.

- A soft headband or colorful scarf (folded down to headband size).
- Put hair into a softly sculpted puff by shaping it with your hands.
- Part hair in the middle and make two Afro puffs if hair is long enough. Use a scrunchie. For added fun, make a zigzag part.
- For a longer-lasting hairstyle, try a double-strand twist:
  - Divide hair into four sections.
  - Clip or braid three sections to contain the hair.
  - Part hair into ¾-inch boxes; twist (using two strands).
  - Apply aloe vera gel to hair to hold ends or, if necessary, use black-fabric-covered rubber bands.

---

7   This ritual is for all caretakers and those for whom they care; this means it can easily be comforting to a father fixing his child's hair, a grandparent working with her grandchild's hair, and so forth.

• Take breaks. Massage her shoulders. Mist her hair and apply aloe or other edge cream as needed. Continue until the entire head is styled. It should last at least four weeks, especially if a silk scarf is worn to bed (or if silk or satin pillowcases are used).

You're Not Finished Yet

Complete the ritual with a cup of peppermint or chamomile tea: boil two cups water; add one peppermint and one chamomile tea bag to each cup; pour water over tea bags to fill the cups. Sweeten with honey, if desired; flavor with lemon or milk (it's your choice).

By now, the two of you should be relaxed and eagerly looking forward to next month's ritual. In the interim, it is a good time to set up a María Lionza altar for next time. On a small table or mantel, lay out a beautiful blue cloth; red, yellow, white, and/or blue candles; candies; and a bubbly drink (she prefers champagne). Let this be an extension of your togetherness time. Have fun shopping for interesting oils, incense, herbs, and floral waters for the next María Lionza Mother and Daughter Hair Ritual. Work together on making it your own ritual that makes hairdressing fun.

Next is some work that is again intergenerational. You can do this for your Queen Mother (elder), she can do it for you, or you can do it for yourself.

Herbal Dyes for Mature African Hair

As we grow older, our hair gradually loses its natural color and turns gray. For some, this process begins as early as their twenties. Many women are not ready for such a big change. Some want to hold on to their natural hair color, while others choose to enhance gray or white hair. Like most dark fibers, brunette or black hair is more resistant to dyes than light fibers or blond hair. The complex hair shaft of kinky and curly hair requires more colorant, and gray hair is very resistant. To top it off, hair grows ¼ to ½ inch per month, making coloring hair a challenge. Shown resistance, we have a tendency to reach for permanent color rather than gentle solutions—this can lead to damage, especially if relaxers or straighteners are also used. This section is written for those seeking natural ways to enrich graying hair. Botanical rinses work with existing color, providing subtle highlights, increased shine, and youthful vibrancy without causing permanent changes.

RED HOT OIL

Add reddish highlights, warm sallow skin, and enliven dingy gray hair. A rich red hue can be created from the roots of the herb alkanet (*Alkanna tinctoria*) and extracted into oil. Red Hot Oil conditions dry hair and colors it simultaneously. Apply it as a hot oil treatment.

⅓ cup cut alkanet root, sifted
⅔ cup sweet almond, safflower, or olive oil

Place the alkanet root in a sterile, dry jar with a screw top. Fill the jar with oil, and set it in a window. Steep 24 hours; swirling periodically. Warm ¼ cup red oil; apply to the hair while warm. Divide the hair into four sections. Part hair ¼ inch at a time and apply oil from roots to tip. Put on a plastic cap, then wrap the head in a towel. Leave on 45 minutes, then shampoo.

Yield: 2 or more applications (depending on hair length)
Shelf life: 1 year

FLAMIN' RED

This recipe features madder root (*Rubia tinctorum*), a relative of alkanet root, which was featured in the previous recipe. Flamin' Red works well on medium- or dark-brown hair. As this is a progressive dye, color intensifies with repeated use.

1½ cups water
⅓ cup madder root

2 tablespoons apple cider vinegar

Boil water, then add madder root. Stir, cover, and reduce heat to medium. Simmer 30 minutes. Add vinegar, then simmer 30 minutes more. Reduce heat to low; steep 30 minutes more. Strain and cool. To use, pour over your head, over a bowl in a sink. This is called the catch method. Squeeze through. Repeat as many times as desired to get the depth of color you seek.

Yield: approximately 12 ounces
Shelf life: use within 24 hours

Henna

One of the strongest hair dyes is henna (*Lawsonia inermis*). People have enjoyed henna since the civilizations of ancient Egypt. As legend has it, Cleopatra had lovely red hair, as did Nefertiti. Henna brings out reddish highlights in the most resistant hair, including graying hair. Henna is not recommended on hair that has been dyed recently with commercial dyes; a chemical reaction occurs, turning hair black. Henna is also not recommended for hair more than 50 percent gray. To use packaged types, follow manufacturer's directions and enhance as follows:

- Shampoo hair first.
- Enhance red tones by using cognac, red wine, carrot juice, cranberry juice, hibiscus tea, or rose hip tea in place of water.
- Tint and scent: add vanilla extract for scent or any combination of ground allspice, cinnamon, or cloves for enriched brown tones. Limit spices to a teaspoon. Avoid use on abraded scalp or by sensitive or allergic individuals.
- To minimize brassiness, use strong black coffee, rosemary, sage, or black tea in place of water.
- For body: add flat beer or hops tea in place of water.
- Quench dryness with the addition of mayonnaise.
- Attract moisture with yogurt, sour cream, honey, or molasses.
- Follow up with a hot oil treatment to counteract dryness.

ROSEMARY (*ROSMARINUS OFFICINALIS*) AND SAGE (*SALVIA OFFICINALIS*) RINSE

This is an age-old formula for blending gray hair into darkly colored hair. It works on the same principle as tea or coffee—the concentration of tannins facilitates desired staining.

1½ cups distilled water
1 teaspoon each dried rosemary and sage

Boil water, then add herbs. Cover, and reduce heat to medium. Simmer 20 minutes. Reduce heat to low and simmer 20 minutes more. Turn off heat, then steep 1 hour and strain. Apply using catch method.

ALTERNATIVE: Use 3 cups strong coffee or black tea. To prepare, brew 3 tablespoons loose Assam, Ceylon, or oolong tea or three Tetley tea bags in 3 cups boiled water. Cool, then apply using catch method.

Yield: approximately 12 ounces
Shelf life: 2 weeks

TOBACCO HERBAL RINSE

Tobacco (*Nicotiana* spp.) rinse is one of the most effective ways of quickly staining graying hair. This rinse adds golden, auburn tones.

1½ cups distilled water   2 tablespoons vinegar
¼ cup dried tobacco

Boil water, then add tobacco. Reduce heat to medium low and cover. Infuse 40 minutes. Remove from heat then add vinegar and steep 20 minutes. Strain. Apply using catch method.

Yield: approximately 12 ounces
Shelf life: 1 month, refrigerated

NIGHTS ON NEGRIL BEACH

This is a natural bluing treatment designed to bring a midnight moonlit glow to graying hair. This will also enrich black hair.

2 cups water
½ cup blueberries
½ cup blackberries

Pinch salt
2 tablespoons powdered alum

Boil water. Add berries, salt, and alum. Cover and reduce heat to medium. Simmer 20 minutes, checking, stirring, and mashing berries every few minutes. Strain through a fine sieve. Apply using catch method.

The Silver Trail

Ever since my very early twenties, I've had gray hairs popping up here and there on my head. I love growing my hair long, and I've also spent a long time dying my hair. As you can see from my recipes, I've done a fair amount of natural dyes that are plant-based. I've also hit up the salon and pharmacy for those easy ready-mixed boxes, which by the way, I found to get me in a lot of trouble.

I had naturally colored coffee-brown hair until I was in my twenties, although even in those years I experimented with things like lemon lighteners, henna, and so forth. I used henna, natural plant dyes, and commercial permanent and semipermanent dyes—but then I decided to bring all that to a halt.

I had grown my hair just about as long as it would go—past my shoulders, to my bra-strap area. I had started going to a natural salon, dedicated to curly cuts like the DevaCurl or Rezo cut, along with the coloring techniques of balayage and the very individualist pintura highlights.

I was consulting with a master colorist and she kept looking at my hair with that look that stirs up the pit of your stomach. Picking up handfuls and letting it back loose. "Your hair is super unhealthy," she finally said. "Why don't you let it be its natural color? You have a gorgeous type of gray. Dye is ruining your hair."

After the shock and horror seeped through my brain, I thought, *What is she saying? We*

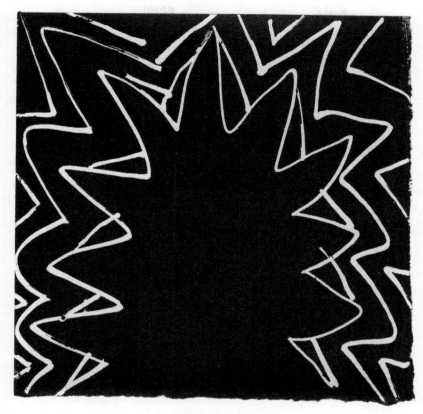

Owia a Repue: Rising Sun
Meaning: Warmth, hope, and strength to face life anew

cut it all off? All my years of new growth, since cutting it all off previously to start fresh from my locs? Surely, she jests! But actually she wasn't. "Let's do a big chop. Let some gray grow in and do another big chop," she said.

What in the world? I thought. This sounds like some S&M BS, I laughed inside. *Cut, chop, and cut chop until all that gray I'd been covering up for decades could show its full face? Ah, no thanks!* Alas, I did get it halfway chopped off. I wanted to see what she was talking about. My stylist was in full agreement. He said my hair was a white-gray. Hmmm, food for thought.

I'm not going to lie. Getting to that place by Uber, then paying for the fancy services, hurt my pocketbook. It was months before I returned, and by then, I had an appreciable amount of this new white-gray my stylist seemed to be anticipating. In between my visits,

I had tried long extension braids with pink and lavender hair added in—several times, so I had a few inches.

Meanwhile, articles were being released and announcements made on the news broadcasts. There is a potential link between hair products—like relaxers (which I hadn't used in eons) and hair dye (my stalwart friend)—and certain types of cancer. These cancers were striking Black and Brown women at higher rates, and for some proved to be deadly. More food for thought.

I'd made an executive decision. It was all coming off—the dyed blackish-brown, I mean. It had been at least fifteen years, but I was ready once again for a fresh start. "Are you sure?" "Are you certain?" Everyone in my life, inside and outside the shop, asked. "Yes, I'm sure."

Afterward, I looked at all my years of hair growth on the floor and had to smile. I was like a sheep that had been sheared. That was a lot of hair on the floor, but I stepped over it and kept on keeping on. I don't look back. I'm looking forward to seeing what lies ahead on the Silver Trail.

I do nourish my TWA (teeny-weeny Afro). I drink lots of water and use a wonderful grapeseed oil and rice water concoction that defines my curls. I oscillate between aloe vera gel to lock in the curls and certain other products I like. I'm happy with my hair; moreover, I'm really happy I don't have to camouflage my hair every 4 to 6 weeks like I had been doing for oh so many years! I'm eager to see how this goes.

HOT SHEA BUTTER HAIR TREATMENT

For most types of hair (gray and white included), shea is a good hot oil treatment, wherein it is melted, cooled slightly, then applied warm to the ends of the hair (where split ends occur) and to the scalp.

Use a clean (art) paintbrush as a handy tool for applying the warmed oil to the scalp. Part the hair in sections as you work. Work quickly, otherwise shea will solidify. Put on a plastic cap, and sit out in the sun, if possible, or under a dryer for 30 minutes. Alternatively, cover head with a bath towel to retain heat. After 30 minutes, shampoo thoroughly and rinse. Shea adds shine and softens.

HAIR POMADE

Africans have been using shea butter as a hair dressing for hundreds of years. This application is recommended for super thick, curly, kinky, or dry hair.

Thin, straight hair would become overwhelmed and weighed down by a shea pomade; locs (dreadlocks) may also appear dull or develop a tendency to attract dirt when shea is applied to them, so it is not recommended for them.

Scoop out about a teaspoon of shea butter into the palm of your hands (use less for short hair and more for longer hair). Place your palms together. Rub gently, using your body heat to melt the shea butter. Once shea transforms from solid to liquid, rub it on your hair. Then style as usual. This is fine as a weekly hairdressing pomade.

BOTANICAL STYLING GEL

A very effective gel can be created from flaxseed or Irish moss since both contain mucilage. I have used both many times with great success. They add body and shine without the flakiness of some commercial products. They also cost a fraction of the price of prepared products from beauty or drugstores.

1 teaspoon cut Irish moss, sifted,
　or ground flaxseed
¾ water

¼ cup vodka
1 teaspoon essential oil, absolute,
　or hydrosol

In a pot, dissolve 1 teaspoon Irish moss or ground flaxseed in ¾ cup water. You will need to adjust the amount by doubling or tripling the quantity if you have long or very thick hair. Bring to a boil. Stir. Add more botanicals or water if needed in the ratio given, then stir again. Reduce heat to medium, and continue to cook 8 minutes. Remove from heat. Whisk in vodka and the scent of your choice. I suggest neroli, rose, lavender, patchouli, or a mixture. Whisk again. Leave overnight. You can apply this to freshly washed hair and it will help define curls. It will also help hold hair into smooth updos or chignons, or you can use it as a setting lotion as you would a commercial lotion.

Just in Time for Mother's Day: Neroli Luffa Soap

The soft nature of neroli lends itself to creating your own handmade soap. As a first step into soapmaking, purchase ready-made blocks of unscented soap called "melt and pour (MP)." These soap blocks, sold by the pound, are prepared using a variety of ingredients: aloe vera, olive oil, shea butter, hemp, honey, or even oatmeal. Follow manufacturer's directions. If you enjoy color, add orange soap chips or even an orange Crayola crayon in the last stages of melting the soap. Add the manufacturer's recommended amount of essential oil (neroli). You can enhance the orange scent further by adding three tablespoons of neroli hydrosol (orange blossom water) during the melting stage.

As a neat alternative, pour melted, scented soap over luffa sponges cut into 1-inch slices and place them in a metal or Pyrex baking dish. Luffa sponge is a vegetable skeleton with unique exfoliating qualities. Most recipes create at least a dozen bars of soap—consider giving some away. Orange blossom soap makes a great gift for Mother's Day and only takes a few hours to complete. Wrap in clear wrapping paper and seal with a festive ribbon.

Ananse Will Appear

When my three children were all under the age of eight, my husband Damian and I traveled Down Under with them for a year. Our youngest, the girl of the bunch, was eighteen months old.

Now let me set the stage. The Northern Territory—Alice Springs, no less—where that leg of my work had led, wasn't just hot; it was H-O-T! My daughter was chilling on her tummy in just a diaper. The rest of us played board games and then were watching a television show. I noticed that our little girl, Olivia, had fallen fast asleep. But then I also noticed something horrifying. A redback spider, one of the most poisonous spiders in the world, was crawling down her back. My husband, Damian, and I saw and looked down at our baby gripped in horror.

What to do?

What to do?

We asked each other and ourselves silently. What instinct told me was not to seek to kill it. Let it crawl, because if I angered it and my aim was off, which it usually was, surely she'd get bitten.

We waited for a few minutes that seemed like hours. And you know what? The spider crawled down her back and off her, onto the floor. Once again the message was coming from the spider. Be patient. It was also encouraging balance and to use my head. It sparked curiosity and generated self-control and self-awareness. Phew! Another lesson from Ananse. These are the lessons of the spider.

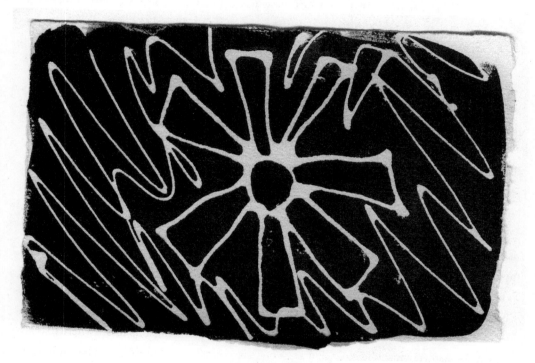

Ananse Ntentan
Meaning: The Spider Web
Ananse Ntentan is a symbol of artistic tendencies, uniqueness,
craftiness, creativity, and the complexities of life

Spring Cleaning Naturally

Lessons of the spider arise in both common and unusual circumstances. One lesson is that we can't just kill living creatures in our home. If possible, and assuming they aren't immediately threatening, we can find clever ways to be rid of them. Meanwhile, we can see what lessons they have to offer us. I'm not encouraging you to live with poisonous creatures, yet everything that crosses your path has a lesson to offer. Folklore says that spiders are lucky. I'm assuming this wisdom is built around the common, everyday spider and the numerous ways they keep other bugs from infiltrating the home.

Mothers and other caretakers do a lot in the home, and they need the treats dispersed throughout this book to nurture the spirit. Now we're going into some roll-up-your-sleeves work. Rather than using commercial products, harmful to you and the earth, as well as to her creatures, here are some ways to work with nature.

Glossary of Natural Home Cleaning Terms

Abrasive—an ingredient that uses friction to wear away wax, dirt, grime, and stains in a process called abrasion.

Acidic—a compound that readily gives protons to other substances. When dispersed in water, acids conduct electricity. Inorganic (mineral) acids include sulfuric, nitric, hydrochloric, and phosphoric acid. Organic acids include acetic, citric, hydroxyacetic, and oxalic acids. Acids aid in housecleaning by breaking down dirt stains and deposits. They are used for resistant, difficult-to-clean projects like cleaning the sink, toilet, and tub, or removing rust, tarnish, and mineral deposits from hard water. Natural acids include Tabasco Sauce, ketchup, tomatoes, milk, lemon, orange, or lime juice.

Active ingredients—ingredients designed to achieve the product's objectives.

Aerosol—substance dispersed by air.

Alkaline—solutions with a pH higher than 7 used to strip wax, degrease, or cleanse soil. Solutions contain more hydroxide ions than hydrogen ions. Reacts with skin, sometimes causing major irritation or even burns. Sodium hydroxide, potassium hydroxide, and sodium carbonate are strongly alkaline.

Allergenic—causing an allergic reaction; irritant.

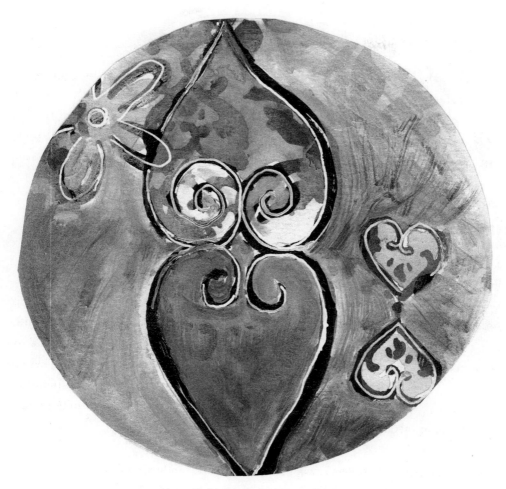

Asase Ye Duru: The earth has weight
Meaning: Providence and divinity of Mother Earth; importance of Earth as sustainer and steward of all life

Anhydrous—an ingredient or product that has had all of its water removed—for example, anhydrous lanolin, which is used to make salves and balms to protect or soothe the skin.

Antibacterial—ingredients that attack bacteria.

Antibiotic—a substance usually made from mold or bacterium that kills microorganisms with the potential to infect or cause disease.

Antifungal—substances that fight fungi.

Antimicrobial—substances that prevent bacterial contamination and the microbial deterioration it allows. Usually small amounts of preservatives are used to perform this function.

Antiseptic—ingredients with the property of destroying disease- or infection-causing microorganisms.

Antiviral—ingredients that fight viruses.

Biodegradable—an ingredient or product with the inherent ability to decompose.

Broad-spectrum—ingredients with multiple cleansing properties.

Buildup—dense deposits of dirt, grime, or wax.

Calcium carbonate—chief mineral that causes hard water; it is a combination of chalk and limestone.

Caustic—strong alkaline substance that irritates the skin on contact.

Deodorize—to remove odors.

Detergent—typically synthetic ingredients that work like soap but are more effective at penetrating minerals, thereby leaving fewer residues behind.

Disinfectant—an ingredient or process that destroys microorganisms with the potential to cause disease.

EPA—Environmental Protection Agency, a government body concerned with environmental safety and pollution.

Essential oil—the aromatic, volatile extract (essence) of a plant. Oils are extracted using cold-pressing or steam distillation.

Neutral cleanser—cleaner that has a pH between 7 and 9, especially important with waxes because high pH can attack wood and dull wax finishes.

Petroleum-based products—as it sounds, products created using petroleum, a nonrenewable energy source.

Phosphate—substance used as water softener.

Sanitize—to substantially remove undesirable organisms like bacteria, preferably without negatively impacting the wholesome qualities that need to be retained.

Saponin—a natural surfactant with detergent-like action found in plants. The word *saponin* is derived from the soapwort plant (*Saponaria officinalis*) because of its strong foaming and lathering action. Saponins are toxic to some fish because of the type of glycosides they contain. Some research suggests that saponins are antibiotic.

Solvent—liquid that dissolves other substances. The two most commonly used in home cleaning are water and alcohol.

Submersion—to soak in a liquid to cleanse.

Surfactant—substance that lowers surface tension of water, modifying the wetting, dispersal, foaming, and spreading abilities of a product.

Tarnish—a thin film or residue that changes or dulls the color of metals.

Volatile—element, ingredient, or constituent that evaporates during drying.

Tools for Holistic Home Cleaning

Chamois—deerskin cloth used for polishing metal and buffing furniture. Availability: can be purchased from automobile supply shops, hardware stores, and art supply shops.

Dust mask—protects respiratory system from fine particles of dust, ground herbs, and resins as well as other materials encountered during product creation and cleaning.

Latex or other protective gloves—protect hands while cleaning.

Rag—piece of cloth; strong cotton works very well. Used for polishing and some cleaning. Cotton rags from old, cleaned clothing like T-shirts works well. Availability: recycle and reuse old clothing, purchase cheap clothing from secondhand stores, or purchase from automobile supply shops, hardware stores, or art supply shops.

Sponge—natural sea sponge or pure cellulose work best. Natural sea sponges are the skeletons of an aquatic, lower invertebrate life-form called Porifera. Uses: to spot-clean areas all over the house including floors, bath, basin, toilet, tiles, and appliances. How to use: sponges that are suspected of containing disinfectants can be sterilized with boiling water (submerge in pan for about five minutes) or by washing in a dishwasher. Availability: widely available in grocery stores, health food stores, and hardware shops. Precaution: sponges that claim to "kill odor" or disinfect surfaces are thought to contribute to the increase in antibiotic-resistant bacteria.

Spout-top bottle (squirt bottle)—to store and dispense homemade cleansing products. How to use: shampoo and conditioner bottles can be used reused by sterilizing first with boiling hot water. Precautions: to avoid confusion and prevent potential injury or dangers, homemade cleanser put in these types of bottles should be labeled like all natural home cleaning products. Availability: most people have these types of bottles from shampoo products or dish detergent ready to be sterilized and reused. Specialty soapmaking and other craft supply shops carry new bottles.

Spray-top bottle—for general cleaning and dispersing liquid ingredients without harming the environment. Availability: some people have these types of bottles from hair care products or dish detergent ready to be sterilized and reused. Specialty soapmaking and other craft supply shops carry new spray-top bottles.

Natural Home Cleaning Ingredient List
Animal

Beeswax—a hard wax made by bees. Uses: homemade furniture polish, floor wax, candles, healing balms, and salves. How to use: melt in a double boiler; or for polish, melt with turpentine; add herbal ingredients and fixed oils as directed by recipe. Availability: purchase from beekeepers (apiaries); candle-making, soapmaking, and general art supply shops. Precautions: since it is usually heated, care should be exercised with formulations, and children should be under adult supervision.

Diatomaceous earth—skeletons of prehistoric algae. Uses: absorbs oil and water; has abrasive qualities. Diatomaceous earth is a very effective nontoxic insecticide. How to use: sprinkle on the spot to be cleansed, then scrub with a sponge or blot with a rag. Availability: specialty shops and online catalogs. Precautions: though considered nontoxic, diatomaceous earth contains tiny particles that can irritate the lungs and eyes. Safety is important, including wearing a dust mask to protect the respiratory system and possibly goggles. While this ingredient kills pest bugs that infiltrate the garden and pantry, it kills the good bugs too, so it should be used with great care and consideration.

Lanolin—oil found in sheep's wool. Sheep are unharmed by the removal of lanolin. Uses: included in leather cleaners and used for healing balms as well as salves. How to use: either directly (placed on a rag) or melted in a double boiler to which fixed oils and essential oils are added as per recipe. Availability: beauty supply shops, herb craft shops, and online.

Shellac—lac is a beetle excretion. Uses: furniture sealant is created when mixed with alcohol, which is used as a solvent. How to use: pour a small amount onto a rag. Treat area, rubbing gently. Availability: art and herb craft suppliers. Precautions: must be used in well-ventilated areas. Wear gloves to protect sensitive skin and a safety mask to limit the inhalation of vapors and help those with respiratory problems.

Fruit

Citrus peel—a natural solvent, deodorizer, and pleasant fragrance. Uses: citrus peel can be simmered to freshen the air, added to potpourris, used as an air freshener, added to homemade incense blends along with spices to freshen the air, and added to cleansing water as an essential oil for disinfecting the bathroom, kitchen, refrigerator and other appliances, floors, and clothing. How to use: dried citrus peel is used in potpourris and air fresheners as well as incense. Fresh peel can be simmered and added to cleansing water. Essential oils are dropped into the solution as directed in recipe.

Grapefruit seed extract—though not registered with the EPA, grapefruit seed extract is a highly touted cleansing aid with antiseptic qualities. How to use: add by the teaspoon to water or other dispersal agents such as vegetable-based soap for cleansing.

Lemon—one of the best natural cleaning ingredients. Can act as an air freshener, a mild bleach, and as an insecticide against fleas.

Lime—aromatic and antiseptic, lime is used in general household cleaning products and as an air freshener.

Orange—aromatic air freshener, deodorant, used in cleaning formulas, especially furniture and floor preparations.

Tomato—the acidic nature lends itself to removing or reducing tarnish on certain metals.

Vegetables

Celery—absorbs odors; can be rubbed on cutting boards.

Corn (meal)—used as a soft abrasive to spot-clean areas, pots and pans, appliances, bathrooms, and kitchens.

Rhubarb—bleaching action.

Vegetable glycerin—used in cleaning recipes as a stain remover and in herbal formulas to help oil mix with water when making creams, salves, or balms.

Flowers

Rose, lavender, orange blossom, and other pleasantly scented waters can be used in home cleaning. Rosewater, lavender water, or orange blossom water is added to the final rinse of wash to scent clothing. Floral waters are sprayed in the air as air fresheners. Bowls of floral water are set out to scent the air.

Houseplants

Houseplants are used to enhance air quality. These plants include aloe vera, English ivy (which attacks benzene, a known carcinogen), fig tree (which attacks formaldehyde in the air), and spider plant (also for formaldehyde).

Herbs

Flaxseed oil (linseed oil)—used in furniture polishes.

Horsetail (shave grass)— high in silica, horsetail is used to scrub and polish pots and pans and for general cleaning that requires scrubbing action. Horsetail stems are used like sandpaper as they are abrasive. How to use: rub a handful of dried stems on surfaces, rinse, and wash with vegetable soap if necessary to remove green staining.

Lavender, rosemary, calendula, eucalyptus, juniper, sage, thyme, angelica root, pine, spruce, and fir—can be brewed in water and infused to create a disinfectant solution as a tea; steep 20 to 25 minutes covered, then strain and use as a general cleanser alone or in combination with soapwort and essential oils.

Soapwort—an important herb for cleaning because it is high in saponin, making it a natural herb for a lathering, sudsing action. Soapwort is used in personal care and herbal home cleaning, floor washes, general cleansing, and the safe cleansing of fragile or delicate fabrics. A tea is made from the herb to extract the lathering qualities. Many plants contain saponins, including yucca, soaptree, papaya, and peach leaf.

Almost all herbs lend to natural home cleaning. View essential oils for individual qualities of herbs in cleansing the home.

Sweet cicely seeds are crushed and added to linseed oil to make furniture polish.

Essential Oils

Antibiotic herbs and essential oils—balsam of Peru, bergamot, cinnamon, clove, eucalyptus, eucalyptus radiata, garlic, German chamomile, hyssop, lavender, lemon, lemon eucalyptus, lime, myrtle, niaouli, nutmeg, onion, oregano, patchouli, pine, ravensara, Roman chamomile, sarriette, tea tree, and terebinth.

Antifungal herbs and essential oils—balsam of Peru, eucalyptus radiata, juniper, lavender, lemon, lemon eucalyptus, myrtle, onion, patchouli, pimento, sage, sandalwood, sarriette, savory, tea tree, and thyme.

Antiseptic herbs and essential oils—bay, bergamot, bois de rose, cajeput, camphor, cardamon, cedarwood, celery, cinnamon, citronella, clary sage, clove, cumin, cypress, elemi, eucalyptus radiata, garlic, geranium, German chamomile, ginger, hyssop, juniper, lavender, lemon, lemon eucalyptus, lemongrass, lime, mandarin, marjoram, myrtle, niaouli, nutmeg, onion, oregano, parsley, patchouli, peppermint, petitgrain, pimento, pine, ravensara, Roman chamomile, rose, rosemary, sage, sandalwood, and wild celery.

Antiviral herbs and essential oils—citronella, clove, eucalyptus radiata, garlic, lavender, lemon eucalyptus, onion, parsley, ravensara, sandalwood, tea tree, and thyme.

Broad-spectrum essential oils—eucalyptus radiata, lavender, lemon eucalyptus, tea tree, and thyme.

NOTE: Pine oil disinfects and deodorizes, but it is a potential allergen so it needs to be used sparingly and always with protective gloves to avoid contact with the skin.

Minerals

Alum—a soft mineral used with acidic substances like vinegar or lemon. Uses: to lift hard-water stains. How to use: sprinkle on spot to be cleaned, scrub, and rinse.

Baking soda—a common mineral made from soda ash that is slightly alkaline and used as a nonabrasive soft scrub for cleaning and to remove or prevent odors. Uses: cleaning clothing, bathrooms (basin, tub, toilet), refrigerators, and garbage bins. How to use: sprinkle on areas to be cleansed or deodorized, like trash cans or drains. Add to the washing machine by the cup (after water is already in to avoid clumping).

Borax—disinfects, deodorizes, and inhibits mold growth. Uses: cleaning the kitchen, bathroom, garbage, basement, ovens, and other heavily soiled areas. How to use: sprinkle on spots to be cleaned, scrub, and rinse. Precautions: individuals with sensitive skin or who are prone to allergic reactions might like to wear protective gloves.

Chalk—nonabrasive cleaner. Uses: spot whitener. How to use: apply to spots that need whitening, wet slightly, rub, and rinse. Reapply or leave on overnight for tough spots.

Cream of tartar—cleans porcelain, drains, and metals. How to use: disperse in water. Submerge metal, soak for several hours, then rinse. Pour directly down the drain and flush with water. Sprinkle on bathroom basins, tubs, or tiles; scrub and rinse.

Pumice—aids the cleansing action of soaps and absorbs moisture. Uses: an abrasive cleanser for hands, hard metals, and hard-water deposits. If using a pumice stone, scrub areas that need to be cleansed. Pumice is also added to hand-cleaning recipes, soaps, and other cleaning solutions in pulverized form, as per recipe. Precautions: this is a strong abrasive, so use with care and discretion, both on the skin and within the home, to avoid scratching or discoloration.

Salt—a non-scratching (to most surfaces) abrasive cleaner with antibacterial qualities. How to use: sprinkle on areas that need to be cleaned, scrub with a sponge or rag, and rinse. Repeat as needed.

Washing soda (caustic soda)—sodium carbonate. It has a high alkalinity (around pH 11) and cuts grease. It is used to clean clothing, removing dirt, oil, and stains, and to neutralize odors. How to use: add to the washing machine during the wash cycle (after water is added to avoid clumping). Sprinkle directly on areas to be cleaned, especially in the kitchen and bathroom. Precautions: this is a potential irritant to the skin, so wear gloves and make sure clothing washed with this is rinsed very well or it may irritate the skin. Use sparingly for allergic and sensitive individuals.

Miscellaneous

Castile soap—olive-oil-based soap; it is liquefied and used as a natural soap base in a wide variety of cleansing solutions. Dr. Bronner's is a name-brand castile soap with multiple purposes. Uses: shampoo, (hand-washing) dish detergent, and cloth detergent. How to use: add suggested amount to shampoo blends along with fixed oils or essential oils as directed. Can also be used straight to wash and cleanse the body and home. Special precaution should be taken to remove soap scum or buildup that may occur by following up with a vinegar rinse.

White bread—absorbs odors in the air when placed in the refrigerator or nearby when working with onions.

White vinegar—acidic natural substance made from a variety of different ingredients during the fermentation process. The acidic action dissolves buildup, removes tarnish from metals, and cleans dirt from organic and inorganic substances. Vinegar helps clean and deodorize laundry and diapers and is good for cleaning the toilet, sink, refrigerator, countertops, windows, and glasses and pouring down drains to discourage clogs.

STAY-AWAY PEST MOJO

A pleasurable spring-cleaning activity is to put away the darker-colored heavy woolens and dense cottons of winter to make way for the lighter silks and linens of spring and summer. Once my warmer clothing is clean and folded, I put them away until fall, and I'm sure many of you do the same. Try including this sachet mojo. Tucked into the closet, the bag is designed to keep insects away that might otherwise bore holes into some of your favorite sweaters. Here is the blend I craft for my entire family.

4 cups dried cedarwood chips
2 cups dried lavender buds
1 cup dried peppermint leaves
2 teaspoons cedarwood
  essential oil
2 teaspoons lavender essential oil
2 teaspoons pennyroyal
  essential oil

1½ teaspoons eucalyptus
  essential oil
1 teaspoon peppermint
  essential oil
½ teaspoon patchouli essential oil
½ teaspoon cassia essential oil

Pour cedarwood chips into a large bowl or stainless-steel stockpot. Bruise the lavender buds and peppermint leaves by hand or with mortar and pestle. Crumbling these herbs releases their essential oils. In a small separate bowl, add essential oils one at a time. Mix with a stirring wand or swirl to combine. Pour this over the herbs. Stir with a stainless-steel spoon, and put the mixture into an airtight container to mature for 4 to 6 weeks. Then put it into small muslin drawstring bags. Hang them in the closet or on hangers, or put them in drawers or storage containers with fall and winter clothing. When you need these clothes again, they will smell clean and maintain their fresh appearance, especially if stored in bins or drawers.

Herbal Home Cleansing with Smoldering Herbs

Egyptians used smoldering herbs to clean and *perfumo* to heal, using indigenous and imported resins and herbs. In the United States one of the most influential incense cleaning methods is called smudging, designed by the Native Americans. Smudging goes well beyond dirt and grime. It is a type of holistic herbal cleansing addressing the spiritual, emotional, and physical aspects of clutter. While many people use sage almost exclusively for smudging, this segment shares some of our other lovely aromatic indigenous herbs, presented in the interest of plant sustainability. The incense herbs discussed are widely available, and many are easily foraged from your own property. Here is how to use them:

- Light the end of a braid of herbs, tamp the flame, and then travel through your home, clockwise, in the four cardinal directions (east, south, west, and finally north), spreading her delightful vanilla scent and inherent wisdom along the way.
- Focus on encouraging the positive vibrations from the smoke to bless your home as you travel carrying the braid.

Indigenous North American Incense Herbs

Balsam fir (*Abies balsamea*)—Seneca blessings incorporate these sacred plants of the northern woodlands. Fir, popularly known as a "Christmas tree," has pleasing, aromatic qualities that are considered cleansing and purifying. Native to Northeastern United States and Canada, balsam fir is used medicinally by the Algonquin, Woodland Cree, Iroquois, Menominee, Micmac, Ojibwa, and Potawatomi. Ojibwa inhale the smoke from the needles to treat symptoms of cold.

Bayberry (*Myrica pensylvanica*)—emits a pleasant fragrance when dried and burned as incense.

Bearberry willow (*Salix uva-ursi*)—prominent healing trees.

Bee balm (*Monarda didyma, M.* spp.)—when dried and used in incense blends, bee balm has a fragrance reminiscent of oranges and mint combined.

Cedar (*Libocedrus decurrens, Juniperus monosperma, Thuja occidentalis*)—commonly called desert white cedar, California incense cedars are the preferred smudging cedars. Cedar is burned for a variety of reasons, including prayer, invocation, and home blessings (for moving into a new home). The tree is believed to ward off illness in the lodge and individuals, so it is used as a smudging incense. Cedar works as a purifier and attraction herb when the wood chips are sprinkled over a hot charcoal block (see mesquite).

Cedarwood (*Cedrus atlantica*)—wood chips can be used as a kindling source for other leaves and branches. Cedarwood is revered for its calming, balancing, ancient wisdom, considered a protective plant that aids focus while bringing clarity. The physical aspects are perfect for spring smudging blends, and cedarwood is antiseptic and energizing.

Juniper (*Juniperus communis*)—a revered tree whose needles, berries, and wood are all useful in smudging blends. Juniper is celebrated because it is a tree that is uplifting, protective, and purifying, and it boosts confidence and energy levels.

The physical uses include as an antiseptic, a diuretic, and a tonic. Southwestern groups have used juniper to ward off illness and ill intent.

Mesquite (*Prosopis glandulosa*)—a fragrant wood that is an ideal charcoal base for burning smoldering herbs during smudging.

Mugwort (*Artemisia vulgaris*)—is a very useful, easy-to-grow alternative to the sage genii listed that is conducive to burning as a smudging incense.

Pine (*Pinus sylvestris*)—pines are associated with endurance, perseverance, focus, trust, and stability. The tree is noted by healers for its anti-infectious, antiseptic, tonic, stimulant, and restorative abilities.

Piñon (*Pinus edulis*)—piñon pine needles are used by Southwestern groups such as the Navajo, Apache, Pueblo, and Zuni in smudging rites, sometimes in place of sweetgrass.

Red willow (*Salix laevigata*)—also called osier or **Pacific willow** (*Salix lasiandra*), it grows in the Western United States. Willows are prized in many tribes and used in ceremony for healing. The Hidatsa people, whose name means "willow," are noted healers concentrated around the Missouri River. They have developed many medicinal and healing uses for willow.

Sagebrush (*Artemisia tridentata, A.* spp.)—wild sage is preferred over culinary sage (*Salvia officinalis* or *S. apiana*) as a smudging herb. Sagebrush has been used traditionally by Western groups to treat colds. Spiritually, sage is considered to be protective of the spirit. It is also known to have antiseptic and tonic qualities to aid our energy levels. Sage is a very popular smudging herb, but **American sage** (*S. divinorum*) is a slow-growing plant indigenous to a small area of the Southwestern United States. American sage, as well as a few other types, is rapidly becoming an endangered species because of its ever-increasing popularity as a smudging herb. Thus, it is important to use the alternatives listed within this section when possible, or to grow and cultivate the herb in your own garden.

White cedar (*Thuja occidentalis*)—is burned as incense by the Ojibwa and Potawatomi people in purification ceremonies. The Chippewa burn it as incense as well, primarily in spiritual ceremonies.

White spruce (*Picea glauca*)—is considered a protective, renewing, grounding, and harmonizing tree that enables us to regain focus and clarity. Other healing properties include being an antidepressant and antiseptic and having stimulant actions.

Smudge sticks—in addition to these traditional native herbs, many people use lavender, hyssop, and rosemary for smudging because they are also holy plants that are widely available, easy to grow, and very fragrant.

The following directions offer guidance to help create your own smudge stick. Try to use homegrown plants or sprigs from trees on your property, bearing in mind that a part of the spirituality of using smudging herbs is that the herbs should not be bought or sold, but instead traded, bartered, or harvested respectfully on your own, thanking the plant for each part taken. If you do not have any trees or herbs available, you might try bartering with a family member or friend.

- Gather available sprigs and branches in the morning after dew has evaporated.
- Cut each herb to between twelve and eighteen inches.
- Bundle the herbs, and then tie with hemp string.
- Bring the bundle inside and hang it upside down away from direct sunlight.
- Dry for several days—the bundle should still be pliable.
- Lie the bundle on a natural-fiber cloth or a newspaper.
- Fold the bundle in half, then roll it until there is a neat six-to-eight-inch-long bunch.
- Bundle using natural hemp string or natural (undyed) cotton string.

Open a door or some windows for good ventilation, then light the smudge stick. Tamp out the flame. Carry the smoking wand clockwise, emphasizing the four directions (east, south, west, and north) through each room in the home. Be attentive to all areas and smudge all corners and crevices. Languish over areas that need cleansing or where unfortunate occurrences and arguments have taken place. Some people enjoy using a found bird feather to spread the smoke as they travel, but your cupped hands are just as effective. This same approach could be used to help purify a new home, a nursery, or even a sick room.

Another style of smudge is achieved by crumbling an assortment of herbs from the list provided and burning them over a mesquite charcoal block or pieces of cedarwood, piñon, or other fragrant wood.

Once you are finished with the cleansing ritual, dampen the smudge stick in seawater or rainwater. Hang it up to dry until the next time.

Additional Uses for Smudging Herbs

Some people find smoke in the home disagreeable even with good ventilation. These are some alternative ways to use smudging herbs in the home.

- Bundle sacred possessions inside a sage bundle between uses, like a healing crystal, mineral, lodestone, or other stone.
- Take a bath containing 3 to 4 drops clary sage, rosemary, eucalyptus, or pine. This is

an ideal way of ridding the body of any negative spirits that may have been encountered or accumulated on the person during smudging. I swear by this type of bath, and this is the way of practitioners of Santería, Candomblé, Vodou, Obeah, Hoodoo, and many other practices inspired by African indigenous religions.

- Essential oils can also work as a cleansing substitute for smudging. Add ½ teaspoon pine, juniper, fir, cedar, or spruce to a wash bucket filled with water. Add ¼ cup unscented castile soap, and mix. Wash countertops, bathrooms, floors, or walls to enjoy the herbal blessings of sacred evergreens during spring-cleaning rites.

In closing, remember the West African notion of iwa-pele (which is about having right character and balance). Always consider balance in any health ritual. That means that, just as you smudge to banish negativity, you will want to add charms, natural amulets, and different types of drawing incenses, and use affirmative herbs like life everlasting, frankincense, and myrrh to invite positive spirit.

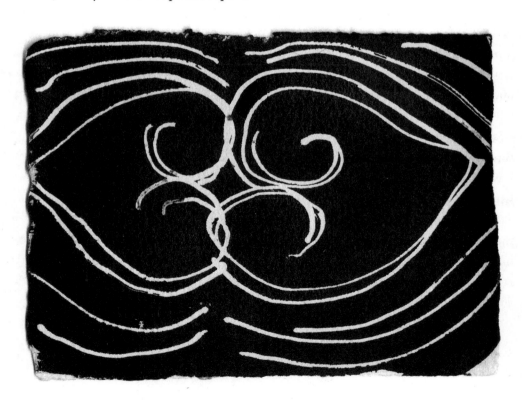

CHAPTER 14

Summer of Vibrant Health

Summer: Magic with Herbs and the Orishas

Oak Moon Bathing Ritual

Summer is a flurry of activity. It is a time of holidays that are important to our holistic health. I am featuring some of those deserving greater attention since typically they go unnoticed. During early June when it is still technically spring, Oak Moon arrives. As you can tell by my lengthy segment on oaks in my book *Trees of the Sacred Wood*,[1] oak is a very spiritual tree with which I feel fully connected. You can connect in a very physical way to oak through its newly opened leaves. This is one of the treasures evident during Oak Moon: the leaves of the tree are a bright, almost crayon green. Shaped reminiscent of an outstretched hand, the leaves feel tender and fresh.

Oak Moon begins around June 10. This hardy tree is steeped in mysticism and holds the spirit of the ancestors, as I expressed through the Angel Oak story of the Gullah people in chapter 10. Across many cultures, oak is revered for its longevity and strength and as a reservoir of perennial knowledge. The sacred tree represents the Great Mother. To absorb some of the nurturing gift of oak, go outside and gather ten pliable oak leaves. Draw a bath

---

1   Reprinted as *The Healing Tree: Botanicals, Remedies, and Rituals from African Folk Traditions* (Newburyport, MA: Red Wheel / Weiser, 2024).

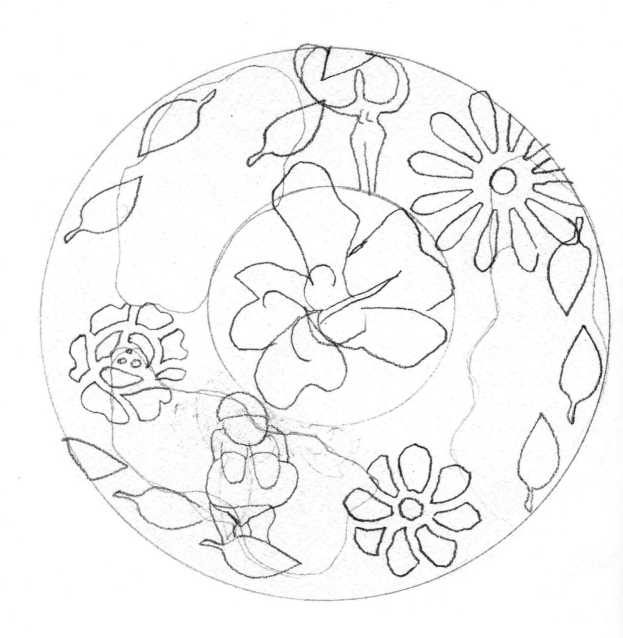

at dusk. Light a white candle with the scent of rain; place this on a safe candleholder. Place seven of the leaves in the tub. Use the other three to wash your body. Wet, then lather up one leaf at a time; wash your body as you recite:

Strength and courage I summon thee
Wisdom of the mighty oak tree
Cleanse me, treat me, and touch my soul
Thereby others I can make whole.

Juneteenth: Working for Freedom

A few weeks after Oak Moon comes a holiday commemorating a heinous event in American history. June 19, which is called Juneteenth, marks the delayed transmittal of the news of emancipation to enslaved Africans held in Texas. Whatever your ethnicity is, it is always good to recognize that you have freedom—and if not, Juneteenth reminds you to work hard at obtaining it.

If there are bonds tying you down, such as debt, addictions, or unwanted relationships, create a list that marks out a strategy that leads toward freedom. Wear white today; it is the color of spiritual strength. Fire is important. For dinner, create a barbecue featuring favorite foods. Be sure to include some tasty roasted tubers and root veggies like sweet potato and sweet onion. Have an extravagant soft drink—it is the tradition to have strawberry soda (see recipe below). As the coals of the fire gain heat and the sun settles in the west, it is time to turn to ritual. It is appropriate to purge things holding you down. Burn old unnecessary papers. Set yourself free from the past by clearing clutter. You'd be surprised how much this improves your mental health!

JUNETEENTH STRAWBERRY SODA RECIPE

Water to make ice
Ice cube tray (especially fun
    shapes with a silicon tray)
Peppermint leaves fresh from the
    garden
1½ pints of organic strawberries,
    thoroughly washed, patted dry,
    hulled, and chopped

4 cups spring water
Between ¾ cup and 1½ cups
    granulated sugar, to taste (if
    strawberries are supersweet,
    you might not need sugar)
½ organic Meyer lemon, washed
    and juiced
16 ounces mineral water

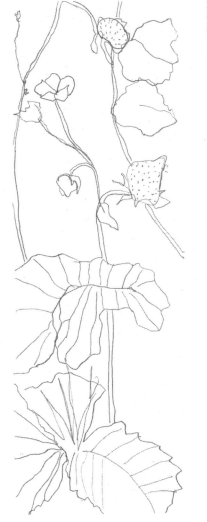

Strawberry herb

Put water in your ice cube trays. Place a couple of peppermint leaves in each tray. Freeze. Then put your fresh strawberries in a heavy-bottom saucepan or skillet. Stir in spring
water and add sugar. Simmer and stir frequently with a
wooden spoon to mix well. Mash with a potato masher. Simmer until there is a strawberry syrup. Strain in a fine-meshed
strainer. Use your wooden spoon to press all juices out. Stir
in the juice of ½ ripe Meyer lemon. Stir in the mineral water.
Drop several ice cubes into each of four small glasses and
pour some of your strawberry soda pop on top.

Freedom from Addiction and the Chains That Bind Mojo

July 4 is the date when the Declaration of Independence was set forward in 1776. One of the more compelling portions of the declaration, particularly in relation to freedom is:

> *We hold these truths to be self-evident, that all men are created equal, that they are endowed by their Creator with certain unalienable Rights, that among these are Life, Liberty and the pursuit of Happiness.*

Clearly though, this beautiful sentiment did not apply to all of us, as it was not until 1863 that the Emancipation Proclamation was written, stating:

> *That on the first day of January, in the year of our Lord one thousand eight hundred and sixty-three, all persons held as slaves within any State or designated part of a State, the people whereof shall then be in rebellion against the United States, shall be then, thenceforward, and forever free; and the Executive Government of the United States, including the military and naval authority thereof, will recognize and maintain the freedom of such persons, and will do no act or acts to repress such persons, or any of them, in any efforts they may make for their actual freedom.*

Later still, the 19th Amendment of the Constitution was ratified, finally giving women the right to at least vote:

> *The right of citizens of the United States to vote shall not be denied or abridged by the United States or by any State on account of sex.*

All the while, there has been a humble root, dug up from the depths of our Great Mother, that Hoodoos of various faiths, colors, and creeds have held close to their person, shrouded inside a mojo bag that is emblematic of freedom and personal rights and which holds the promise of happiness. High John the Conqueror (*Ipomoea jalapa*), is more than a simple tuber; it is held tight in a *hand*, also called a mojo bag, as a symbolic representation of breaking free of the chains of slavery. High John, a relative of both the morning glory and the sweet potato, represents the slave who could not be held in chains, who fights the endless war against enslavement until freedom is obtained.

We all suffer from one type of slavery or another. Today, create a mojo, utilizing the power of the natural amulet, High John, along with the stone hematite (known to strengthen the system and help one break free of addictions) and various supplemental natural ingredients that do the same. Get yourself a red flannel (a bag with a drawstring closure) and add in a High John the Conqueror root. Add a clear, charged, powerful-feeling hematite stone. Put a pinch of kosher salt into the bag and a few Devil's shoestrings to keep evil at bay. Slippery elm, lemongrass, and eucalyptus are also known to aid in freedom, so throw in a little pinch of each. Roll the bag on the ground a few times so the herbs crumble and are well mixed. Finally, add a few drops of rose oil to feed the herbs, stones, and minerals so they stay powerful. Now you've got yourself a *"freedom from addiction and the chains that bind"* mojo bag, so walk mindful of freedom.

Midsummer Attraction Work

As you approach midsummer, you are bound to become a little more frisky, romantically inclined, or at the very least outgoing. Some people know just what to do to make their nature rise so that they are attractive to others. In case you need a few pointers, here are a few herbs sure to do the trick.

- Dab pure sandalwood oil straight onto pulse points to attract people of the opposite sex. Sandalwood also calms nerves, is relaxing, and eases sexual inhibitions.
- Men, especially in the Middle East and North Africa, find gulhina—that's right, the perfume oil of the henna plant—a surefire way to become more attractive. It is used the same way as sandalwood oil.
- In Hoodoo and some other paths, folks who want to attract those of the same sex adore lavender. If that is your desire, dab some onto a few of your chakras.
- Southerners have taught us that the plants that grow so readily in their region can add a touch of magic to the love life. Slip a dried magnolia leaf or two between your mattress and box spring or under your futon to keep your lover close and faithful.

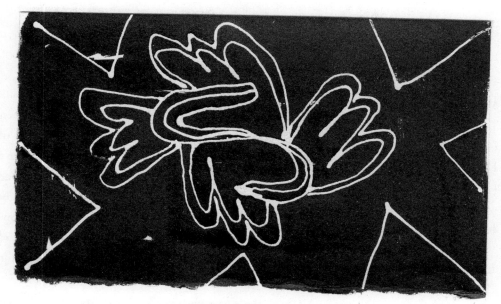

Bi Nka Bi: No one should bite another
Meaning: Symbol of justice, social justice, fairness, equality, equity, freedom, peace, and unity

Little John, Justice Herb

July 28 is the day the 14th Amendment was enacted. The 14th Amendment promises equal protection and due process of the law. This is a great time to engage the herb discussed in chapter 5 that is beloved by Hoodoos. It is called Little John. Little John (*Alpinia galanga*), also called galangal, is an herbal symbol of fairness and justice in legal proceedings. Sometimes equal protection and justice, though promised, unfortunately, are not granted, so we need extra help from the domain of the spirit. Here are a few ways Little John, a relative of ginger, can be used as a chew or charm in spellwork:

- Put a cleaned piece of Little John into your mouth. Chew it until soft. Try not to swallow.
- If you are supporting a court case or are on trial, spit the Little John fluid outside the courthouse.
- If you want only good outcomes to legal proceedings by mail, spit the Little John juice near your mailbox.
- If you want a lawsuit you've been informed of by mail to end peacefully, spit on the envelope and bury it either at a nearby crossroads or on your personal property.

- To positively influence the court, keep Little John on your person inside a red mojo bag, along with some calendula flowers, deer's tongue, and oregano.

Working Basil's Magical Green Energy

The fields and forest are bustling with every possible type of green by late July. Green is symbolic of verdant earth, abundance, Osayin's herbal delights, and the fecundity of Earth Mother. An easy-growing summer green is basil. It is always nice to find new ways to utilize it so that it doesn't go to seed. Try this green scented floor wash to harvest the abundance that is your destiny. Add 2 cups fresh basil to a large cauldron of boiling water (use a stockpot if necessary). Remove the cauldron from the heat. Add 1 ounce pyrite chips to the cauldron, cover, and set outside overnight. Strain, being careful to remove and save the pyrite for other spells. Add 8 drops holy basil essential oil. Put a bowl of fine sea salt in the center of the room you are blessing. Clean surfaces with the wash using a natural sea sponge with your dominant hand, concentrating on your desires the entire time. Sprinkle some of the fine sea salt on stains as you work. Open the doors and windows if possible so the spirits can aid your work. Good fortune should flow your way.

Ogun Protection Dust

With doors and windows ajar, people coming and going with the breeze, one's attention might turn to natural protection magic in the summer. You can build your psychic armor utilizing the protective energy of orisha Ogun's warrior magic. Borrow this traditional formula from the Hoodoos to add to your repertoire of potions protective of the home and hearth, and take time out of your busy day to make and use some of the fierce protective dust. Gopher's dust is designed to protect your space from *hants* (disruptive spirits) and negative human energy. Mix equal parts sulfur (brimstone), sea salt, cayenne powder, and black pepper (powdered), and you'll have homemade gopher's dust. (Make enough of the powder for the job at hand.) You'll want to spread this in a protective ring around your property. If it is an apartment, loft, or condo, make enough to spread out in front of your door. This dust protects the home, blowing forcefully toward bad energy spread by intruders with malicious intentions.

Late Summer, Sun Ra Invocation

As the sun pierces your consciousness and you struggle through those "dog days" of summer, it becomes easy to understand the ancient Egyptian respect for the sun god, Ra. Inevitably, sunny days have helped you enjoy the fruits of summer and perhaps brought some romance with them along the way. As I have said about the rain, it's best to go with each season. Shield your skin with an excellent sunscreen, but open the spirit to Ra. Pay tribute to sun god Ra for his blessings in the way he likes best. In ancient Egypt, myrrh was burned at high noon to please him. Put a few small chunks of myrrh on a white charcoal block placed on a fireproof surface outdoors. Use your hands to gently brush the smoke upward toward the heavens as you chant:

In honor and praise I send this smoke toward you
Thanks for the blessings and the sunny days too
Sun Ra, great god, emblem of the sun
I honor and praise you for all that you've done.

A Day of Peace

Summer has many themes. It is the season of freedom, justice, and peace. September 21 is the International Day of Peace. In a war-torn world, this day has all the more meaning. Try invoking the spirit of Egyptian goddess Ma'at on this day, whose primary purpose is to ensure fairness, justice, and peace. Ma'at is one of my favorite goddesses—her business is spiritual fairness and justice. She weighs the hearts of the gods and goddesses against an ostrich feather, creating a scale of equality. If equilibrium is struck between the feather and the heart, the god lived a good life and can pass on for a fruitful afterlife. However, if the heart is too heavy, the opposite occurs. Use Ma'at's magical tool to bring clarity and peacefulness into your life. Touch all your ceremonial tools with an ostrich feather today (if unavailable, it is fine to use a peacock feather as a substitute). Touch your correspondence, particularly legal papers, judgments, or liens, with the feather of Ma'at so that people will deal with you in a just manner, ensuring peace and freedom.

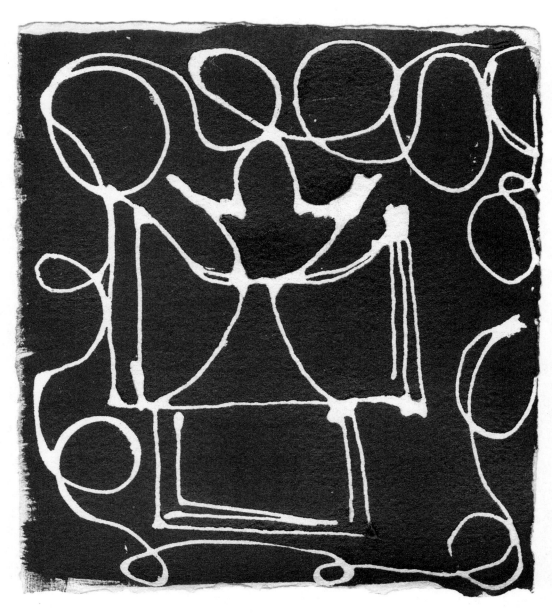

Gye Wani: Enjoy yourself
Symbol of celebration and enjoyment

Roasting African-Caribbean Fruit and Vegetables

In the spirit of Gye Wani, let's do some roasting. All over the African diaspora, we enjoy roasting food outdoors. This is the way of indigenous people. It takes little, if any, equipment when you get right down to it, and for the most part, it is enjoyable as it's outdoors. We are going to turn our attention to Africans in the Caribbean and check out some ideas for the good ole BBQ.

This is just a partial list of gifts of the Motherland that are wonderful additions to outdoor meals:

Banana—place on grill with skin intact. Turn until deep brown all the way around. Cut open to reveal baked banana. Serve with cold whipped cream with a touch of cinnamon for contrasting temperatures, color, and flavor.

Roasted corn—put corn with husk and silk intact on grill away from flames. Turn periodically for about 15 minutes. Shuck corn and remove silk. Eaten as is, roasted corn has a rustic, smoky flavor. Tasty toppings range from the expected butter and sea salt to the more interesting squeeze of lemon or lime. Also try a dash of ground red pepper or harissa, a splash of hot sauce, or a sprinkle of grated aged cheese.

Grilled pineapple—peel pineapple and slice it widthwise in ½-inch slices. Place directly on the grill. Sear each side about 4 minutes. Eat as an accompaniment to seafood or as a dessert.

Roasted squash—you can roast summer squash, such as patty pan or chayote, as well as zucchini or hard-shelled winter squash like butternut, delicata, or acorn. Summer squash should be clean and dry. It can be cooked whole, sliced and added to kabobs, or chopped and cooked inside foil with olive oil and seasoning to taste. Summer squash is cut in half, seeds and insides removed; brushed with corn, peanut, or olive oil; and seasoned with lemon, sea salt, and pepper. Ground ginger or cinnamon goes well with winter squash. Place prepared winter squash halves in foil. Put them on the barbecue grill. Roast until tender, about 35 to 40 minutes.

Roasted sweet potato—scrub the potato, rinse it, and pat it dry. Prick it with a fork, wrap it in foil, and place it on the grill. Turn periodically. It will cook in about 30 minutes on a medium grill. Test for doneness; it should feel soft. Cut open, carve an X shape on each half, and squeeze and fluff the potato. Serve it warm with butter, sea salt, and fresh ground pepper. Cinnamon and cayenne will add a nice warmth on a chilly eve.

STUFFED PAPAYA ROAST

This is my adaptation of a hearty Caribbean dish, chock-full of antioxidants, vitamins, minerals, color, and a pungent curried flavor. This dish is perfect for those who want to reduce meat intake.

4 to 6 pounds ripe papaya
½ teaspoon sesame oil
1 teaspoon coconut oil
2 cloves garlic, minced
½ pound mushrooms
Pinch sea salt
Freshly ground pepper
2 cups vegetable broth
2 cups coconut milk

1 teaspoon cumin
1 teaspoon turmeric
½ teaspoon harissa powder
2 cups white or brown rice
½ cup mozzarella cheese
½ cup parmesan cheese
2 teaspoons butter (vegan butter or coconut butter is a good substitute), chopped

Preheat oven 350°F. Use a stainless-steel cooking sheet (line it with parchment or apply coconut oil if you're worried about sticking). Cut papaya in half. Scoop out and discard seeds. Wash, then pat papaya dry with a towel; place it on the pan and set aside. Meanwhile, heat sesame and coconut oils in a cast-iron skillet on medium. Add garlic to the skillet. Wipe off mushroom thoroughly, and chop coarsely. Add to garlic, and sauté the two ingredients. Add pinch of sea salt and freshly ground pepper. Add mushroom/garlic blend, broth, milk, cumin, turmeric, harissa, 1 teaspoon of the oil mixture, and the rice to the rice cooker. Turn to "cook." When rice mixture is done, pour it into a mixing bowl. Add half of each of the cheeses. Stir. Stuff the flavored rice into papaya shells. Top with the remaining cheese and dot with the butter. Bake 30 to 35 minutes or until bubbly and the tops are brown. Serve hot with salad.

Coconut, the Flesh Fit for Obatala

Obatala, wise man, elder, orisha of all orishas, prefers the pure white flesh of coconut as an offering. Many may look at the stubborn brown hull and wonder how to get inside. Here are tips for selecting, opening, and creating basic milk and other delicious treats from the coconut.

Selection—choose a coconut with a chestnut-brown hull that is smooth with no apparent holes or mold. Shake and listen for the sound of liquid. If it still contains water, it will be moist and tasty.

Opening the nut—bore two holes in the eyes using an ice pick or sharp knife. The eyes are the dark-brown spots at either end of the coconut. Pour coconut water into a bowl. You can add this to your bath or beauty recipes or use it in rituals and ceremonies that honor appropriate orisha. See "Coconut (*Cocos nucifera*)" in chapter 10. Hit the hull on a hard surface sharply a few times—it should crack open. You can also hit the nut with a mallet or hammer. Once it cracks open, scoop out the flesh, which is called coconut meat, to use in the recipes that follow.

Making coconut milk—heat 1½ cups water in a kettle on medium-high heat. Meanwhile, grate the coconut flesh and put it in a sieve over a large bowl. Just before the water comes to a boil, slowly pour the water over the grated coconut in the sieve. Press the coconut meat with the back of a wooden spoon. Remove sieve. Pour this liquid into a Pyrex measuring cup with a spout. Repeat this step 3 to 4 times. This makes about 1¼ cups rich coconut milk.

Coconut cream—to make coconut cream, bring 1½ cups full-fat milk almost to the boil. Go through the steps above (to make coconut milk). Coconut cream is a bit denser, with a full-bodied, sweeter taste, just right for desserts and drinks.

Toasted coconut—remove coconut from hull with a sharp knife. Shred the coconut. Add 1 tablespoon olive oil to a cast-iron skillet. Add a pinch of sea salt if desired. Toss until medium brown. Use this as a topping for fruit salads, yogurt, or cereal, or eat it alone as a snack.

Reflecting on Oshun

As we are about to move on to cultivating beauty physically, orisha Oshun can surely show us the way. This is more of a musing than a practical ritual, although if the opportunity presents itself—go for it! Oshun abides by the riverside, a place rich in African and African American lore. To invoke her spirit and pay homage to her sassy ways, you will need to work with a partner.

- Begin by setting out a brass or ceramic candleholder.
- Place a few cinnamon-, honey-, or orange-scented candles on the candleholder.
- Light the candles.
- Gaze into the fire and reflect on the beauty and mystery of Oshun.

In unison with your partner, say the praise poem:

> *Barewa lele* (The beautiful one emerges)
> *Umale* (The spirit-god)
> *Arele umawo* (One of the family reincarnated)

Repeat until you are both relaxed and comfortable.

- Spread honey on each other's lips and elsewhere if you'd like.
- Share the honey between you.
- See where this leads.
- Afterward, look around you and see which of Oshun's gifts appeals to you. Collect a few items such as tumbled glass, driftwood, or river rocks. Bring these back to your altar at home.
- Gaze at these items, remembering Oshun is not only goddess of love, sensuality, and sexuality; she is also protectress of women and children and has been known to alleviate menstrual disorders; help us heal from physical, sexual, or psychological abuse; and help us increase our fertility.

Love, Sensuality, and Beauty

Iemanjá is mermaid orixá of the Afro-Brazilian path of Umbanda. She is the Brazilian manifestation of Yemaya-Olokun, who I speak of so often as she is my patron orisha. Iemanjá is so revered that she is seen as an incarnation of the Virgin Mary by a culture that is largely Catholic. She is the one to turn to when you are near the sea, her home. Try this midnight invocation.

In warm weather, devotees petition Iemanjá for good fortune by the seaside. Our minds frequently turn to her during the summer months when so much love and natural beauty surround us. People come bearing gifts for blessings during the coming year. In Hoodoo we conjure helpful spirits to assist in our daily lives and spiritual work. Whatever path you follow, you might like to appeal to Iemanjá during one of your visits to the seashore this summer. If so, try this:

Begin this work just before midnight on a waxing moon. Go to the seaside, carrying talcum powder, a light-blue and a white candle, rum, fragrant flowers (lily, gardenia, rose, or jasmine), a cigar or pure tobacco (with a charcoal block to heat the tobacco), a large seashell, and matches in a basket or bag. If using tobacco, light the charcoal block and place it inside the seashell atop a mound of sand. Quietly make your plea to Iemanjá as you light the cigar or tobacco and candles. Arrange these items on the sand. Sprinkle some of the talcum powder in a protective white circle around the seashell, candles, and smoldering cigar (or tobacco). Pour some of the rum on the ground inside the circle. Cast the flowers out to sea. Sprinkle the talcum powder on the foam of the sea as well—all the while imagining that you are powdering the spirit of Iemanjá. Sit down, gaze upon the fire and smoke, listen, and look hard as you breathe deeply; see what messages Iemanjá has for you.

Hydrosols for Intimate Apparel

During the summer it is a very appropriate time to experiment with washing your intimate apparel, silks, and scarves with hydrosols in the gentle essences of blossoms. Put an adequate amount of spring water, rainwater (if you live in an unpolluted area), or tap water of the recommended temperature. Add ¼ cup soapwort infusion (see "Make Your Own Botanical Shampoo" in chapter 13; soapwort is used traditionally to cleanse valuable textiles). Next, add ¼ cup of your favorite hydrosol. Qualities of the three most popular hydrosols to consider:

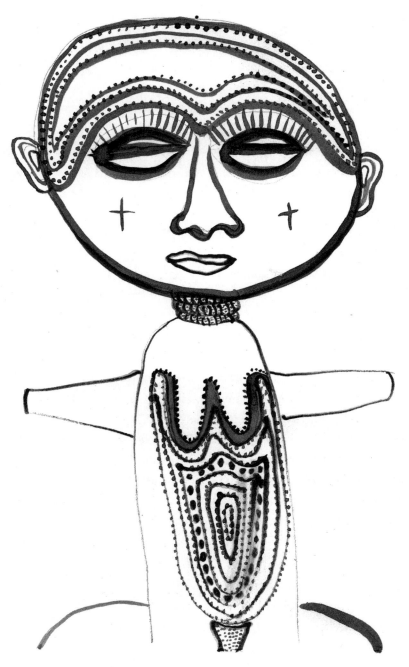

Asante fertility figure

- Lavender is relaxing and unisex.
- Neroli builds confidence in sexuality and in recovery from embarrassment.
- Rose lends energy, is stimulating, and aids the adventurous spirit.

Swish clothing in this water gently to work up lather. Soak 20 to 30 minutes, rinse, and hang up to dry.

BAY RUM COLOGNE

This old-fashioned charmer makes a good Father's Day or graduation gift. It gets better with age, so you can make it in the summer and store it properly to give as a winter holiday gift as well. Either way, the special man in your life will enjoy the scent, love, and care that goes into this gift.

20 drops clove bud essential oil
100 drops bay leaf essential oil
6 ounces 100-proof vodka or
    Everclear, divided
6-inch piece cinnamon

1 teaspoon whole Jamaican
    allspice
4 to 5 bay leaves
⅓ cup pure witch hazel tincture
1 teaspoon aloe vera

Mix essential oils with half of the alcohol or vodka. Stir with a stirring rod, or swirl. Leave 48 hours. Crack cinnamon stick into small pieces. Crack allspice balls and bay leaves with a mortar and pestle. Add the rest of the vodka. Stir and let sit another 48 hours. Add the witch hazel. Store the mixture in a dark bottle in a cool, dark location. Mature 2 to 4 weeks, swirling bottle daily to avoid separation and settlement. Add aloe vera, then strain. If too strong, add more witch hazel.

ROSE GARDEN DUSTING POWDER

1¼ cups cornstarch
¼ cup baking soda
½ cup ground dried pink rose
   petals
¼ cup ground dried lemon peel

6 drops attar of roses
4 drops geranium essential oil
4 drops lime essential oil
2 drops lemongrass essential oil

Mix dry ingredients in a nonreactive bowl. Drop in attar and essentials oils, stirring with each addition. Pour into a dusting powder box. Apply with a powder duster. If this type of packaging is unavailable, pour through a funnel into a shaker-topped powder bottle. Add a few grains of rice to stop ingredients from clumping. Shake on the body and bed, or inside shoes or drawers.

GENTLE BREEZE SOLID PERFUME

¼ cup beeswax pastilles
¼ cup fixed oil (argun, moringa,
   or grapeseed)
1 teaspoon lavender essential oil

½ teaspoon rose geranium
   essential oil
¼ teaspoon patchouli essential oil

Melt wax on low in a double boiler. Add fixed oil, and stir. Add essential oils. Stir slowly—with a stirring wand, if possible. Let cool but not solidify. Pour into a 4-ounce double-walled jar with a screw top. Dab on pulse points or chakras.

Bringing Eden Home
Lavender Honey

Trust me, it sounds strange, but you'll end up loving this as I do. It is comforting and soothing and helps you relax. The perfect nonalcoholic way to unwind is to add a teaspoon of this to your favorite relaxing tea like chamomile, catnip, or even lavender tea.

Fill a sterilized jar loosely with lavender blossoms and leaves. Pour your favorite type of honey on top, filling the jar completely. Cover and let steep away from sunlight for six weeks.

Alternative: Rose Honey
Same directions, but replace lavender with fragrant, organic rose petals, making sure the plant itself is disease free.

Ambrosia Fruit Salad

Though it goes by different names in the diaspora, fruit salad is a much-loved warm-weather treat in Africa and throughout the diaspora. Inevitably at our barbecues or picnics, someone would show up with a tempting salad called ambrosia, or "food of the gods." I have tossed this one together for you, which utilizes some of the blessed health foods of the Caribbean, the Americas, and Africa discussed in depth in part II. All fruit must be carefully selected at the peak of its flavor—this is what takes the most work, for the rest is just peeling, chopping, stirring, and good eating. When shopping, you get hints of the flavor because even when uncut the fruit should emit a highly aromatic sweetness that is reminiscent of the taste. The color should be rich. Avoid moldy or dried-out fruit. Brown spots on the banana suggest sweetness, yet the skin should still be rather smooth and tight.

AMBROSIA FRUIT SALAD

½ pineapple
2 mangoes
3 bananas
1 extra-large slice watermelon
⅔ cup pitted and halved fresh cherries

½ cup plain yogurt (with live cultures)
1 teaspoon orange blossom honey (optional)

Peel the pineapple, mangoes, and bananas. Cut the pineapple and mango into cubes, and place them into a bowl. Slice banana about ½ inch thick. Remove pits from the watermelon. Cube the melon and add it to the bowl along with the cherries. Mix yogurt and honey (if using), add this yogurt mixture to the fruit, and stir well. Serve chilled.

Melon Tips

Muskmelon, cantaloupe, and honeydew should feel soft near the stem and smell very much like you expect them to taste—these are signs of the melon being ripe and tasty.

MELON BALL AND MINT SALAD

1 small round sugar baby
watermelon
1 muskmelon

1 honeydew melon
1 tablespoon peppermint leaves

Cut melons in half. Remove seeds and excess fibers. Scoop out melon flesh using a small melon ball tool with a twisting motion. Add the multicolored balls to a chilled serving bowl. Toss gently to mix. Garnish with thinly chopped fresh mint. Serve alone for breakfast or lunch, eat after a main meal as dessert, or enjoy anytime of the day as a healthy snack. For a light meal, balance with protein, adding an ice-cream scoop of cottage cheese or plain yogurt to ½ cup salad per person. Serves at least 4 (more depending on the size of the melons).

Sautéed Summer Delight

My mother and Aunt Edith made this basic country dish with produce fresh from their gardens, filling in what we didn't grow ourselves with produce from local farmers. I added the ginger and colorful red pepper because they are healthy and enhance the look as well as the taste of this dish. When you become involved with gardening, it is surprising how very abundant a little patch of earth can be. Sautéed vegetables with lots of tomato is a wonderful way to keep up with the output of your gardens, so nothing goes to waste.

SAUTÉED SUMMER DELIGHT

1½ cups okra
1 cup patty pan squash
2 cups tomato
1 green bell pepper
1 red bell pepper
1 small onion

2 cloves garlic
Cold-pressed olive oil spray or
   1½ tablespoons liquid olive oil
½-inch piece of ginger
Sea salt
Freshly ground pepper

Wash the okra, squash, tomato, and bell peppers. Remove stem of okra and cut them into ½-inch slices. Remove stem of patty pan. Peel and chop tomato coarsely. Mince onion, garlic, and peppers. Heat pan to medium high. Add olive oil and allow to heat a few minutes. Add onion and sauté until translucent. Add pepper and ginger, turn the heat down to medium, and cook 5 minutes. Add garlic, salt, and pepper, and cook 3 minutes. Add okra, patty pan, and tomato, and stir. Cover, and reduce heat to medium low. Braise 20 minutes. Serve vegetarian with rice or as a side dish. Serves 4 to 6.

Memories and Healing

Healing sometimes needs to be of the spirit. Sometimes, as in the case of this peach cobbler recipe, food becomes a reservoir, holding experience, memory, and special connection. Many of my people have passed on, but their foods and colorful recipes are an important way of reconnecting with our experiences together.

Remembering Ma's Peach Cobbler

My ma, Margie Marie, was strong and radiated warmth and beauty. When I was a little girl, I was certain that she was *the* most beautiful woman in the world. I remember the day she cooked pork chops when I was ten. It was autumn, and we had recently moved to a house in the country from East Orange, a suburb of New York City. We ate overlooking the greenish-black lake, trimmed by evergreen conifers. It's been over thirty years, but Lord, I can still remember the taste of that meal. Pork chops dipped in a seasoned cornmeal batter, deep-fried and served with hot mashed potatoes, creamed gravy made from the pan drippings, hot and sour collard greens with fatback, and buttermilk biscuits. The dessert was Margie's deep-dish peach pie, made from local South Jersey peaches and served à la mode with Breyers vanilla ice cream.

I can still hear them in the kitchen.

PEACH PIE À LA MA

Preheat the oven to 375°F. Parboil 10 to 12 scrubbed, ripe but firm peaches, then set aside to cool.

Blend some shortening and flour with two butter knives till nice and crumbly. Take water you've chilled in the freezer and sprinkle it by the teaspoon over the flour to moisturize it lightly. Roll out the dough on a floured surface till it's about ¼ inch thin.

Cut two circles slightly larger than the pan. Place one circle of dough in the baking dish and prick it gently with a fork. Prebake for 5 minutes.

Meanwhile, peel and slice the peaches. Drizzle them with some sugar, lemon juice, flour, and a bit of cinnamon.

Remove the piecrust from the oven. Cover with seasoned peach mixture. Dot lightly with butter. Cover with remaining crust. Crimp edges, and prick with a fork.

Three-quarters of the way through baking, Aunt Edith, who had her own soul food restaurant, puts her hands on her ample hips and suggests brushing the top side of the crust with some milk.

Sprinkle a little more sugar, chile, then toss you some cinnamon and nutmeg lightly over the milk. Put it way back in the oven; bake till the crust is golden brown and the peaches are bubbly.

Serve warm with cream or softened vanilla ice cream.

Get Juiced: Purees, Juices, Smoothies, and Other Summer Concoctions
The Songhai Healthy Beauty Way

The idea of blending elements of cultivated society with ingredients of a completely wild origin is an ancient concept recorded in the Songhai Empire of ancient Africa. The Songhai see the landscape filled with numerous spirits living in all aspects of the natural world. They believe these diverse entities can come together for the greater good of humans. As such, the Songhai understand that illnesses and disorders are curable using combinations that bring together wildcrafted and harvested flowers and cultivated roots, stems, and flowers with products associated with farming, like milk, cheese, grains, and eggs. A healing synergy develops by bringing together these disparate elements of nature.

Next you will find several recipes that incorporate the Songhai philosophy. These nurturing formulas are affirming, emollient, softening, and wholesome in a holistic manner.

SONGHAI SMOOTHIE

This multipurpose smoothie is fragrant, soothing, emollient, rich, and even tasty. Designed for sun-parched skin, it embodies the Songhai way of blending elements of nature. Songhai Smoothie is enriched by vitamin-imbued strawberries and alpha-hydroxy acid (AHA; an ingredient you'll find in quite a few of these recipes), and buttermilk because it nurtures sensitive skin. The emollience of peach flesh and peach kernel oil, creamy coconut milk, soothing chamomile, and relaxing oat straw makes this the perfect health brew. The only problem is whether to drink it or apply it to the body——I suggest a bit of both.

1 small ripe peach
⅓ cup washed and chopped
   strawberries
½ cup coconut milk

1½ cups buttermilk
1 tablespoon cut and sifted oat
   straw herb
1 chamomile tea bag

Preheat the oven to 170°F. Scrub, peel, and finely chop peach; reserve the kernel. To begin to release the peach kernel's oil, crush the pit with a mallet on a cutting board or in a strong mortar with a pestle. Add this to a baking dish. Combine the chopped peach and strawberries in a bowl, and pour milk over the fruit, add herbs and chamomile tea bag, and stir. Pour this mixture into the baking dish, add chamomile tea bag, cover, and infuse mixture in an oven set at 170°F for 2 hours. Remove from oven, and whisk mixture. Pour through a fine sieve, then press herbal and fruit material resting inside the sieve with the back of a spoon to extract the healing medicine (being careful to keep the chamomile tea bag intact). Set sieve aside. Whisk, then repeat straining and squeezing process. Dab smoothie on face and neck using a cotton ball. Leave for 5 minutes. Rinse well with cool water. This is a comprehensive treat, so there is no need for further treatment. Songhai Smoothie cleanses, tightens, and moisturizes.

Yield: 16 ounces
Shelf life: 48 hours

Alternative Uses:

• Pour this in your bath for a luxurious moisturizing soak.

• Sip smoothie throughout the day, as it is tasty and nutritious.

Benefits of Freezing Fruit

Freezing ripe fruit helps save money because foods spoil more quickly during warmer months—especially if you don't have air-conditioning and live in a hot, humid area. Freezing helps you save time and money, enabling you to buy in bulk from food co-ops and prepare the food in advance. The freezer works wonders to enhance smoothies. Chipped ice adds body and a welcomed chill. You can freeze peeled bananas in plastic freezer bags or containers. Freshly picked berries freeze well and add great fiber and fresh taste to smoothies. Peaches and apples should be blanched in boiling water, coiled, peeled, cored, sliced, and then frozen. Keep these on hand so they are ready to whip up into a smoothie when the mood strikes you. Having them prepared and ready to go makes it easier to start the morning on a healthy foot—a time when you may feel weaker and lack the energy needed for time-consuming food preparation.

SALAD CRÈME FACIAL

When we are out and about during the summer months, people pay a great deal of attention to our skin and complexion. We don't want to appear dull or shiny. This combination of ingredients corrects many skin disorders and sloughs off dull skin. The bleaching action of the buttermilk makes it an especially helpful fading ingredient for unwanted freckles, scars, uneven pigmentation, or discoloration. Buttermilk, rich in alpha-hydroxy acid (AHA), gently removes dry skin and an ashy appearance in the process. Buttermilk encourages cell renewal, which slows the appearance of wrinkles, tightens saggy skin, and brightens overall appearance. The lipids in buttermilk attract moisture so your complexion will gain a healthy glow but will not appear greasy. Cucumbers are astringent, further alleviating a tendency toward a shiny nose or gleaming forehead. The North African native plant lettuce is excellent for cleansing skin prone to breakouts and acne. Carrots contain healthy doses of vitamins A and E, antioxidants that check aging skin and encourage a youthful glow. You will be amazed, as I have been, to watch your old skin flake off after a few days, to be replaced by a new layer of rosier skin. Salad Crème Facial is only recommended for combination and oily skin.

2 carrots
½ cucumber

1 cup iceberg lettuce
2 cups buttermilk

Preheat oven to 170°F. Scrub carrots and cucumber; rinse them and the lettuce. Spin the salad vegetables to remove debris and excess moisture. Peel carrots and cucumber. Cut the cucumber in half, and scoop out and discard the seeds. Shred the vegetables by hand or in a food processor, then add them to an ovenproof bowl or baking pan. Cover with the milk. Steep 2 hours, stirring occasionally. Drain by pouring through a sieve placed over a catch bowl. Pour this Salad Crème Facial through a funnel into a sterilized cobalt or brown bottle. Cap, and store in the refrigerator.

To use, pour a small portion of the crème onto a cotton ball or square. Dampen face with the soaked cotton. Leave on 3 to 5 minutes. Rinse with cool water, and pat the skin lightly with a towel to dry. Use this instead of soap morning and night.

Yield: approximately 12 ounces
Shelf life: 1 week refrigerated

3-IN-1 RECIPE: ISLAND LASSI

When enslaved Africans were freed in the Caribbean, there was still a drive for a very inexpensive labor force. Since many of the colonizers began to import indentured servants from areas they had colonized in Asia, thousands of Indians were brought to the islands, and with them many distinctive dishes merged into what is now considered Caribbean cuisine. Island Lassi is inspired by the East Indian drink mango lassi, which serves as a cooling companion to spicy foods and a smooth background to complex spices. It is a cooling fusion of dairy products and fruit, fitting into the Songhai philosophy of health as well. The enzymes of fresh mango are softening. I have developed this recipe to be adaptable for hair and skin care. It detangles, moisturizes, and smooths rough ends. Lemon adds shine. If you decide to use the essential oils, they will leave traces of an alluring aroma. Cardamom, one of my favorite pods, is earthy, unique, and spicy; peppermint is lively, green, and stimulating to the scalp. Both must be used in moderation to avoid irritation.

1 ripe mango, peeled
Juice of ½ lemon
½ cup whole-milk yogurt

4 drops cardamom essential oil
4 drops peppermint essential oil

Slice mango in your preferred manner. Add to blender. Add juice of the lemon and the yogurt. Blend on medium for about one minute or until smooth. Pour through a fine sieve over a nonreactive bowl. Drop in essential oils, and mix well. After shampooing, pour over hair, covering all strands well. Massage and rinse.

Yield: approximately 6 ounces
Shelf life: 24 hours refrigerated

Alternative Uses:

• Double recipe. Use half as a conditioner and the other half for a moisturizing bath.

• As a beverage. Follow all directions but be careful to omit essential oils. Drink chilled as an appetizer, dessert, or breakfast drink.

HEALTHY NAILS

Wash your hands. Rub the tips with lemon to naturally whiten them. Soak your clean fingertips in warm soy milk for 10 minutes. Wash again. Rub cuticles with full-bodied nutritious oil like baobab or melted cocoa butter (wax). Rest hands on a washcloth; let nails soak in the oils for an additional 10 minutes.

SUGAR FOOT SCRUB

The sugar, cornmeal, and flaxseed meal in this recipe slough off dead skin. The AHA in the buttermilk encourages vibrant new skin growth, making this a great way to get feet in sandal shape for summer. The combination of sandalwood and neroli delights the senses and tones the skin, while providing a tantalizing scent to the scrub. Baobab oil has superior moisturizing abilities.

½ cup sugar
¼ cup yellow cornmeal
2 tablespoons flaxseed meal
3 tablespoons buttermilk

1 tablespoon baobab oil
5 drops sandalwood essential oil
3 drops neroli essential oil

Add ingredients one at a time to a bowl. Stir to moisten dry ingredients with the milk and oil. Slather on soles, tops of feet, and between the toes. Scrub gently. Rinse well. To seal in moisture, apply black cocoa butter or shea butter to extra-dry feet afterward or a lighter oil such as sweet almond, argun, or baobab for normal skin.

Juicing

Once upon a time, juicers were rare in the home, thought to be too expensive, cumbersome, and difficult to clean. No more! Today juicers start at well below a hundred dollars and come with a few removable, easy-to-clean parts. I received one for my birthday and find it indispensable. There are books and articles featuring fancy recipes, but my husband and I do a delightful health ritual with juices and it's simple. Ice in the glasses, juice of the color and type we feel we need and have available, a toast to good health, and then down the hatch.

Produce tip: For optimal health benefits, use organic vegetables and fruits from your garden or your community. Make sure they are very clean.

Get started by juicing some of these six accessible fruits and vegetables. These are my juicing favorites:

Carrots—the antioxidant wonder child. Typically inexpensive and easy to grow, carrots yield a beautiful, sunny orange-colored juice with a rich yet exceedingly sweet taste.

Cucumber—very easy to juice. Scrub the skin, cut in half lengthwise, and juice the entire vegetable. It's nice for early morning and is good combined with other fruits and vegetables.

Celery—fiber-rich, with a nice crisp, bright taste. Good to add to tomato, cucumber, and carrot for salad in a glass.

Pear—juices well. Very sweet, pear is great alone or added to other less tasty fruits and vegetable juices.

Tomato—because of all the water it contains, lutein-rich tomato yields a great deal of juice. Tomato juice is invigorating, especially when combined with a little hot sauce, ginger, or garlic.

Apple—as with most fruits, it makes a sweet juice the children love. Experiment with all the different types of apples available during the summer and fall months.

Fresh herbs such as parsley, oregano, and peppermint (leaves, not stem), and the green watercress work well added in small portions to vegetable juice blends.

VEGETABLE 8 DRINK

4 plum tomatoes
2 carrots
2 stalks celery
½ cucumber, sliced lengthwise
¼ beet

1 tablespoon chopped
   watercress
1 tablespoon chopped parsley
¼ cup washed spinach

One at a time, juice the tomatoes, carrots, celery, cucumber, and beet. Roll together the greens and herbs, and push them through the juicer.

Optional: Add clove of garlic or ½ inch peeled ginger for zip. For a spicy taste, add ¼ teaspoon dried cayenne pepper or freshly ground black pepper. To brighten tastes, add juice of a lemon wedge.

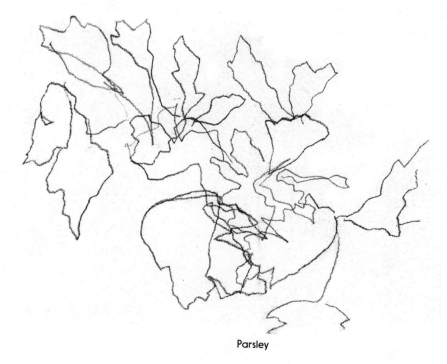

Parsley

Smoothie

Smoothie is a name for pureed fruits, though you can do the same to some vegetables. The beverage combines liquid, such as orange juice, apple juice, or water, with pieces of chopped-up fruit. You'll notice certain fruits are missing from the juicing list though some of them are juicy: watermelon and other melons, bananas, mangoes, peaches, pineapples, blueberries, raspberries, and strawberries. And you may wonder why. Soft fruits and vegetables make out better in the blender than the average juicer. They will most likely get wasted, caught up in the fiber filters, and render very little juice. The exception is if you have an industrial-grade juicer. Some of them can juice just about anything. I like to mix soft fruits with ice cubes and juice (orange, grape, or apple) in the blender to make a basic smoothie. Then if I have lots of energy left, I'll juice some apples and pears and add that to the smoothie as it is being blended. Another good approach is to skip the ice cubes and instead use frozen fruit. This adds more concentrated flavor and makes the drink very cool and refreshing. You can add honey and fiber (flaxseed meal or wheat germ) to smoothies. On the islands, Puerto Rican rum is often added to pineapple-juice-based smoothies to make daiquiris, piña coladas, and other alcoholic beverages. Experimentation is fun and yields surprising results!

BAHAMA MAMA

½ cup coconut milk
½ cup guava juice

1 frozen banana
1 cup pineapple

Add ingredients to the blender. Blend on medium low for 15 seconds, medium high for 15 seconds, and high for 10 seconds. Drink immediately.

Yield: two 8-ounce servings

SOFRITO

Pureed raw vegetables, fruits, and herbs make this practical yet tasty sauce used in Puerto Rico and elsewhere in the diaspora. I add sofrito to basic stock for hearty bean dishes, flavorful rice, and pasta sauce. Sofrito also provides a way to amplify tastes in otherwise bland soups and stews.

1 sweet Vidalia onion
1 red bell pepper
1 orange bell pepper
1 green bell pepper
4 cloves garlic
1 cup fresh cilantro
2 beefsteak tomatoes or
  5 plum tomatoes
1 banana pepper, seeded and
  cored

¼ jalapeno pepper
½ cup recao leaves (if you can't
  find these at your botanica or
  local market, just add an extra
  ½ cup cilantro instead)
Pinch of sea salt
Dash of freshly ground black
  pepper

Peel onion. Wash peppers, and remove seeds and core. Peel garlic. Wash and spin cilantro in salad spinner. Scrub tomatoes. Add all ingredients to the blender. Puree until smooth. Add to stock for sauce with rice, bean, or pasta dishes. This will freeze well in a plastic bag or container. Smaller portions can be frozen in ice cube trays and used in smaller increments as needed.

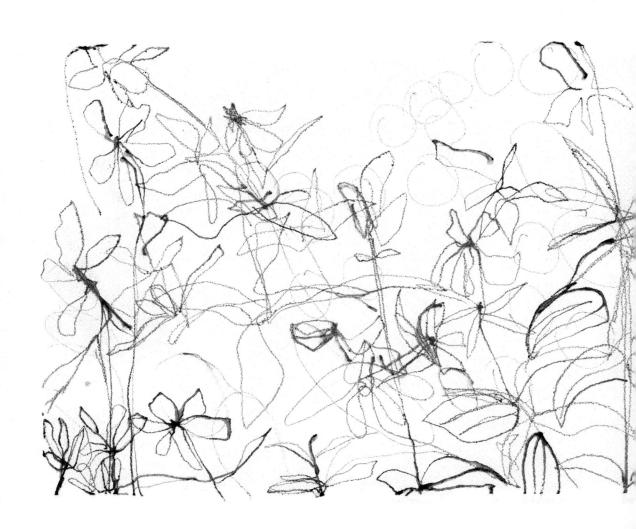

Juice and Smoothie Additives

- You can enhance these juices with honey as a sweetener and antibacterial agent, as we discussed in depth in chapter 4. Other bee substances, like royal jelly and bee propolis, can be added to juices (see pages 70–73).
- A teaspoon or two of maple syrup can be added as a sweetener.
- Spirulina and ground kelps, explored in chapter 9, are a favorite addition to vegetable juices.
- A clove of garlic, some onion, or a bit of ginger, as I've mentioned, adds energy and immunity-boosting power. Black pepper and cayenne pepper add warming power and energy, especially useful for vegetable juices with a dash of sea salt.
- Ground flaxseed adds vitamins, minerals, and fiber.
- Wheat germ adds fiber.

A variety of cold-pressed oils have additional phytonutrients. I recommend borage or evening primrose oils for women transitioning into menopause; pumpkin seed or rose hip seed oil for those who suffer with acne and breakouts; and hempseed, flaxseed, or olive oil for just about anyone working to improve their health.

Ice Fun

We like to cool off in the summer. Frequently, iced drinks pave the way. Have fun with ice.

- Buy ice trays with heart, flower, star, or other shapes.
- If you grow herbs abundantly like peppermint, sage, rosemary, oregano, lemon verbena, and lavender, you know that you need to pinch them back frequently so they don't flower. Flowered herbs are not as flavorful or rich, and the leaves don't have as much of the medicinal content. You can preserve summer herbs in ice cube trays quite easily. Pinch back, wash, and tamp dry with a paper towel. Chop finely. Place in an ice cube holder. Cover with a bit of spring water. This can later be dropped into broths, soups, stews, and sauces.
- Add small organic edible flowers to water, freeze, and add to drinks. This gives a poetic, romantic feel to an otherwise ordinary drink. Edible flowers include violets, rose petals, and the wonderful, bright orange nasturtiums.

- Icing tea. The secret to good iced tea is picking flavorful, fresh tea leaves and being very patient. Out of the numerous herbs discussed in this book, I recommend either the South African honey bush or rooibos, American/Caribbean hibiscus, peppermint, and rose hips with or without the addition of quality black tea. Dried herbs give off more concentrated flavor and medicinal content than fresh herb leaves. Use more of the tea than you would if drinking it hot, as it will be diluted later by the ice. Let the tea steep and cool for at least 15 minutes. If honey is desired, add it while the tea is still very hot. You don't need any sweetener with the South African bush teas. When the tea is completely cooled, strain and serve over ice.

SOURSOP ICE CREAM

I first tasted this in Australia on an exotic fruit tour. It is heavenly. And really, soursop itself tastes like ice cream eaten as it is. These ingredients come together to enhance the soursop's naturally creamy taste with a hint of tartness from the lime and a dash of ginger for spice. You'll find yourself returning for more.

1 soursop
¼ cup water
Juice of ½ lime
½ teaspoon vanilla extract

1 can condensed milk
½ teaspoon ground ginger
1 tablespoon sugar

Peel soursop and remove the seeds. Press soursop flesh through a fine sieve over a bowl. Add water to the soursop, and place this in the blender. Add lime juice, vanilla, condensed milk, ginger, and sugar. Blend 20 seconds. Pour this into a conventional ice cream container or ice cube tray, then freeze until the ice cream reaches the desired consistency. Makes 1 quart.

CUCUMBER WATER

This is easy and cool for a hot summer day—no need to say more. Try it; you are sure to enjoy its simplicity.

1 English cucumber   ½ gallon spring water

Scrub, peel, and slice cucumber thinly. Put the slices in a pitcher. Add the spring water. Put in the refrigerator for at least 1 hour before drinking.

Alternative Waters

You can substitute the cucumber for thinly sliced lemon or lime for a zesty water. This type of water is preferred for those beginning or ending a fast and is recommended as a way to deter sinus buildup.

GINGER BEER

This inexpensive spicy drink is enjoyed in West Africa and the diaspora, particularly in Jamaica. I like to do this slowly, beginning in the early morning, using a slow cooker. This way, the drink has the opportunity to brew slowly and the complex flavors meld well if cooked slowly in a slow cooker. Those without this tool can use the oven on the lowest-possible setting and steep in a covered pot.

2 4-inch gingerroots   ⅔ cup sugar
6 cups boiling water   2 6-inch cinnamon sticks
Juice of 1 lemon or lime   3 whole cloves

Wash and peel gingerroots. Grind the gingerroot in a food processor or blender (add ¼ cup water to blender first) or pound it with mortar and pestle. Put ginger in the slow cooker. Pour boiling water over the pulp. Cover, heat on high for 2 hours. Strain to remove pulp, then mix in remaining ingredients. Brew in the slow cooker for another couple of hours. Strain again. Allow to cool, then serve over ice. Dilute with water if desired.

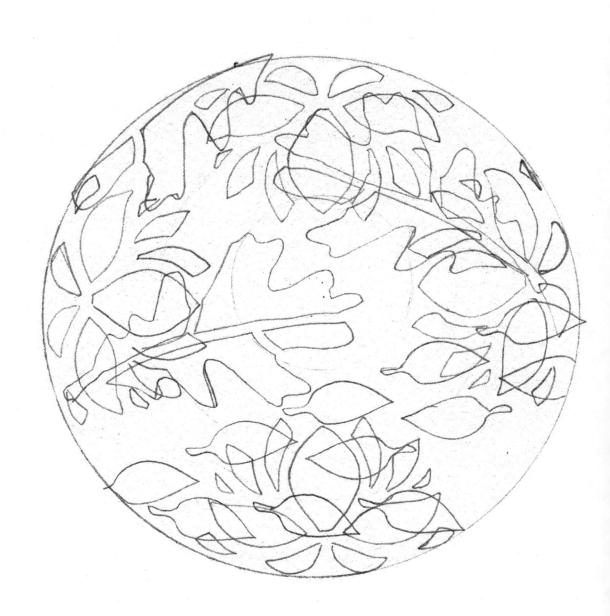

CHAPTER 15

Harvesting Autumn

Fall West

Daily, the sun rises in the east and sets in the west. Here, west is correlated with autumn for many reasons. It is the time we are pulling in; our year is older, more settled and predictable. At Hallows' Eve (Halloween), we see huge spider webs on people's homes. These are to connote creepiness, but knowing the lessons of Ananse as well as we do at this point, they are also indicative of other things. Webs are an indication of the cunningness of spirit and the intricate nature of life and how it is connected to death.

Autumn has always been an inspirational time for me as a painter and writer. Warm-colored leaves take flight, performing an ephemeral modern dance across a curtain of cool blue sky. Beyond the curtain, dramas are played out in the heavens, and these have been preserved by the griot in various mythic tales. Not only is the fall a season for revisiting myths and legends, it is a very magical time of the year. Apart from sparking all manner of creativity, autumn is the season for reflection and divination. This is a season when we can set aside time for looking upward and examine the message held behind the veil that separates spirits, ancestors, and humans. In the busy season that is the prelude to the "holidays," it is easy to forget the nature spirits and ancestors; autumn is a designated time to remember those who have journeyed to the great beyond.

No, I am not stepping out onto a limb here either. Look around you each fall: What do you see? Images of graveyards, ghosts, cobwebs, fortune tellers, sorcerers, witches, and decay—people dressed as though they have traveled through various parts of history, different spaces, and distance places. Let's face it—autumn is one of the most mysterious, spiritual, mystical seasons of the year.

In a mundane way, collectively as humans we seem to be aware that autumn is a time of change. Flickering leaves become a metaphor for the dynamic quality of the ever-changing characteristics of life. We know that it won't be long until Mother Earth's palette shifts from fiery red-orange to the cooler side of the color wheel dominated by gray, blue, brown, and black. Not long till that time when trees are stripped to their bones and birds leave for warmer climes.

In our region, this season of quiet austerity lasts for many a moon. Personally, autumn is also a time of reflection and continued mourning. It is the season when I lost one of the brightest lights in my life. My mother loved autumn; in fact, hours before she died she was busy taking photographs of the trees across the lake from her home, hoping perhaps to inspire a painting by me.

This is a bittersweet time. We are blessed with the harvest of ripe fruits and vegetables; the air is electric with fiery orange, red, and yellow leaves; and sadly, our days grow shorter. Fall is time to begin the journey inward, into ourselves and into our homes. Fittingly, we celebrate Thanksgiving for our wonderful blessings, a harvest celebration derived from cultural sharing between Native Americans, European Americans, and African Americans.

I like to open our Thanksgiving up to friends and new family members as an opportunity to share their favorite dishes. My son-in-law brings a mean Puerto Rican rice from his heritage. It is wonderful. We also have had a young Yoruba woman come and bring jollof rice. In my mind's eye, it didn't seem like it would go with the rest of the menu, but once I tasted it, I couldn't have cared less about that. I love it, and so does my family.

Interestingly, jollof rice is named for the Wolof of the great Wolof Empire of the fifteenth to eighteenth century. This is a new, definite tribal affiliation my family has, on the southern edge of the Sahara of Western Nigeria. My soul had been hankering for something from the Motherland, something different from the dishes I grew up with—jollof rice is it!

Many people also observe the advent of fall through celebrations like Autumn Equinox and All Hallows' Eve—two ancient nature-based observances that mark the passage of the seasons with an awareness toward the cyclical aspects of all forms of life.

Building altars is a very moving autumn activity. It is a tender way to keep your ancestors in your home during the holidays, rather than falling into a depression over their absence.

In parts of Nigeria, the Yoruba people celebrate Awuru Odo, a biennial celebration akin to Día de los Muertos in Mexico. Many traditional cultures that have maintained elements of earth-based spirituality celebrate the ancestors and remember them in a lively/interactive way. The departed are not relegated to an isolated cemetery; instead, they are invited to be a part of the family's daily life.

Thanksgiving affords a wonderful opportunity for engaging with the ancestors in this manner. Try setting a special place at the table with food and drink. Prepare specific favorite foods for loved ones, and then leave an empty chair as an invitation for the departed spirit to join the meal.

Nighty-Night Sleeping Potion

Early fall is a flurry of activity. It is an unofficial new year, with back-to-school being a peculiar type of holiday all its own. Back-to-school carries over to businesses in many different ways; thus, whether you are in school or have children or not, this time of the year becomes a new beginning for all. And anyway, the animistic-based agrarian cultures that built their annual calendar after the harvest season began their New Year at the end of fall, not in early winter as our New Year is currently.

With the winds of change blowing and holidays upon holidays piling up, autumn becomes a very stressful time. In many ways, it is visually disorienting as each day during the height of fall, the world around you becomes noticeably different. The flurry of activities and desire sets in, particularly for those of us in the temperate zones getting things finished before winter or before the "holidays" arrive.

We become increasingly overwhelmed trying to squeeze so much activity in, that we get little sleep, especially not high-quality sleep. I heard of this Jamaican brew that helps offer some solace and build a peaceful night of sleep. This brew takes advantage of the calming quality of warmed milk and the exotic cardamom pod. This simple sleeping potion hails from Jamaica—you can add a shot of rum to it or take it straight. Take one white cardamom pod for each person and grind it in a mortar and pestle—this releases its medicine. Remove and discard the large parts of the husk. Add crushed pods to a clean cauldron or pot. Add 1 cup milk (cow's milk or goat's milk; soy milk is OK too) for each person. Warm this brew, but do not let it boil. Strain to remove cardamom. Add ⅛ teaspoon vanilla extract for each person. Pour into cups. Sprinkle top with nutmeg or another spice with a tranquilizing effect on the nerves. Before you know it, you'll all be nodding off to a sound night of sleep.

Blood Moon Ritual

Images of the moon assert themselves in popular culture. They are iconic and featured in October's horror films and beyond. Let's turn our attention to engaging very directly with the moon.

Blood Moon begins the first week of October. On the eve of the third day of Blood Moon, prepare and ceremoniously pour a libation to celebrate the earth and sky. All participants should wear white (or silver) robes or gowns and jewelry containing carnelian or moonstone with silver accents. The spiritual leader of the group should clean a chalice with rosewater, then dry it. Each member will prick his or her finger with a sterilized needle and add three drops of their blood to the chalice. Pour a cup of red wine into the chalice. Slice a ripe pomegranate in half. The leader squeezes the juice into the chalice and adds 1 teaspoon honey. Each member of the circle can stir the potion with a thet or magic wand. Go outside and form a circle holding hands. The leader lifts the chalice, gives humble praise to the auspicious Blood Moon, brings it down, takes a sip, and passes the chalice clockwise around the circle. Each member also toasts Blood Moon.

The other moon of autumn is appropriately named Harvest Moon, which begins around Thanksgiving. Knowingly or not, most people salute this moon through fellowship with friends, family, and seasonal foods such as cranberries, pomegranates, corn, sweet potato, and other root vegetables.

Oya, Orisha of the Winds

Many people are drawn to the seductive orisha Yemaya-Olokun, for their connection to the sea is romantic, or to orisha Oshun, who symbolizes refinement, sensuality, and fine art. During the fall, my attention turns fully to orisha Oya. Oya is an orisha that can but shouldn't be romanticized. She is tough, containing tumultuous energy and awesome physical force. Oya's domain is the cemetery. She is fierce and held responsible for swift actions, tornadoes, storms, quarrels, restlessness, change, and renewal. Oya is the essence of the winds of the four directions—in short, between our delving into the spiritual realm and our considering cemeteries and the physical experience of winds, Oya is orisha of autumn in temperate zones. You may wish to engage her energy or at the least pay homage to her during the fall. Here are a few particulars about her that are useful to know:

- Her color is reddish-brown or rust (such as rusty nails); she is what are considered "earth tones."
- Parts of the body system she is affiliated with include the lungs, bronchial passages, and mucous membranes; she enables foot track magic, magical powders, and dust to take effect.
- She enjoys offerings of red wine, purple grapes, eggplants, plums, chickweed, comfrey, and mullein. Mullein is used as a substitute for graveyard dirt because it is one of her corresponding ewe (herbs). You could also add a bit of chickweed and comfrey to your Oya Graveyard Dirt.
- Her consort is the thunder orisha Shango. The two guard the cemetery and must be appeased or feted in manners concerning their sacred space.

Oya Altar

Each autumn I toast her with her favorite drink, red wine, and build a special altar to her containing cornmeal, ears of corn, some tobacco, an animal's horn, beautiful ripe eggplants, and a couple of quirky sweet potatoes. These are displayed outdoors on a simple table where spicy, orange incense featuring crushed orange peel, frankincense, myrrh, and patchouli is burned in her honor. Next to this, a libation is poured to her consort, Shango, which consists of lightning water gathered during a thunderstorm. Shango also appreciates the tobacco that is included.

Graveyard Dirt

With all the engagement of the egun and ghede (ancestors), as well as visits to the cemetery, you will need to be attentive to Oya and Shango. You may also desire graveyard dirt as it is a useful altar material used in spiritual healing work—as well as for evil, which we will not engage in here. Graveyard dirt is a central component in the Hoodoo's bag of tricks. The lessons of the Santería are especially informative in terms of how to gather and use this ritual dirt. It is gathered from specific gravesites for special reasons:

- Dirt taken from a young child's grave is believed to contain innocence or sweetness.
- The gravesite of an elder that lived a long, happy, generous life supplies dirt with wisdom and compassion.

Here are some other places dirt can be gathered from:

- Dirt is gathered from racetracks for gambling luck.
- Dirt from a courthouse is used to influence the outcome of a court case.
- Dirt from foot tracks of certain animals is used to harness some of their energy.
- Dirt gathered from a specific person's foot track is used to affect that person.

Motherland Ritual

Gather about a cup of fertile soil (potting soil is fine). Put it in a pretty bowl on your altar. Pick out a few ripe gourds and squash of various colors, shapes, textures, and sizes, and place those on your altar as well, along with lightning water. If you are not the type to keep an altar, place these items on a nice cloth on your mantel or a windowsill. With this humble rite, you are giving thanks for the harvest season while preparing for the challenge of winter. Your preparation has begun early—blessed be!

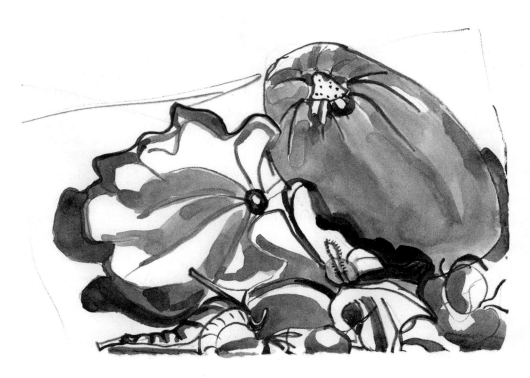

Health and Soil

Mud can be applied to beestings, an all-too-common occurrence with the harvest season and with apples fully ripened and flowers in full bloom. Mud, particularly that with high clay content, is applied to the sting and will draw it closer to the surface. From there, it can be removed with tweezers.

MOTHERLAND FACIAL

1½ cups watermelon with seeds (which yields some Kalahari seed oil)

1½ tablespoons rhassoul (earth from the Atlas Mountains of Morocco)
1½ teaspoons aloe vera gel

Add all three ingredients to the blender. Puree on medium for 15 seconds, then medium high for another 15 seconds. Test consistency. If too thin, add another teaspoon rhassoul; if too thick, add another ½ teaspoon aloe vera—until the consistency feels right for you.

Apply to the face, neck, chin, and upper chest. Allow mud mask time to set (about 30 minutes). Then wash it off completely with warm water. Spray face with rose or neroli hydrosol. Moisturize if desired with an African oil such as sweet almond, baobab, or argun.

Now let's move on to the abundance of ways to use the fruits of the harvest. These recipes utilize some of the autumn's most nutritious foods as well as staple foods that offer comfort and solace during this time of change.

AUTUMN FRUIT SALAD

Whether you grow apples yourself or visit a farmers market, the world seems to be brimming with apples of many shapes, tastes, sizes, and colors each fall. I like to mix and match tastes including Gala, Granny Smith, strawberry, and Pink Lady to make this salad, also called a Waldorf salad after the hotel in Manhattan. Eating the foods that grow within your village is good for the soul and for the community as a whole. I recommend local produce if at all possible for this recipe.

6 apples, washed, peeled, cored, and chopped (local apples recommended; squirt with lemon juice to retain color if desired)
1 cup dried cranberries

1 cup chopped walnuts
3 stalks celery, cleaned and minced
½ cup yogurt
Honey and ground cinnamon (optional)

Add apples, cranberries, walnuts, and celery one at a time to a large serving bowl. Stir in yogurt until everything is well coated. Sweeten with a drizzle of honey and add a dash of cinnamon for color if desired. This is a salad people of all ages will love!

Apple Cider Vinegar Tonics

This is a favorite in my extended family.

- Take apple cider vinegar by the teaspoon three times a day to add energy and aid sluggish digestion—and just to feel good!
- Vinegar is an excellent multipurpose, biodegradable home cleaner as discussed in chapter 13.
- Vinegar is an excellent skin tonic as well. Try adding ¼ to ½ cup apple cider vinegar to your bath—especially after a workout. Vinegar softens the skin and gets rid of body odors.
- Diluted vinegar (1 tablespoon vinegar to 6 ounces distilled water or hydrosol) revives tired complexions and lifeless hair.

Working with Spices

OK, I admit it, I am an avid spice lover! Spices are one of the wonderful contributors to the herbal kingdom, especially beloved in Africa and the Caribbean. In the United States the use of hearty spices is catching on, especially as we work to reduce our salt intake. I say, step out of the ordinary because after a while the ordinary becomes truly boring. I have seen fear and foreboding on the faces of my sisters as they speak of trying anything different in their sweet potato pie or alternate ways of preparing sweet potatoes. The pie is good—the sweet potato is even better on its own—but neither recipe is sacred. I have used cardamom—one of my favorite spices, by the way—in sweet potato pie with great results.

Spices do more than just enhance the taste of food; they enhance the quality of life. Later in this chapter you will revisit foods used as seasonings that can significantly improve your health. For now, here are two spice blends that some will consider essential for autumn cooking.

AUTUMN FRUIT/VEGETABLE SPICE

I find this spice blend useful for enhancing the taste of sweet potatoes, winter squash, sweet potato pie, and spicy gingerbreads. Making this early in the fall sends a wonderful aromatic energy into the air and helps shorten your workload later during holiday cooking, when this really comes in handy. When you use whole nutmegs, you are getting two herbs in one, as the mace is connected to the shell of the nut. Though nutmegs look like a formidable spice to grind, they are actually quite soft as they are filled with essential oil, which makes grinding easier.

2 6-inch cinnamon sticks
3 nutmegs

½ teaspoon cloves
3 to 4 allspice balls

Break cinnamon sticks into small pieces, then grind each ingredient after blowing a healing breath very gently into the blend for a meaningful spiritual harvest. To grind the spices, use a perfectly cleaned (odorless) coffee maker or a cleaned and dried mortar and pestle. Use this blend sparingly as it is very strong and much more effective as a spice than the store-bought type, which is typically quite old, having been on the shelves for months or even years! Store in a labeled airtight plastic or glass container (ziplock bags do well in a pinch for short periods of time).

TURKEY/CHICKEN RUB

¼ cup dried sage
¼ cup dried rosemary
2 teaspoons dried lavender buds

1½ teaspoons multicolored
  peppercorns
1 teaspoon coarse sea salt

Grind these ingredients in a mortar with a pestle until fine. Store in a labeled airtight plastic or glass container (ziplock bags do well in a pinch for short periods of time). Rub this over a whole turkey or chicken. You can double this recipe or triple, depending on the size of the poultry served.

RAINBOW BEAN STEW

2 cups sofrito (see recipe on
  page 401)
8 ounces crushed tomatoes
1 cup each black beans, red
  beans, pink beans, and pinto
  beans
1 teaspoon cold-pressed olive oil
1 onion, minced
4 cloves garlic, minced
¼ banana pepper, seeded
  and cored

½ red bell pepper
½ chili pepper
½ cup water
1 tablespoon balsamic vinegar
½ teaspoon coarse sea salt
1 teaspoon black peppercorns
1 teaspoon dried rosemary
1½ teaspoons ground cumin
1 teaspoon gingerroot powder
1 teaspoon ground turmeric
⅛ teaspoon chipotle pepper

Add sofrito, tomato, and all the beans to the slow cooker, and turn it to high. Begin heating oil in a cast-iron skillet on medium high. When oil is hot, add onion. Cook until translucent. Then add garlic, and cook for a few minutes; stir well to mix the flavors. Mince the banana pepper, the red bell pepper, and the chili pepper. Add them to the skillet, and sauté about 5 minutes. Add the water and vinegar, cover, reduce heat to medium, and braise for 10 minutes. Meanwhile, add salt, pepper, and rosemary to mortar and grind with the pestle until fine. Mix in the remaining ingredients, then stir this blend into the onion, garlic, and pepper mix, and combine well. After 2 to 3 minutes of warming the spices, add this entire blend to the slow cooker, and stir well. Cook until warmed through—about 2 hours. Serve with rice, salad, and corn bread. Serves 8 hearty eaters. Feel free to freeze leftovers because this can make several meals for small households.

PUMPKIN SOUP

2 teaspoons grapeseed oil
1 tablespoon butter
1 Vidalia onion, minced
½ teaspoon sea salt
½ teaspoon freshly ground
  white pepper
1 cup chopped shallot
1 teaspoon ground ginger
⅛ teaspoon ground white
  cardamom
⅛ teaspoon ground cinnamon

32 ounces vegetable broth,
  divided
24 ounces pumpkin puree
  (canned is fine, but make sure
  there are no added spices)
1 cup orange juice with pulp
1 cup half-and-half
Yogurt and hulled toasted
  pumpkin seeds for garnish
  (optional)

Heat the oil and butter in a cast-iron Dutch oven on medium high. Add onion, salt, and pepper, and sauté until translucent. Add the shallot, ginger, cardamom, and cinnamon, and reduce heat to medium. Cook until onions and shallot begin to brown, then reduce heat to medium low. Add 8 ounces of the broth, and whisk in the pumpkin puree; cover and cook for about 20 minutes. Measure out the rest of the broth (24 ounces), the orange juice, and the half-and-half. Add a bit of the pumpkin/onion puree to a blender, along with some of each of the liquids; puree and return to the pot. Continue to work in batches until all the pumpkin has been pureed with some of the broth, orange juice, and half-and-half. Once the mixture is all returned to the pot, heat thoroughly on medium low (about 10 minutes). Be careful that ingredients never come to a boil, or they will separate. Serve this filling meal with a dollop of full-fat yogurt and a smattering of (hulled) toasted pumpkin seeds, if desired, and add some bread on the side.

ROASTED ONIONS WITH BALSAMIC VINEGAR

This is a savory side dish that goes well with vegetarian casseroles, meats, and roasted vegetables. My mouth waters just thinking about this—savory and sweet: an autumnal delight!

3 Vidalia onions, peeled and
halved
1 tablespoon olive oil
¼ cup aged balsamic vinegar

1 tablespoon brown sugar
Pinch fine sea salt
½ tablespoon freshly ground
mixed peppercorns

Preheat oven to 400°F. Brush onions with the olive oil. Put in a shallow baking dish, and cook for 10 minutes. In a separate bowl, mix vinegar, sugar, salt, and pepper. Add this mixture to the baking dish, and cook for 15 more minutes until onions feel tender. Eat hot as a side dish.

CORN BREAD

1 tablespoon salted butter
¼ cup unbleached wheat flour
¾ cup quality yellow cornmeal
2 tablespoons sugar

2 teaspoons baking powder
1 cup 2% milk
¼ cup canola or corn oil
1 organic and/or free-range egg

Preheat oven to 400°F. Put butter in a cast-iron skillet and place it in the oven. In a large bowl, mix the flour, cornmeal, sugar, and baking powder. In separate bowl, whisk together milk, oil, and egg. Pour into dry ingredients and mix just enough to blend. Swirl butter around in the skillet so it is coated well, then scrape the batter into the skillet. Bake 20 minutes or until broomstraw inserted in center comes out clean. Serve warm with honey, jam, or your other favorite spread. Serves 8.

Autumn Season of Life

When humans and other animals enter the autumn season of life, they are what is called middle-aged. We all age differently, thus we all hit middle age at diverse points according to our biological clocks. Looking around us at our animal companions, it is easy to see aging almost at the speed of light, as generally their lives are much shorter than our own.

Middle age is a time when many people first realize the importance of healthy living in connection to the body. Throughout this book, I have shared numerous ideas for using herbs, natural products, and whole foods for optimal health. This last segment of wellness is dedicated to autumn in terms of life stages and will review the main points of *Motherland Herbal*.

- Drink adequate fluids—the recommended 8 cups of water per day really does wash some of the potential illness away.
- Eat foods high in antioxidants—these foods are typically brightly colored and include many soul foods such as sweet potatoes, watermelon, collard greens, and other greens.
- Listen to your body; this requires spiritual connection to signs, symptoms, dreams, and messages that may give you early warnings that something is wrong.
- Eat lots of fiber, which prevents waste from stagnating in the body. High-fiber foods include oatmeal, flaxseed meal, yams, sweet potatoes, whole grains, and seeds.
- Another way people of African descent have traditionally purged waste from their bodies has been through the use of clay—eating small amounts of dirt. This is thought to bind free radicals and pull them out of the body. The types of clays used are of the purest type available; otherwise this exercise is counterproductive.
- Reach out for nuts and legumes as the people in Africa do. Peanut, which is actually a legume, is a wholesome, inexpensive, versatile food that is a good source of protein. Black-eyed peas, cowpeas, black beans, limas, and pinto beans—those foods that have time-honored traditions across the diaspora in our kitchens—are all very wholesome, especially when prepared either vegetarian or using poultry instead of the more traditional pork. Almonds, pecans, and walnuts, among others, are wholesome snacks with heart-healthy oil. The coconut is a large and versatile nut; drink the milk, cook with it, eat it as a snack. Getting nutty may end up saving your life!

- Reduce refined sugar, reduce fats, and reduce salts. This is just common sense and can curtail the tendency to develop numerous health problems, including the biggies: cancers, heart disease, and stroke. You can defeat these enemies by eating more whole foods. Love cookies and cakes? How about switching over to more of an emphasis on fresh fruits of the Motherland? In South Jersey we ate lots of melons and tomatoes, just washed and sliced. Africans in the Caribbean eat plenty of pawpaws, mangoes, soursops, bananas, melons, and plantains. These foods are not just more wholesome; they are also satisfying to the appetite for a longer time than processed sweet foods.
- Exercise! And if you hate to exercise, make it fun. I enjoy dancing, as do many people of color. Dancing is a part of our traditional culture. If dancing isn't for you, think about what it is that you like to do. One of the best forms of exercise is weight-bearing exercise. The weight-bearing exercise most of us have to do each day is walking. Increasing the distance in small increments yields health benefits and reduces the tendency to pick up excess pounds during midlife. Swimming is another excellent activity. It is so gentle that those with rheumatic ailments can benefit, as well as those with certain types of physical challenges.
- Consensual sex with a loving partner gives a sense of well-being, self-confidence, and holistic satisfaction. Many people find creative ways to pleasure themselves. It is important to maintain a healthy sex life in midlife and beyond. Widows/widowers, divorcées/divorcés, and other single people striking out into new relationships should always trust their intuition and spirit when building new relationships and use condoms to avoid one of our biggest life threats, HIV/AIDS, as well as STIs.
- Be mindful of your spiritual health. Scientific tests have shown that those who have a sense of community and belonging tend to live longer and remain happy. This goal can be met in a variety of ways: friendship, spiritual fellowship, mentoring, and earth stewardship are just a few.

Women's Concerns

At middle age, women notice many changes in their bodies. Starting at the age of forty, you should be getting mammograms. Well before that, you should have started self-exams.

I am going to spare you the startling statistics concerning disease in women of midlife. I find these statistics tedious, and we know people of color are often not adequately represented in scientific testing. I urge you to build on the wisewoman knowledge in terms of your health—that gut, that granny knowledge that you have built on to get to your middle age. Watch, listen, read, meditate, and work hard to stay grounded and centered. Learn to doctor yourself, as has been the way of our people. And if you are very good at it, share this skill with others, particularly those of the younger generation. When you have alarming symptoms, of course you need to go straight to your alternative practitioner, ND, or MD.

Midlife Women and the Four Directions

One of the main reasons there is a parting of ways in terms of discussing the physical health of women and men is our reproductive organs. This is what largely separates us as humans as well. As our breasts head south (headed only the goddess knows where), we notice our body, like the Earth Mother, continues to evolve and change. One of the more challenging aspects of midlife is the rite of passage into cronehood called menopause. For many women this crossroad begins as early as the forties with what is called perimenopause: not exactly menopause but headed quite quickly in that direction. Whereas a great deal of health advice is aimed at the physical aspects of a woman's midlife, my advice is from more of an African holistic perspective, using the theme of the crossroads and the four directions that stem from it. Consider the four directions as you consider midlife.

North: Mind and Spirit

As women approach midlife, they begin to really examine their lives and goals and assess their placement in the world. Many traditional women have children or share in the raising of other children. As these children depart, some women suffer with what is called empty nest syndrome. This is an unsettling time when adjustments must be made for a new direction and path, which defines the place in the world. For other women, there may be significant changes with work. The new guard is noticeably different: working women must learn to change, evolve, or move on. Others still begin to examine their romantic relationship or lack of one. Generally in midlife we consider what we have had. Though there is more talk of midlife in terms of the physical body, just as important to our well-being is what is going on up north with our mind and spirit.

Recommendations:
- Affirmations
- Meditation
- Journaling
- Paying attention to dreams
- Developing or refining interests

These are spiritually sustainable midlife activities, particularly if you have felt that you never had time for such activities in the maiden and mother stages of life.

East: Looking Ahead

East concerns what we have and what we desire for the rest of our lives. It is important to organize time and resources so there is more time to seek pleasure and meaningful activities. Taking care of the self has never been more important. Women (even those who do not raise children) are usually cast by relatives, the community, or their work environment in a mentoring or nurturing capacity toward others. This is good and bad in terms of getting to know your soul's purpose. Here is what else you can do:

Recommendations:
- Do some soul searching.
- Organize and remove clutter.
- Discard or donate physical objects that lack meaning.
- Challenge your relationships; work to strengthen, change, or reinforce them.
- Make time for your health: focus on eating well, resting, exercising, and strengthening your spiritual connection to the earth or a group.
- Make plans—working hard to keep them realistic—for your finances, your relationships, and a replenishing vacation or retreat.

South: Reproductive Organs

Women in long-standing relationships may feel a reduced interest in sex that is part physical, part mental, and part spiritual. This varies according to the situation. Women who have followed a traditional path may feel that their sexuality is of little consequence now that they are no longer of childbearing age. For those who have suffered with infertility while wanting a child, this feeling can become almost too painful to bear. Then there are others—lesbian, straight, or bisexual—who simply no longer feel that their appearance is sexy. This is in large part due to images in the media, movies, and advertising—or rather, the lack thereof—of vibrant middle-aged women. Last but certainly not least, there is an abundance of physical complaints that crop up for some as the result of menopause. The symptoms vary and can include depression, lack of sexual drive, hot flashes, and feeling cold, tired, achy, and irritable. Women in midlife should feel the power they contain and yield it to approach discomforts of the mind, body, and spirit.

Recommendations:

- Be proactive, not reactive. Take control, take responsibility, and strike out to make a change.
- Educate yourself about the mind/body/spirit connection of midlife and well-being.
- Seek healthful foods rich in antioxidants, incorporate homemade juices rich in minerals and phytonutrients, drink herbal teas with phytoestrogens, and add a whole-food-based multivitamin to the diet.
- See a health professional for regular pap smears, breast exams, and annual physicals; seek out the advice of an empathic professional health provider about reputable treatments for any serious symptoms.
- Make a conscious effort to work at relationships by reading, watching videos, and talking with your lover or friends and learning to love the self you are becoming.
- Ending on the proactive note, don't feel that you are a victim of your body; do everything in your power to have the body you have always dreamed of. Most likely this is going to involve some type of weight-bearing exercise like push-ups, sit-ups, or weight training. Perhaps this is the best time of your life to join a gym, start going to the community center, and partner with your lover or a friend to begin to work out together.

West: Heart Health

Yes, the heart is on the left or west side of your chest. As we explored in depth in chapter 8, the heart is so much more than an organ in ATRs. It is the seat of spirit and compassion. It is where we feel sorrow, pain, joy, and love. When once heart disease was more the domain of men, today we share the heart burden with them—equality of this sort, I am sure we could do without. Since the west is such a loaded territory, particularly for women, there are many ways of tending to it.

Recommendations:

- Try to pinpoint what makes you happy and set out to do it. This sounds incredibly simple, yet it may be the single most difficult midlife goal to accomplish.
- Do something good for your heart in a spiritual way. Reach out to your loved ones. Don't hold in your feelings; share and express them. This will lighten the heart.
- Laugh—that's right, engage in comedy. Watch funny films, go to a comedy club, buy a book of jokes, and learn the art of joking in a healthy way. Laughing also lightens the heart.
- Eat heart-healthy foods; drink the heart-healthy juices and herbal teas explored throughout this book. Watch your cooking methods; reach out to braising, roasting, and steaming. Forget about fast food unless it is a prepared salad or smoothie— yes, they are very fast. Otherwise, slow cooking is the way to go. The slow-cooking technique preserves fleeting nutrients that are cooked away during frying and boiling. A busy cook's best friend is a slow cooker. As you've noticed, I even make healthy drinks in the slow cooker. They are also great tools for those too busy to stand over the stove and create dishes that require enormous amounts of time. Using a slow cooker just requires planning ahead, something I have stressed throughout this part.
- Kick the empty-nest feeling by finding alternate ways of nurturing. During midlife, many women turn to gardening, tending houseplants, window boxes, and if there is the space, a communal or personal garden. Then too, there is that spiritual garden I shared with you earlier in chapter 2. Another way of nurturing is looking out for the elders in the family and the community. Give of yourself—and this doesn't just mean money, though that certainly helps some situations if there is money to spare. Giving can be in the form of helping the spiritual development of those who are less developed

on their spiritual path. Nurturing may take the form of sharing family lore, community history, cultural folklore, and healing traditions through an apprenticeship program or community teaching. Some women will take in animals, form animal shelters, or feed wild animals like deer, ducks, and birds—or even squirrels. Others will develop a very specific animal fancy that leads to raising show pets or striking out on a wild safari. There is no end to nurturing. If nurturing is your way of keeping your heart healthy, it does not need to end after childrearing.

Midlife Men and the Four Directions

I have always been feminine in a traditional way. I loved ballet as a girl, I love flowers to this day, and I enjoy all that is fragile and delicate about life. I am also very involved in the women's spirituality movement and goddess study. My ideal life would have been to grow up in a family with lots of sisters and to raise six daughters, but this was not the plan of the goddess. Sometimes when you are too much one way, the spirit throws in a curve so that you strike the ever-important iwa-pele ("balance") through duality. I have lived among many males as a girl; growing up, for the longest time, I was the only girl in the family. And now too, my house has many more males than females. In the larger ATR movement, there is attention to the spirituality of men as well. We see in African communities a type of pervasive negative image of Black men that is more stereotype than truth, and we are acting against that taking root. Anyway, long story short, those of us truly involved in spiritual development and holistic health embrace men and realize they have been shortchanged.

As a mother raising three boys, I know personally it is a difficult battle to raise tender, caring, spiritual males in a society that wants them to be thugs—or at least more of the warrior of the village. Basically, people are people: there are warrior women and there are men who love to do ballet, cook, and garden—this is the truth, but not the cultural understanding. The story of men develops with boys, and really with babies, who should be taught to appreciate fragility, nurture delicacies in life, and keep an open heart. Most everything I have said about women's four directions goes for men, with a few exceptions. Still, this part will go beyond what was offered for the health of women, catering specifically to the holistic development of men.

North: Mind and Spirit

There is a preponderance of spiritual advice and spiritual outlet for women of all ages. The stereotypical image of someone meditating, doing yoga, or attending spiritual services is typically a woman. Men, on the other hand, are cast in leadership roles, leading spiritual and politic movements, as well as holding leadership positions in the workforce. These images are in a constant state of flux, like life itself, and as I have said, these are images more than reality, which is far more diverse. Still, being cast in the role of leader, provider, conqueror, and warrior is taxing to the ori, the seat of the north (mind and spirit).

Recommendations:

- Attack stereotypes.
- Are you too shielded to be who you are? What would happen if some of the armor were to come off?
- Examine what is beneath your shell; visualize it and set it free.
- Is your position who or what you are? Is it a small part of what you are, or is it not you at all?
- Soul-searching is an important element of the four directions of midlife:
  - Who are you?
  - What have you always wanted to do?
  - How can you accomplish those things?

East: Looking Ahead

Planning or looking to the east is a very important activity for both men and women. Traditionally, men have a tendency to work, fight various battles, and work some more. By midlife, many men question this limited way of traveling through life. Men who carry on through life without facing up to the east sometimes die prematurely in terms of their soul's purpose. It is important for men to make connections, stay connected, and create and maintain healthy goals throughout life. The midlife crisis that occurs when some men dump their partner who is of the same age for a younger person is often a way of looking back instead of facing the east.

Recommendations:

- Assess your life; if it is not as you hoped it would be, set out to make changes.
- Banish stereotypes from your mind, body, and spirit. This might mean changing your physical image.
- You can live longer and happier by being yourself, especially when it is not harmful to anyone including you.
- Make plans, realistic and dreamy plans; visualize your future—if you can dream it, you can be it!
- You are more than a number; if you want to live a fulfilled, wholesome life, work toward that as you have worked at other things in life.
- Keep your affairs in order, financially, health-wise, and in terms of friendships and relationships.
- Build toward a happy future.

South: Reproductive Organs

At midlife, men typically get a series of wake-up calls, with many of the messages coming from down south. Men find sexual expression taking a bit longer; they may feel blockages of a mental or physical sort, or experience irregularity, sluggishness, and impotence. Relief is important. Those who need medicine should seek it out. On the other side of the coin, happiness doesn't just come from a bottle of pills like the Viagra commercials suggest. You can still dance the salsa with your loved one without a pill and take long, romantic walks on the beach. In fact, exercise and sharing reinforce your holistic health. If you have a serious disease, then of course you need medication. Today, the majority of men do experience some type of prostate problem or another that leads to sexual difficulties and discomfort; sometimes this suggests an underlying serious illness like prostate cancer.

Recommendations:

- An impeccable diet works wonders; eat healthy whole foods from the Americas, the Caribbean, and Africa.
- Include homemade vegetable and fruit juices in your diet; a juicer is an invaluable investment in your health.

- Eat nutritious snacks like nuts, dried fruit, trail mix, and berries.
- Be vigilant about fiber and water intake. Keep toxins and waste from stagnating as these give illness the opportunity to take root.
- Learn to trust and listen to your intuition; if something feels wrong, it may well be.
- Build a good relationship with a health professional.
- Be diligent about testing for cholesterol, prostate cancer, and blood pressure; do stress tests. Know your real numbers, not just the statistics that defeat your sense of well-being.
- As a preventative, drink herbal teas that build strength, energy, virility, and a strong reproductive system; highly recommended is saw palmetto for prostrate and kola nut for energy (see pages 254 and 248).

West: Heart Health

Men's heart health is of major concern, particularly in midlife. Just as I have mentioned in the women's heart section, the heart as a concept has to do with soul's purpose. Heart, soul, and spirit—however you describe it, it has many needs.

Recommendations:

- Men's hearts, like women's hearts, need love.
- The heart is strengthened by conviction.
- The heart maintains health by sharing and being open.
- The heart's strength grows when men love others, whether those in their family or community.
- Falsely considered more of women's work, men's hearts strengthen through building and maintaining friendship and camaraderie.
- Find and share interests to be open, commune, and maintain or obtain lightness.
- Stay positive! Negativity is self-defeating and can actually shorten your life. Seek happiness that has nothing to do with money. Spiritually fulfilling happiness is easily within anyone's reach.
- As is true with women, men need to work hard, maybe even harder, to stay grounded and centered. Meditation, yoga, dancing, swimming, and weight lifting can shave years

off your biological clock and lengthen your life, while also enhancing the quality of your life right now.

Bones and Joints: People and Their Animal Companions

We have explored the health of people using the lesson of the crossroads and the four directions that are natural to life on earth. Animals are not backdrops to our daily dramas; we intersect at various crossroads daily. This varies in form depending on where you live, but even in the most urban areas, dead and live animals are a part of daily life. Dead animals means the leather, suede, and meat sold in grocery stores. Though taken from live sheep, wool apparel keeps sheep energy close to our skin. In ATRs various charms and game hunted for feasts are important aspects of holidays. Live animals are in our homes, zoos, reserves, yards, trees, and conservatories. Birds are the chanteurs that bring joy to many neighborhoods, while squirrels—though they can be pests at times—bring vitality and busy animal spirit to otherwise dry suburban or urban areas.

The animals' environment, whether they live indoors or out, benefits from the use of whole foods, botanicals, natural products, and biodegradable household cleaners. Moreover, whenever possible, and with the permission of your holistic veterinarian if your animal friend is ill, share some of the herbal teas and whole foods discussed in this book with your animal companions. Introduce whole foods in small amounts if she is not used to anything beyond commercial foods. Many types of birds (wild and domestic) enjoy fresh fruit, honey, nuts, and seeds. An occasional spray with calming, pure hydrosol such as rose or lavender seems to help an agitated caged bird settle down. Dogs and cats who experience emotional upsets benefit from the very gentle tincture Bach Rescue Remedy, a flower essence that is added to their water—just a few drops will do. There is a whole array of flower essences with very specific qualities to address various emotional challenges in humans and other animals. I have given my puppy chamomile and peppermint tea to help him settle into our home when he was first adopted. I added just a small amount to his regular drinking water. He is a huge dog but loves tiny blueberries added to his meat-based food. Our dog, as do many others, loves (large) raw bones. Of course, everyone knows cats love catmint, also called catnip. They love some of the other herbs as well and adore certain fruits like cantaloupe, discussed in chapter 4. I have quite a challenge keeping our cats off the cutting board when I am preparing mushrooms. My cats love all things that smell of the forest, especially game. We make an effort to give them appropriately sized raw bones as well as raw meat, and their health shines in return. I do this now, when they are still young, in an effort to help them maintain healthy dispositions and organs and especially agile joints during what we hope will be a long and happy life.

As I said though, use your judgment and patience when introducing new foods to animals. And if the idea overwhelms you, reach out for the newer food formulas that are organic and contain sunflower seed meal, flaxseed meal, healthy oils, and little if any grain. There are also freeze-dried organic meat-based foods for cats and dogs, wild game foods, and meat-and-bone food prepared then sold by numerous suppliers. One such online supplier of holistic products and organic foods for dogs, cats, and birds is Waggin Tails.[1]

Too often, we forget that we are simply animals ourselves. Animals of all sorts are important to sustainable life on earth, just as the plants are essential to the ecosystem.

The lessons of this book concern crossroads, particularly the meeting ground of mind, body, and spirit. We have to look at where we came from and realize where we are headed. No one is exempt from this discussion. We need to learn to live with nature, respecting the Motherland and learning our role in ensuring sustainable life on earth.

I want to end with our joints because they play such an important role in helping us move forward. "Us" is not human-centric; "us" includes our animal companions as well as those in the wild. We are all joined together as creatures of this earth. Joint issues arise from use, basically from living and moving forward. Joints affect us all.

As we age, we become more keenly aware of our joints. In our animal companions, this is noticed much more quickly than in the human life span. With some animals, like large dogs in particular, joint struggles can begin as early as two years old. In midlife, humans and animals hear creaking and snapping almost as though we need oil. We make jokes about feeling rusty and needing some lubrication.

Wear on the joints is called osteoarthritis. Osteoarthritis is influenced by inflammation. Natural anti-inflammatory foods, especially those with coumarin, which we have discussed, alleviate this type of joint discomfort. One of the biggest natural NSAIDs (nonsteroidal anti-inflammatory drugs) is ginger—a very popular ingredient in African, American, and Caribbean cooking. NSAIDs are making the news these days after some

---

1   http://www.waggintails.com.

of the pharmaceutical types like Vioxx have met with some controversy. NSAIDs block the formation of inflammation, inducing substances similar to hormones. Ginger blocks prostaglandins and leukotrienes, while also breaking down inflammatory acids within the joint's fluid. Turmeric and cloves also help. The combination of ginger, turmeric, and cloves is used to make curried dishes so popular in Jamaican, West African, and Caribbean cuisine. Frankincense, the beloved East African resin, shows some potential benefits as well. Several companies are busy developing and marketing supplements with natural ingredients that work like pharmaceutical NSAIDs. One company called New Chapter has developed Zyflamend, which combines extracts of ginger and turmeric with other antioxidant, anti-inflammatory herbs. Another company from Europe is bringing ginger and galangal together with herbs we have explored. Wonder why you've never heard of these? These supplements meet with resistance for economic and political reasons—it has been suggested that special-interest groups from the pharmaceuticals community block reporting on them. You should keep an open mind, cook with these ingredients, and seek out reputable sources of these ingredients prepared as dietary supplements if you are seeking relief using natural sources.

Other ways to reinforce the joints and defeat painful inflammation are also food-based. A hallmark of African American soul foods, oily fish such as mackerel and salmon, help a lot, especially when combined with ginger. Other fish that strengthen joints as well as bones include herring, sardines (with the bones), and tuna. Cutting down on omega-6 oils found in corn oil, safflower oil, sunflower oil, and margarine also helps combat joint pain. It is also very helpful to stay mindful and listen to the body so that you find any allergic triggers.

Glucosamine and Chondroitin

Two of the natural supplements to gain more recent international attention are glucosamine and chondroitin sulfate. These are natural and found in the body. Glucosamine is an amino sugar believed to play a role in cartilage formation and repair—it gives cartilage elasticity. Glucosamine is extracted from seafood tissue. Chondroitin comes from shark cartilage and similar sources.

People report pain relief—and animals appear to benefit—from glucosamine and chondroitin sulfate. According to the Arthritis Foundation, the two help mild to moderate osteoarthritis. Pain relief similar to that from NSAIDs such as aspirin and ibuprofen is experienced after 6 to 8 weeks of use. If relief is not felt by that point, even after sustained use, chances are it never will be, and thus use should be suspended.

Recommended Dosage:[2]

- 1,500 mg glucosamine
- 1,200 mg chondroitin
- Use for at least 6 to 8 weeks consistently. The supplements should be obtained from a reputable herbal dealer and should not contain other additives (which can confuse the results).

Side Effects:

- Soft stool
- Gas

Contraindications:

- People taking blood-thinning medications and blot-clotting agents should consult with their health care professional.
- Those allergic to shellfish may have adverse reactions but not always because of the source. This requires consultation with a professional as well.
- Diabetics must also check in because the supplement is a sugar.

As we grow older, bones become an increasing concern. We work to avoid broken bones and brittle or weakened bones. In various areas of this book, I have hit upon bone-strengthening foods and herbs. Remember to consume the calcium-rich foods—such as collard, mustard, and turnip greens, as well as kale, fish, and dairy products—that have sustained people of the Motherland for hundreds of years. Vegans or those intolerant to dairy can still build calcium reserves through vegetables as well as the numerous types of milk on the market enriched with calcium, including rice milk, soy milk, oat milk, and al-mond milk, in addition to fortified orange juice. Health experts advise those building their

---

2   Katey Davidson, "Glucosamine Chondroitin: Uses, Benefits, Side Effects, and Dosage," Healthline, May 10, 2021, https://www.healthline.com/nutrition/glucosamine-chondroitin-benefits-and-side-effects.

calcium stores to cut down on alcoholic beverages, coffee, and salt. Eating soy products like tofu and seitan helps strengthen the bones, as do boron-rich pineapple and peach.

Our most common animal companions, cats and dogs, benefit from some additions to their diets that are also enjoyed by humans. Many newer formulas for middle-aged to elderly cats and dogs include ample human-grade whole foods including fruits, vegetables, and fibers like flaxseed or sunflower meal. Glucosamine and chondroitin are given as supplements and are sometimes added to the food formula itself. Contemporary breeders and holistic veterinarians stress an animal-specific diet for dogs and cats that is rich in raw meat and raw bones (appropriate to breed size), as this is what their ancestors thrive on in the wild. I have tried this with my own animal companions with very good results.

Many dogs are developing allergies, and indeed our dog has allergies to corn and wheat, a dominant product in many dry foods. This may sound indulgent but the two grains actually make his hair fall out in huge patches—not a pretty sight. Our dog, like many others in our community, thrives on a protein-rich, meaty diet with the addition of some blueberries, yogurt, flaxseed meal or oil, glucosamine and chondroitin, garlic, a little ginger, and some olive oil. The most prominent coat conditioner featured in cat and dog health food formulas is avocado meal. (See more on avocado on page 223).

The human food dogs, cats, and birds do not tolerate at all is chocolate. It can be deadly, so avoid leaving it around where they can get at it. Onions are dangerous for cats, while parsley is harmful to animals with kidney conditions. I recommend the following three books for definitive information on herbal health for your animals: *Encyclopedia of Natural Pet Care* by C. J. Puotinen,[3] *Dr. Kidd's Guide to Herbal Dog Care*, and *Dr. Kidd's Guide to Herbal Cat Care* by Randy Kidd.[4]

Healthy Teeth, Gums, and Supporting Bones

In middle age, poor dental hygiene built over the years comes to roost. Suddenly, yellow teeth from smoking and drinking certain beverages, such as coffee, become very apparent. Throughout this book, I have shared ways to use whole foods and herbs for dental hygiene. For example, black tea stains and gradually yellows the teeth because of the high amount of tannins it contains; yet tannins also have many positive functions, as you will

---

3   C. J. Puotinen, *Encyclopedia of Natural Pet Care* (New Canaan, CT: Keats Publishing, 2000).
4   Randy Kidd, *Dr. Kidd's Guide to Herbal Dog Care and Dr. Kidd's Guide to Herbal Cat Care* (Pownal, VT: Storey Publishing, 2000).

see below. Strawberries have a natural bleaching effect, lightening the stains on teeth, as do citrus fruit, though use these in moderation so as not to strip enamel. Sage leaf from the garden is an easy-to-use tooth freshener—just wiping the leaves across the teeth cleanses. Chewing peppermint leaf freshens the breath. Broad-spectrum cleansing agents in neem, tea tree oil, and myrrh make an excellent trio for fighting gingivitis, an inflammation of the gums, and periodontal disease, a more serious, low-grade bacterial infection of the gums, bones, and ligaments supporting the teeth. The tannins in green tea, bay, eucalyptus, oak, fir, and juniper tighten surrounding tissue and cleanse the teeth, combating many types of gum disease. Chewing various roots and twigs for dental health is a way of life in Africa. Herbs such as neem twig, licorice root, and marshmallow root are natural dentifrices. Antibacterial and antiviral agents in echinacea, bloodroot, calendula, lavender, pine, and aloe are helpful for deterring gum disease. Look for toothpastes that contain combinations of these herbal ingredients. Taking a multivitamin helps maintain good teeth throughout life. Vitamins C (Ester-C) and E, in particular, play an important role in dental health, as does the antioxidant coenzyme Q10, which is being added to some natural toothpaste formulas.

Finally, don't be taken in by the urban folklore that dry commercial foods clean animals' teeth. Ask yourself, Does eating a bowl of crunchy cereal in the morning replace brushing your own teeth before setting out into the world? I don't think so. Dogs' and cats' overall health benefits from having their teeth brushed at home as well as some attention from a veterinarian dentist. Teeth, and the bones that support them, need to be kept healthy to assure quality of life. Periodontal disease frequently leads to serious illness, especially in cats. Moreover, would you eat every single meal from a box or a can? Most likely not. Why do this to your animal companions?

Herbs that are used in cleansing the teeth of animals include thyme or parsley tea. In closing, all animals need to have healthy bones, good teeth, quality food, and lots of water. I suggest giving your animal friends purified water or some of your own spring water whenever possible so they consume fewer toxins.

In the end, whether bird, mammal, or reptile, we are reduced to our bones. We know that Africa is the Motherland of civilization because of the ancient bones that rest in her soils. Understanding the integration of mind, body, and spirit in African holistic health requires that we see ourselves in relation to the environment. No one is too young, old, big, small, or different to embrace a holistic lifestyle.

We end this holistic story with middle age. I am hoping that building on healthy habits throughout your life will help you and your animal companions live a long, healthy, sustainable life in accord with the earth and her needs well beyond middle age. It has never been more important to stick together as creatures of the earth, unified with the spirit of the environment.

Ashe!

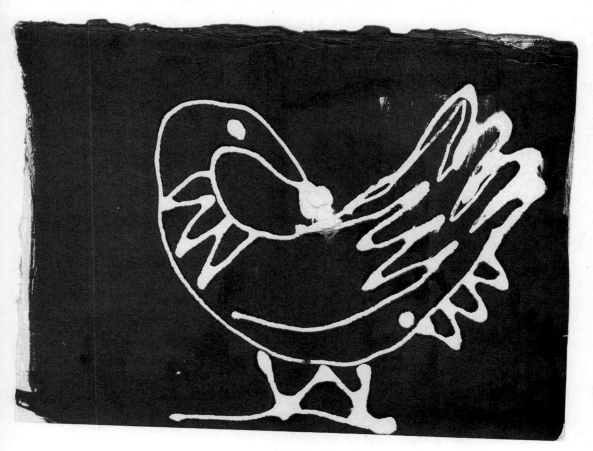

Sankofa
Literal meaning: It is not taboo to fetch what is at risk of being left behind.
Every experience in life should leave you wiser than when you met it.

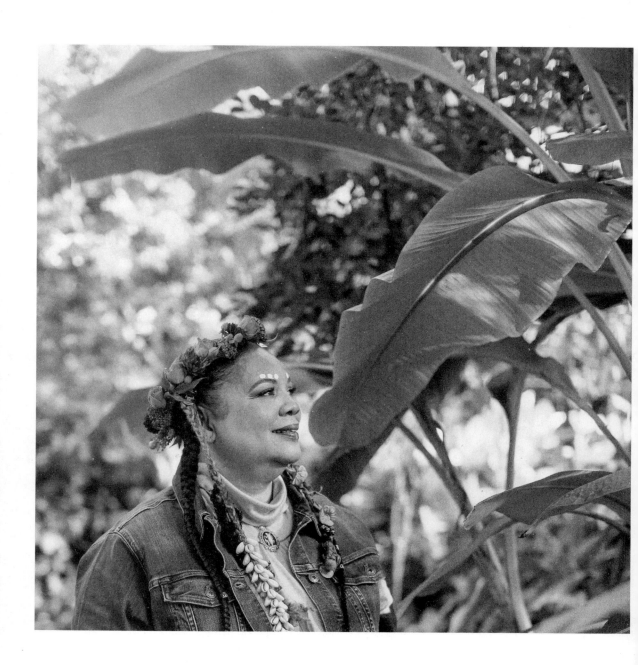

ACKNOWLEDGMENTS

Every book is a snapshot of a time fixed in space. It is also a collaborative effort shaped by numerous editors and the publishers. *Motherland Herbal* had its inception nearly twenty years ago. In that time, it has grown, been trimmed, and areas were cut. Much like a plant, it is alive and needs those things. A book like this is blessed by relationships, discussions, travel, retreats, networks, and colleagues. In short, *Motherland Herbal* is a beautiful synthesis of various aspects of my personal and professional life, left eventually to stand on its own in the sunshine because of all that has gone into it over time.

On the professional front, I want to thank Ericka Phillips and Stephanie Tade of the Stephanie Tade Agency for seeing the light in this book and finding it a home where it could flourish.

I owe a debt of gratitude to the incredibly complex, on-point, and collaborative spirit of the HarperCollins/HarperOne Group publishing team. I was delighted to exchange ideas with Publisher Judith Curr on the vision for the book's unique cover and contents. From its first day of possibility at Harper One, there was the ebullient Sydney Rogers as acquisitions editor for my title when it was seeking a home. It was a joy to work with Sydney during the early editorial stages of the book. Stephen Brayda, the art director, is a visionary wiz who made the visual dream of *Motherland Herbal* a stunning reality. I appreciated the unending editorial guidance of Gabi Page-Fort every step of the way. Maya Alpert and I have worked so closely together on this book. Maya, thank you, thank you, and thank you a million times more. And there are so many other folks at Harper that have blessed the efforts of the book with their hands and heart, including Laina Adler, Lisa Zuniga, Suzanne Quist, Yvonne Chan, Bonni Leon-Berman, Mary Grangeia, Marta Durkin, Ashley Yepsen, Melinda Mullin, Nina Gomez, and Rhya Mills. I appreciate your talents. I see the light in you.

My family has been constantly there as good listeners, sounding boards, encouragers royale, and all that you could hope for from what the word "family" promises. I thank the love of my life, Damian: reader, trusted listener, and synchronous supporter of *Motherland Herbal*. Ian Diego, for being an excellent reader of the text and helping things along with concise and meaningful comments. Thank you, Booty! My spirit twin Livvy showed up in her white chariot just when spa time or a lengthy girl's lunch was in order to get back in the flow. Liam, I appreciated your gentle suggestions, heartfelt reads, and support. Colin and Xeno, your energy at Sunday dinners spiced up my writings come Monday, without fail, as did Lauren's, Maria's, Ra's, and Zara's openness to trying new things. To my little brother, Mike, your encouragement on an almost daily basis was deeply valued. Rene and Rod, our childhood memories inspired large swaths of this story. I appreciated the way Liz, my sister-in-law, put health theory into daily practice. Thanks to my sisters- and brothers-in-law for deep listening from across the ocean and across the country; what you have to say always feels authentic. Mum, you see and foresaw. You show how it should be done, as a living example.

Obviously, I could go on and on, starting yet another book. I want to thank Jan, Iya Sobande, Judika Illes, and Najah Lightfoot for deep conversations. The Queen Mothers: Ye Ye Luisah Teish, Prophetess Mary Ayodele, Sanovia Muhammad, and Osunnike Robin Scott-Manna Anke, merci beaucoup, for shining your elder wisdom my way.

Still, I stand on the shoulders of my ancestors, without whom there would not be a *Motherland Herbal*. I thank you all and your vibrant attending spirits, Ma, Daddy, Grand-pop, Grandma Edwina, Grandma Lucille, VaFawn—all heart to you, from you. Love and appreciation to my myriad cousins, legendary aunts, and uncles. Your being and stories are interwoven with *Motherland Herbal*. Yemaya/Ologun, Ashe, ashe, ase'o!

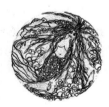